Modern Methods
in the History of Medicine

Modern Methods in the History of Medicine

edited by

EDWIN CLARKE

Sub-Department of the History of Medicine
University College London

220024

THE ATHLONE PRESS *of the University of London*
1971

Published by
THE ATHLONE PRESS
UNIVERSITY OF LONDON
at 2 Gower Street London WC1

*Distributed by Tiptree Book Services Ltd
Tiptree, Essex*

*Australia and New Zealand
Melbourne University Press*

*U.S.A.
Oxford University Press Inc
New York*

© *University of London* 1971

ISBN 0 485 11121 7

Printed in Great Britain by
WESTERN PRINTING SERVICES LTD
BRISTOL

Preface

At certain times in the development of a discipline it is necessary to survey past achievements, to appraise the present situation, and to attempt a forecast of the future. For history this is an occasion for its practitioners to assess its purpose and its role in contemporary research and teaching, to consider its content, and to evaluate its methods and techniques. Each generation of historians will wish to do so but during the last few years there has been an unusual amount of activity in this direction, so that considerable changes are taking place in the traditional subject as inherited from the nineteenth century. There have been, of course, endless books on 'the meaning of history' and on 'the philosophy of history' but of particular note are those dealing with new ways of approaching, interpreting, collecting, handling, and presenting historical data. The pioneer work of Lucien Febvre and Marc Bloch is of special importance and the journal founded by them, *Annales*,[1] has helped to propagate interest in the application of new methods and techniques to historiography; demographic, economic, climatological and other aspects have been presented in its pages and more examples of this type of article are planned for the future. There is also Schove's interdisciplinary studies,[2] and the very recent *Journal of Interdisciplinary History*,[3] the foundation of which stems from the series, 'New ways in history' published in *The Times Literary Supplement* during 1966.[4] Among books which are concerned with the various ways of tackling history, *Approaches to history* (1962)[5] is especially noteworthy.

Historians of science have also been discussing changing trends and the need for fresh approaches to their area of study. Problems in the historiography of science were discussed at Dr A. C. Crombie's conference held in Oxford in 1961,[6] and the annual serial, *History of Science* (Cambridge), has published several articles on them. Kuhn's contribution[7] is of special significance and together with that of Agassiz,[8] it constitutes what Buchdahl has claimed to be '...a revolution of the historiography of science'.[9] Historians of technology too are assessing their subject carefully[10] and historians of pharmacy likewise have recently turned their attention to historiography.[11]

It would therefore seem appropriate that the history of medicine should receive similar attention. Medical historiography has, of course, been discussed on many occasions[12] and at times attention has been drawn to new ways of dealing with it.[13] More frequently, however, the traditional methodologies have been discussed; an excellent survey of them is to be found in Artelt's *Einführung*.[14] Related aspects have also come under consideration frequently,[15] but so far no one has attempted an extended scrutiny of new research problems constituting new methods and techniques applied to medical historiography. It is perhaps paradoxical that individuals who are well aware of the changing face of medicine itself, mostly seem less cognisant of modern trends in discovering, interpreting and presenting its history. They often consider medical history methodologically to be a static field and they continue exclusively to adopt conventional attitudes, which have of course contributed so much in the past and will continue to do so in the future. But as Philip Guedalla has said concerning history in general, 'History does not repeat itself, it is historians who repeat one another', and similarly many years ago Sudhoff described the history of medicine as '...an accidental science, devoid of well-considered revision and method',[16] and to a certain extent this is still true today.

The following collection has therefore been planned as a survey of some of the more recent methods and techniques which can be employed in the history of medicine; although several are already accepted and well-established, others are quite new. Hopefully they will supplement and complement the traditional ways of history and it is intended that each contribution should indicate an area of promise which needs further exploration and exploitation. With this in mind, a list of possible topics and contributors was drawn up towards the end of 1966 and some of the possible authors were solicited. Shortly thereafter George Rosen's Presidential Address to the American Association for the History of Medicine, which had been delivered on 13 May 1966 and which described potential research in the history of medicine, became available,[17] and it was very gratifying to discover how similar the contents of this list were to the research suggestions he enumerated. Thus most of the problems mentioned by him are discussed in this book. The compilation is not, however, intended to be complete and certain advances unfortunately could not be represented; historical demography based on parish registers and similar records, the psychological impact of disease, population mobility, and other topics which will be of considerable importance to the history of medicine in the future, are obvious omissions. If ever there is a need for another edition or volume, these subjects could be included, as well as a follow-up on the research proposals discussed below.

It is intended that this book fundamentally should be provoking and, if possible, inspirational. It will serve a role of the greatest importance if it stimulates active studies in the parts of medical historiography with which it deals. Perhaps it can be thought of best as a manifesto, indicating some of the pathways to be explored '...which', as Rosen observes, 'appear to have important and fruitful potentialities for future research';[18] these are not just new research problems in medical history but they often represent in addition fundamental innovations. Moreover, by focusing on some of the more essential components of the subject, this work may help to define the history of medicine as a more clear-cut discipline. Emphasis can then be laid on what should be its central theme, the evolution of scientific and social concepts in medicine as they relate to human health and disease. Furthermore, scientific methods of handling its data will help to introduce a measure of precision necessary in the history of a subject which is a science as well as an art and a reliable increase of accuracy cannot fail to do good. By these means it is hoped that the book will induce a higher overall level of scholarship in the history of medicine so that the status and respectability of the subject as an academic discipline may be more widely appreciated and more firmly established. There are multitudes of tasks for individuals from many disciplines, united in their wish to pursue truth with impeccable learning and workmanship.

Although written nearly two hundred years ago, Voltaire's pertinent comment concerning history in general is also appropriate for the history of medicine today:

'...One demands from modern historians more details, better verified facts, precise dates, authorities, and more attention to customs, laws, morals, commerce, finance, agriculture, population. It is with *history* as it is with Mathematics and Physics. The field has increased prodigiously. It is as easy today to make a collection of newspapers as it is difficult to write history.'[19]

This book is an attempt to supplement the industry of many scholars already active in medical history. To do so it aims to help stimulate a critical, scientific, and versatile medical historiography, by means of an increased range of methods and techniques, enhanced accuracy and the production of good history. At the same time it may assist in creating a more precise form for the subject and a greater sense of purpose and thrust. If it achieves these objectives the efforts of its contributors will be amply rewarded.

University College London   E.C.
14 July 1970

REFERENCES AND NOTES

1 *Annales. Économies. Sociétés. Civilisations* (Paris). It is now in its 25th year of publication and the most recent issue (No. 6, November–December 1969) is devoted to 'Histoire biologique et société'.

2 E.g., D. J. Schove, 'Eclipses, comets and the spectrum of time in Africa', *J. Br. astr. Ass.* 1968, 78, 91–8.

3 Edited by Theodore K. Rabb and Robert I. Rotberg with associate and consultant editors. It is planned to publish 'articles of innovative historical significance by historians, sociologists, economists, psychoanalysts, etc.'

4 7 April, 28 July and 8 September 1966.

5 H. P. R. Finberg (ed.), *Approaches to history*, London: Routledge and Kegan Paul, 1962.

6 A. C. Crombie (ed.), *Scientific change*, pp. 795–878, London: Heinemann, 1963.

7 T. S. Kuhn, *The structure of scientific revolutions*, Chicago and London: The University of Chicago Press (Phoenix book), 1962.

8 J. Agassiz, *Towards an historiography of science*, The Hague: Mouton & Co., 1963 (History and theory: studies in the philosophy of history, 2).

9 G. Buchdahl, 'A revolution in historiography of science', *History of Science* (Cambridge) 1965, 4, 55–69, see p. 69.

10 See for example, D. S. L. Cardwell, 'The academic study of the history of technology', *History of Science* (Cambridge) 1968, **7**, 112–24 and M. Daumas, 'L'histoire des techniques: son objet, ses limites, ses methodes', *Rev. Hist. Sci. (Paris)* 1969, **22**, 5–32.

11 A. Berman (ed.), *Pharmaceutical historiography. Proceedings of a Colloquium ...January 22–23, 1966,* Madison: American Institute of Pharmacy, 1967.

12 A recent article (G. B. Risse, 'Historicism in medical history. Heinrich Damerow's "philosophical" historiography in Romantic Germany', *Bull. Hist. Med.* 1969, **43**, 201–11) considers earlier methods and this, together with 'An exhibit on the history of medical historiography', *Bull. Med. Hist.* 1952, **26**, 277–87 and G. Miller, 'Backgrounds of current activities in the history of science and medicine', *J. Hist. Med.* 1958, **13**, 160–78, cover most of the literature. Other representatives of this large field are: K. Sudhoff, *Essays in the history of medicine,* edited by F. H. Garrison, New York: Medical Life Press, 1926; J. C. Hemmeter, *Master minds in medicine. An analysis of human genius as the instrument in the evolution of medicine together with a system of historic methodology,* New York: Medical Life Press, 1927; H. E. Sigerist, 'Probleme der medizinischen Historiographie', *Sudhoffs Arch.* 1931, **24**, 1–18; idem., *A history of medicine,* vol. I, *Primitive and archaic medicine,* pp. 17–37, New York: Oxford University Press, 1951; O. Temkin, 'Henry E. Sigerist and aspects of medical historiography', *Bull. Hist. Med.* 1958, **32**, 485–99.

13 Sigerist (1951, ibid., note 12, cited above) in particular enumerated several; see also G. Rosen ('The new history of medicine. A review', *J. Hist. Med.* 1951, **1**, 516–22) who reviews this book. A few of the other authors are: R. H. Shryock, 'The historian looks at medicine', *Bull. Hist. Med.* 1937, **5**, 887–94; G. Rosen, 'A theory of medical historiography', *Bull. Hist. Med.* 1940, **8**, 655–65; B. Aschner, 'The utilitaristic approach to the history of medicine', *Bull. Hist. Med.* 1943, **13**, 291–9; G. Rosen, 'Critical levels in historical process. A theoretical explanation dedicated to Henry Ernest Sigerist', *J. Hist. Med.* 1958, **13**, 179–85; O. Temkin, 'Scientific medicine and historical research', *Perspectives Biol. Med.* 1959, **3**, 70–85; I. Galdston, 'The pathogenicity of progress. An essay on medical historiography', *Med. Hist.* 1965, **9**, 127–32; E. H. Ackerknecht, 'A plea for a "behavioristic" approach in writing the history of medicine', *J. Hist. Med.* 1967, **22**, 211–14.

14 W. Artelt, *Einführung in die Medizinhistorik. Ihr Wesen, ihre Arbeitsweise und ihre Hilfsmittel,* Stuttgart: F. Enke, 1949.

15 E.g., I. Galdston (ed.), *On the utility of medical history,* New York: International Universities Press, 1957; J. B. Blake (ed.), *Education in the history of medicine. Report of a Macy Conference...June 22–24, 1966,* New York: Hafner, 1968.

16 K. Sudhoff, 'Tendencies and aspirations in medical history', in op. cit. above, note 12, pp. 53–60, see p. 56.

17 G. Rosen, 'People, disease, and emotion: some newer problems for research in medical history', *Bull. Hist. Med.* 1967, **41**, 5–23.

ix

18 G. Rosen, ibid., p. 5.

19 M. de Voltaire in [D. Diderot], *Encyclopédie*, vol. 8, Neufchastel, 1765, article on 'Histoire', pp. 220–5, see p. 225, col. 2, under 'De la méthode, de la manière d'écrire l'histoire, et du style'. Also in *Œuvres complètes de Voltaire. Nouvelle édition*, etc., vol. 19, *Dictionnaire philosophique*, vol. III, section IV, p. 365, Paris: Garnier Frères, 1879.

Contents

1 The Historiography of Ideas in Medicine

OWSEI TEMKIN

It has become acceptable among historians of science to profess a predilection for the historiography of ideas, and even to claim that the history of science is a history of ideas. At first glance, there seems to be justification for this claim. The scientist, and this includes the medical scientist, is concerned with facts and with theories. He asks whether they are true or not. By contrast, the historian of science is concerned with the thoughts that refer to facts and theories, be they true or not. Or, as it has been phrased, the scientist studies nature, while the historian of science studies the scientist's mind.

In its exclusiveness, however, the claim is not tenable. The history of science studies not only ideas; it also studies the lives of men and of books; it studies institutions and many other matters that are not in themselves ideas. This is even more true of the history of medicine, which goes beyond the history of its basic and clinical sciences and deals with great physicians, hospitals, medical colleges, diseases and epidemics, quacks, drugs, and surgical operations, and with the peoples' thoughts on health, disease, and cure.

The historiography of medical ideas is but one aspect of the history of medicine. This aspect is not easily separated from others, for 'idea' is itself a vague term. About fifteen years ago, George Boas remarked that 'by last count' the word idea had 'some forty-two distinct meanings'.[1] Such terms as 'idea', 'concept', 'notion', 'thought' are often used synonymously. Since thought existed in early medicine, and since men were interested in others' thoughts then as well as now, there was already a historiography of ideas. The nature of the interest taken in ideas has changed and so have the historical categories under which they are conceived. But the changes have not necessarily destroyed what went before; older forms of studying ideas are still alive and cannot be omitted from an account of the historiography of ideas in recent decades.

We have to go back at least to Aristotle and his pupil Menon, fragments of whose doxographic work have come down to us.[2] From them we learn what ancient Greek physicians thought about the causes of disease. Probably the collection was meant to serve Aristotle in evaluating these opinions for the truth they contained. At any rate, this purpose is manifest in the famous preface of Celsus to the first book of his *De medicina*.[3] A short outline of the history of medicine from its mythological beginnings to Celsus' own days is followed by a detailed exposition and discussion of the tenets of the three medical sects: dogmatists, empiricists, and methodists. The treatment is not only chronological but also shows the clash of opinions, as well as Celsus's own judgement.

The ancient beginnings survived in the great textbooks of the history of medicine from Daniel Le Clerc[4] on. We take it for granted that the old—and the not so old—systems of medicine and the theories of individual physicians down to Paul Ehrlich should be expounded, though no longer as live issues, but as thoughts of former generations. With books like *The growth of medical thought*,[5] where ideas are presented in distilled form, so to speak, we become aware of the long way we have travelled from very old beginnings. Some of the changes undergone and problems encountered on this way will be the subject of the following pages.

II

What Antiquity initiated for medical systems and comprehensive theories it also initiated for opinions on particular topics. The works of Soranus and of Galen are replete with critical remarks on what other physicians thought. Through the scholastic tradition this continued into the seventeenth and eighteenth centuries, when authors would discuss the different hypotheses of the function of the gall bladder, or the nature of hereditary disease.[6] Here, then, was a place for the display of learning, of critical acumen, and of observational evidence. Albrecht von Haller (1708–77) showed a remarkable blend of all three. The following brief passage from his *Elementa physiologiae* exemplifies what many a modern medical scientist may be content to require of a history of ideas. It appears in the chapter dealing with the refraction of light by the lens of the eye.

I do not know whether or not Kepler was the first to discover the refractive nature of the crystalline lens and whether Felix Plater took it from him. This was Scheiner's source, and Aemilius Parisanus defended this nature of the lens as something new. But already at Vesalius' time there were [persons] who placed the organ of vision in the retina, and he himself demonstrates, though obscurely, that he does not believe it to be in the lens. For the Ancients took the lens for the organ of vision, which is easily refuted, since when the lens is destroyed by the extraction of a cataract, vision survives and is not much poorer.[7]

In this example it is the scientific and practical validity of the ideas that matters. Characteristically, Haller, in the analytical index to the volume, labelled the paragraph containing the passage quoted 'Inventores', i.e., 'discoverers' of the refractive power of the lens. Haller wrote from an 'iatrocentric' point of view, to use a felicitous phrase of George Rosen's,[8] and he did not credit the ideas with a life of their own. Life was given to them by the Romantic movement around the turn of the eighteenth to the nineteenth century. What emerged, particularly in Germany, was a historiography of ideas in medicine still iatrocentric but conscious of dealing with more than scientific assertions.

III

The names of Herder, Goethe, Fichte, Schelling, and Hegel represent an intellectual movement with a strong feeling for the individuality of nations and periods, for development in organic life and in history through inner, 'genetic', forces, a feeling underpinned by an idealistic metaphysics in which 'the idea' and 'ideas' united nature and mind. 'The idea', wrote Hegel, 'is the adequate concept, that which is objectively true, or the true as such.'[9] And again commenting on contemporary works dealing with the history of art, of law, or of religion, he told his students: 'in our time this manner of conceptual history (*Begriffsgeschichte*) has been more developed and has been brought to greater prominence...For like Mercury, the guide of souls, the idea is in truth the guide of nations and of the world, and it is the mind (*Geist*), his rational and necessary will, which has led, and leads, the events of the world.'[10] Scientists (K. E. v. Baer) now spoke of species as 'thoughts of creation'[11] and historians (Ranke) thought of states as 'Ideas of God'.[12]

As an example of how history of ideas in medicine could be approached around 1840, we cite C. A. Wunderlich (1815–77). Himself an outstanding clinical scientist, he was yet consciously connected with the romantic view of history. Wunderlich rejected as antiquarianism the show of erudition which examined remote problems of remote periods. Physicians needed a confrontation with the relatively recent past, with which they were still engaged in a debate. On the other hand, he encouraged a kind of historical study which, he thought, was being neglected. 'Individual doctrines, specialties, therapeutic methods, should be subjected to historical investigation.'[13] By showing the genesis of certain theories, medical maxims, and assumptions, thoughtlessly accepted, their hollowness could be demonstrated. 'History of this persuasion', he wrote, 'will be little concerned with finding out the peculiarities of famous men and strange times; rather it will trace the origin of the ideas (*Ursprung der Ideen*) that govern the thought of today. It will reveal how science was formed. The illusory in theory and practice is bound to melt before it, and room can be made for a more thoughtful view of things.'[14] In the same year, 1842, Wunderlich began the publication of an article on fever. The first part of this article discussed opinions on fever from Hippocrates to his own days, whereas the rest was devoted to his scientific research. Wunderlich's method was relatively simple. The older medical literature was scanned for hypotheses and theories, and for observations and experiments supporting them. The findings were critically connected so that the reader came to understand the present situation in this particular area, as well as the mistakes that were made and should be avoided. Ideas of the past were not simply accepted or rejected but were scrutinized for the viable elements that had entered into the progressive development of the understanding of fever. In the introduction to his essay, Wunderlich set forth his philosophical views.[15] Ideas develop, in analogy to the formation of ever-higher species and the development of their foetuses. In all of them the modified surviving characteristics of more primitive stages can be recognized.

In France, the historiography of ideas in the person of J. E. Dezeimeris took a no less aggressive turn than in Germany. If

Wunderlich is an example of the historiographer of medical concepts, Dezeimeris in the twenties and thirties represents the historiographer of medical ideologies. This term would, of course,
already apply to Celsus and his successors, and Dezeimeris actually
takes up the history of some ancient sects, especially methodism.
But he is concerned less with the details of the sect as it once
existed than with its 'spirit', i.e., the essence of its doctrines, in
which he finds the early formulation of physiological medicine as
taught in his days by Broussais.[16] Speaking of medical doctrines in
general, he says: 'To go back to the origin of these great thoughts,
which form the basis of medicine, in order to obtain a bird's eye
view of the developments they have undergone through the work of
the centuries, this perhaps is, of all exercises of the intellect, the
most apt to enlarge it and to bring order to its concepts.'[17] Thus to
Dezeimeris, the internal history of medicine becomes predominantly
a history of medical themes. He distinguishes the internal history
(*l'histoire intrinsèque*), which is the art and science of medicine in its
development, from the external history (*l'histoire extrinsèque*), which
comprises all things external to medicine which have influenced its
course. Both are needed, though they must not be confused. 'To
write only the internal history would mean writing the complete
history of the science, but a history without life, a body without soul.
To limit oneself to the external history would mean not to say even
the first word about the real history of the science...'[18]

   The metaphors of 'internal' and 'external' have found a strong
echo in our own days in the sociology of knowledge,[19] and we shall
have to come back to them. For Dezeimeris' intellectual disciple,
Bouchut, 'nothing is truly useful', as far as history is concerned,
'but the history of the ideas by which men are guided...To enumerate the doctrines, indicate their principles and the transformations
which they have undergone in the course of the centuries, to relate
the lives and the works of their principal exponents, this is the aim
of my teaching and of this book.'[20] Yet in spite of these words,
Bouchut's book was more and less than the twentieth century would
expect of a history of ideas. As the title indicated, it was also a history of medicine with much information about the lives and works
of the authors mentioned and many comments on the truth or
falsity of their opinions.

   The ways represented by Wunderlich on the one hand and by

5

Dezeimeris and Bouchut on the other were neither mutually exclusive nor restricted to national boundaries. *Anatomisme* was one of the doctrines whose history Bouchut sketched,[21] and Rudolf Virchow's famous essay on *Morgagni und der anatomische Gedanke* would find its place within this category. Virchow's essay is remarkable because in his person were united a scientist who contributed greatly to the advance of anatomical thinking and a historian who was able to trace the abstract idea of anatomical thought.

Among the French contributions to the historiography of ideas rather than of ideologies there might be cited passages from the works of Claude Bernard and Genil-Perrin's book on the history of the idea of degeneracy.[22] Genil-Perrin's work shows how far, in some cases, this historiography had advanced shortly before the outbreak of World War I. He looks for the mother ideas (*notions mère*) of degeneracy in ancient cosmogonies and in the works of Greek philosophers. Though mainly concerned with psychiatry, he does not stop there but also touches on manifestations of the idea in forensic medicine, anthropology, artistic life, and social thought. Genil-Perrin illustrates the impossibility of dividing the historiography of ideas into a succession of clear-cut stages. More frequently we are dealing with new emphases and tendencies rather than with new creations.

IV

Until World War I, medical historiography by and large was in the hands of medical men: scientists, clinicians, practitioners. There were a few who could completely devote themselves to the subject, but their number was extremely small. New methods of historiography were slow to enter into the horizon of medical historians, and the names of Dilthey and Max Weber were hardly encountered in their writings. On the other hand, interest in medicine was almost non-existent among general historians, with the exception of philologists whose work was largely limited to the edition of texts.

Since World War I, a change has taken place, slowly at first, but accelerating after World War II. The number of those actively interested in problems of medical history but without ties to medical practice or science has increased. This, in turn, has facilitated detachment from an exclusively iatrocentric interest in medical ideas. More than before, ideas have been examined within the framework of the times and circumstances of their flowering.[23]

Henry E. Sigerist's essay of 1928 on William Harvey may serve as an example of the trend.[24] The very title is significant; the essay tries to assign Harvey's place in the intellectual history of Europe rather than in the history of medicine. Historians frequently had investigated Galen's opinions on the movement of the heart and those of Harvey's predecessors who had challenged Galen's anatomy and had insisted on the necessity of a pulmonary pathway. There were discussions of Harvey's originality, even his dependence on Aristotelian philosophy had been analysed in detail by Curtis,[25] though for a long time his book did not receive the attention it deserved. Without in the least challenging the greatness of Harvey's work, Sigerist characterized it as a phenomenon of the 'baroque'. As baroque art had introduced movement into the static art of the Renaissance, as Galileo had worked out the principles of dynamics in physics, so Harvey had made anatomy dynamic and had employed not only experiment but also a quantitative method.

Sigerist made due acknowledgement to the historian of art, Heinrich Wölfflin.[26] The history of art is especially prone to show the harmony of thought and expression during any given period.[27] There is not only an artistic style, there is also a style of thinking. It may not be inappropriate to designate as 'stylistic' the attempt to lift ideas out of their medical isolation, to place them in a contemporary context side by side with kindred ideas from other disciplines or spheres of life.

The heuristic value of such an approach is obvious and has not been exhausted yet. Problems easily suggest themselves. For instance, psychiatry in the second half of the nineteenth century was much preoccupied with the idea of degeneracy, to which Morel had devoted a classical work.[28] The impact of Morel's ideas can be traced, and has been traced, not only on medicine and anthropology but on literature as well, and so has his dependence on other medical philosophers, notably Buchez.[29] One may also remember that Morel's book appeared in 1857, the year in which Baudelaire published his *Fleurs du mal*. There seems to be good reason to study in detail Morel's work within the framework of the general idea of decadence, especially in France.[30] Morel wished to effect a prophylaxis of degeneration in society by means of public health measures,[31] a

7

proposal which suggests the question how close theoreticians of public health in the mid-century came to the notion of degeneration.

The stylistic approach has its dangers. It is not easy, on the basis of analogies, to decide whether one is dealing with ramifications of the same idea or with superficial similarities without a real inter-connection. To continue with the preceding example: although, in pathology, the notion of degeneration was old, the role it played in Virchow's cellular pathology is, nevertheless, noteworthy. Is it mere chance that this coincided with the elaboration of Morel's ideas?[32] Here we are faced with the more troublesome question of what constitutes real interconnection of ideas, or the unity of an idea expressed by different persons in different fields. The search for the common denominator is threatened by the danger of attributing mysterious powers to the spirit of a period or of a century, an unconscious relapse into Hegelian metaphysics.

Such dangers form a shortcoming of any stylistic approach that does not proceed to an examination of the psychological and social influences connecting ideas or allowing them to exert an impact upon the human mind.

V

The problem of influences on or by ideas has much occupied philosophers of history, such as Arthur O. Lovejoy and George Boas.[33] Lovejoy pointed out that ideas need not be emotionally neutral, that they can represent moods of thought and metaphysical pathos. By way of a medical example, we may offer the proposition that man and animals are alike. Apart from all theoretical discussions of the proposition, people will be found to tend towards either a positive or negative attitude. Some are likely to welcome any demonstration of the effect of drugs on animals as suggestive for man, whereas others will be sceptical from the very beginning. In individual thinkers, it may be extremely difficult to account for such intellectual predispositions. In addition, there is the much broader issue of how far ideas are linked logically, and how far irrational factors, be they psychological or social, account for their origin, their spread, their modification, and their decline.

Here again, as in the case of the stylistic approach, William Harvey's ideas offer a convenient example. Few issues have been discussed with equal intellectual vigour in recent years, and even after the appearance, in 1967, of Walter Pagel's monumental work,[34] the debate still continues.

Harvey attempted to demonstrate the absurdity of the Galenic scheme of heart and blood. Logically, this demonstration culminated in the famous estimate, in chapter 9 of *De motu cordis*, of the quantity of blood expelled by the left ventricle with each systole and in half a minute, a quantity which could not be accommodated by the body unless there existed a circular motion of all the blood. This is a classical instance of a new idea clashing directly with an older set of ideas by proving the latter impossible. Ideas here are chained logically, and it would be scientifically most satisfactory if the modifications of ideas could be ascribed to logical or observational mistakes demanding new observation, experiment, and hypotheses. We would remain in the realm of ideas, and it would agree with the habit of scientists to present their own work in this manner.

Only a prejudice in favour of irrationalism will deny that logic can ever be the power linking ideas.[35] But it is certainly justified to ask whether the logical connection really caused the origin, the change, or the disappearance of the idea in question. Attention has been drawn to the difference between the actual process leading to scientific results and the final presentation of his work by the scientist. Usually, no account is offered of sudden insights, or of the disorder in which thoughts and observations may have followed one another, and much is omitted as irrelevant.[36] If this holds true for the modern scientist, there is good reason for wondering how Harvey arrived at his theory. He is said to have started on the way by puzzling over the function of the veinous valves.[37] This means that we have to consider Harvey as a person, not merely as a disembodied mind. How far consideration may go is indicated by a recent controversy over the political associations in Harvey's work. In 1628, when *De motu cordis* appeared, Harvey was physician to King Charles I. In this book, the heart is compared to the sun and to the monarch, and on the biological side its formation is said to precede that of all other organs. Later, in his *De generatione* (1651), Harvey gave primacy to the blood over the heart. By then the monarchy had been replaced by the Commonwealth. Had Harvey's shift from heart to blood been influenced by the change of the political regime?[38] Did politics enter, as they did in the case of

Rudolf Virchow, where a connection between democratic republican ideas (which placed political virtue and vice in the citizen) and cellular pathology (which placed health and disease in the cell) is plainly evident?[39]

Influences are notoriously difficult to establish. How far is our behaviour dictated by the ideas we profess?[40] In a book on the healing power of nature, Max Neuburger reviewed the opinions for and against the idea of nature as the healer of disease.[41] Theoretically speaking, those who believed in the idea ought to have followed an expectant course in therapy, whereas the therapeutic activists should have come from among the mechanists, who denied nature any benevolent or malevolent intention. But, as Erwin H. Ackerknecht has shown, this was far from always being the case.[42]

Attempts at finding influences of a psychological nature in specific cases go together with some kind of belief in what influences man. To a large measure we rely on the everyday psychology by which we judge men and their actions, or we indulge in speculations based on a psychological theory. These are notoriously uncertain criteria for past ages. For many years Lucien Febvre has insisted on the necessity of explaining man's mentality within the effective life and the general beliefs of his time.[43] Trevor-Roper quite recently has made it clear how absurd it would be to expect a contemporary of the European witch craze to harbour the thoughts of an intellectual of the nineteenth century. Neither Johan Weyer nor any of those opposing the almost indiscriminate persecution of witches had the outlook of a modern psychiatrist, even though they may have judged many of the accused mentally ill.[44]

Recognition of influences which, at a given time, act on more than one individual is implicit in such expressions as *Zeitgeist* or 'intellectual climate'. More recently, sociologists of science have cited in evidence for social causation the multiple appearance of the same discovery, 'multiples' in the language of Robert Merton.[45] The independent discovery of inhalation anaesthesia by Crawford W. Long in Georgia and by Wells, Morton and Jackson in New England in the early 1840's is a well-known medical example. Though discoveries are not necessarily ideas,[46] both are spoken of as being 'in the air', or 'ripe for their time', expressions which bear witness to our readiness to see in ideas not merely individual strokes of genius. Thus, in Germany, a turn from idealistic speculative

thinking to positivistic research with a materialistic bias is notice-
able in medicine during the decade preceding the revolution of
1848, a period of political, economic and social unrest. Or, to turn
to the impact of ideas on social events, the philosophical movement
of *idéologie* seems to have been a catalyst for changes in clinical
medicine towards the end of the French Revolution.[47]

Another factor to be taken into account is the adequacy (or lack
thereof) of an idea in relation to what it is to describe, explain, or
postulate. In medicine this means above all the adequacy of an idea
in relation to the existing public health situation. Broussais' idea of
the ubiquity of gastroenteritis is more clearly understood if the
prevalence of typhoid fever and dysentery during the Napoleonic
wars is remembered.[48] Similarly, the idea of degeneracy appears
less arbitrary if account is taken of the state of public health in
French cities[49] around 1850, the fact that general paralysis was
prevalent yet its specific nature not yet recognized, and that the
laws of heredity were still unknown.

The interaction of ideas, diseases, and social developments falls
under the general heading of the interplay of internal and external
factors in medicine to which Richard H. Shryock has devoted much
attention.[50] One illustration may suffice here. The surgeon who has
to suture wounds, to set fractures, to open abscesses, remove
tumours, naturally has to consider anatomical structures and anatomical changes. By means of percussion and auscultation the surgical point of view was extended to internal medicine. This could
happen around 1800, because of the rise of the surgeon to influential
professional status during the eighteenth century, obviously an
external factor.[51]

Further studies in the mutual relationship between medical ideas
and external events, paying particular attention to the possible
mechanisms, social and psychological, by which the two sides
influenced each other, would be desirable. The objection that we all
carry our unconscious biases with us need frighten us no more than
it frightens the natural scientist. Our task and that of our critics,
present and future, is to assure as much objectivity as possible. If
we are told that objectivity is altogether a chimera, we ought to
remember that this dictum is no more than a variety of the radical
scepticism which defeats itself by maintaining as true that truth
cannot be found.

The above remarks may not be out of place here, in order to ward off the accusation that the historiography of ideas leads to historical relativism.[52] If medical ideas are treated merely as phenomena or products of their time, their medical truth too might appear to be restricted to their respective periods. Hippocrates' idea of disease, it will be argued, was different from our idea, but it was as true for his time as ours is for us, the two ideas having no connecting bond. Obviously this would run counter to the search for scientific truth. But the danger does not lie in searching for the historical meaning and circumstances of the development of ideas and their 'otherness' from us. On the contrary, by comprehending what the Hippocratics meant by disease we are bound to broaden our understanding of the concept of disease. The danger lies in the assumption that cultures, periods, or social classes are closed, self-centred entities, an assumption which, in the final analysis, would make historical studies senseless. Moreover, there exist themes in the history of medicine, e.g., empiricism, which recur at different times,[53] and where the style of the period merely seems to affect their formulation. Many medical ideas live through the ages and not only in their particular age. Dezeimeris and Bouchut here come into their own. There is considerable educational value in demonstrating to medical students how old ideas have survived in modern dress, provided that forced analogies are avoided. The need of the body for regulation of its temperature has been recognized since ancient times. But this does not yet allow us to equate Galen's vital pneuma with oxygen.

VI

The philosopher, Scott Buchanan, thirty years ago, said of contemporary medicine that it had 'a record maximum of knowledge and a minimum of understanding, to say nothing of practical and philosophical wisdom'.[54] If this was the situation in 1938, it is no longer so, for today medicine is eagerly inquiring into its own concepts. Even a cursory look at a current bibliography of medical history conveys the impression that in recent years the history of 'concepts' has come to demand a good deal of attention. Since intellectual comprehension is through concepts, they and their history extend over everything that is observed, thought, and done in medicine. *Concepts of medicine, La formation du concept de réflexe aux XVIIe et XVIIIe siècles, Entwicklungsgeschichte des Krankheits-begriffes, The concept of insanity in the United States* are titles of some books which carry the word 'concept'.[55] Others, like *The historical development of physiological thought*,[56] largely deal with the history of concepts, while still others, like *The meaning of poison*, use a different word.[57] The number of articles falling into this category is large and their variety is very great. The history of the idea of disease and of concepts related to neurology and psychiatry seems to predominate, but even the concept of such a circumscribed pathological entity as 'chronic glomerulonephritis' has found its historical investigator.[58]

The impression is hard to avoid that the history of concepts has become fashionable since World War II. In many cases, the word 'concept' (or 'idea') is inserted in a title which formerly might have done without it or which might have used such terms as 'doctrine' instead.[59] But fashion or not, the trend expresses an interest in meaning rather than in material realities. In order to find an explanation for this phenomenon, we must consider a variety of aims involved.

When we write the history of a concept, such as inflammation, we may follow the genetic approach into our own times. Or we may deal with a concept with which we no longer operate, for instance, 'temperament', which hardly plays a major role in medicine today. Incidentally, this will remind us of the need for distinguishing the history of concepts from the semantic history of words. The Greeks used the word *krasis*, the Latins *temperatio* or *temperamentum*, and the Arabs *mizāj* for the same concept, yet all these words also have a history of their own. To say that the concept behind the words matters rather than the vicissitudes of the words is a truism, which, however, should not make us overlook the importance of knowing the words in which concepts appear in different languages. To get at the root of a concept, reliance on the etymology of a word in any one particular language can be very misleading. 'Physician' is derived from *physicus* and refers to the natural philosopher, whereas the French *médecin*, derived from *medicus*, refers to the healer. The concept of the physician obviously is not exhausted by either derivation alone.

But the development of a concept may appear determined not by necessity but by choice among a number of possibilities. The critic may then question whether what is presently current is necessarily the best, or he may try to determine the historical point at which an idea took a decisive turn. This leads directly to the historical analysis of a concept, where the aim is to lay bare the ingredients that have entered into our medical thinking, though we may not be aware of them.

What do we mean when we say that a person has been 'infected'?[60] Does it denote a mere 'chance' encounter of our body with pathogenic micro-organisms? Is it an 'invasion' on their part? Is it a 'struggle' between the body and the micro-organisms? Is it simply a special kind of 'poisoning' as Virchow claimed?[61] We may not be conscious of these or similar images, which does not prove that they are not operating at some level of our mind. The full meaning of a concept can be grasped as little without its history as the adult body can be understood without its ontogeny and phylogeny.

Now when we speak of 'our' mind, the meaning of this expression is not self-evident. In the case of physicians and scientists, medical books, journals, case histories, lectures, dealings with patients, procedures of medical societies, letters to friends, and other documents will show the concept as it is consciously formulated, or unthinkingly used. If 'our' mind refers to a broader group, possibly a whole nation or a generation, the coverage will have to be broader too. 'Our' concept of the physician's task is not defined by doctors only, but by the layman as well. The less scientific a concept is, the more must the opinion of non-scientists be explored. That goes for the current use of concepts, as well as for their use in the past. Great philosopher as Plato was, his writings do not suffice to tell the historian what the Athenian people of his time thought insanity to be. In the historical analysis of medical concepts the inclusion of evidence for their *modus operandi* is particularly important.

The suspicion arises that to some extent, our situation is similar to that of Dezeimeris, Wunderlich, and Virchow. They were writing history of ideas at a time when medicine was undergoing decisive changes in its outlook, a time when points of view (*Standpunkte*, to use a term of Virchow's) were to be chosen.

With all else in our life medicine shares very rapid changes of its external and internal conditions. What has been happening within the last decades is so well known as to make elaboration unnecessary. While the ever-accumulating knowledge of disease and of the means of its prevention and cure have rendered the knowledge of earlier times insignificant, this very accumulation has posed new problems. Computer methods, to be useful in the diagnosis of disease, require clarity about the relationship of disease and its symptoms. Where classification of disease poses difficulties, as it does in psychiatry, the question arises as to the nature of that which is to be classified.[62] In both cases the concept of disease, and thereby the history of the concept, comes under discussion.

Health, the counterpart of disease, needs equal clarification if health is not merely to be the absence of disease. If we are to promote health, we must know what we mean to promote. In psychiatry the existence of differing schools of thought has stimulated the discussion of the ideas that gave rise to them. In fields where scientific progress has been most rapid it has sometimes been accompanied by the introduction of psychological terminology into the description of supposedly strictly chemical and physical processes. The use of metaphors is nothing new; scales have long been called 'sensitive'. But when human behaviour is to be explained in terms of machines, it matters with what properties the machines have been endowed, and we need to know what the terms are supposed to mean.[63]

When dealing with the history of ideas, man's intellect is in its true milieu where thought meets thought. This makes the history of ideas an exciting enterprise. Beyond this, asking why others thought as they did challenges us to ask why we think as we do. For this question there is great need in medicine, whose progress now affects peoples everywhere for better or, sometimes, for worse. Because as a whole the situation is unprecedented, guidance is expected from insight into how we happen to be where we are, not only in our knowledge and our institutions but also in our thinking. Just because we are so greatly concerned with what we think, the explicit historiography of ideas is but a small part of the concern with ideas in almost all historical approaches to medicine today. As in other disciplines, the historiography of ideas is an aspect rather than a branch of the history of medicine.

NOTES AND REFERENCES

1   G. Boas, 'Some problems of intellectual history', Boas *et al.*, *Studies in intellectual history*, pp. 3–21 (see p. 3), Baltimore: The John Hopkins Press, 1953.

2   W. H. S. Jones, *The medical writings of Anonymus Londinensis*, Cambridge: University Press, 1947.

3   Celsus, *De medicina*, prooemium 10; Spencer's translation, vol. 1, p. 7 (Loeb Classical Library, 1935).

4. D. Le Clerc, *Histoire de la médecine, où l'on voit l'origine et les progrès de cet art, de siècle en siècle ; les sectes, qui s'y sont formées ; les noms des médecins, leurs découvertes, leurs opinions, et les circonstances les plus remarquables de leur vie*, nouvelle édition, The Hague, 1729.

5   L. S. King, *The growth of medical thought*, Chicago: University of Chicago Press, 1963. Books like H. Schipperges, *Ideologie und Historiographie des Arabismus*, Wiesbaden: Franz Steiner Verlag, 1961 (*Sudhoffs Arch. Gesch. Med. Naturw.* Beiheft 1), refer to the evaluation of the thought of a particular period.

6   F. Glisson, *Anatomia hepatis*, c. 18: Fallopii sententia examinatur, Amsterdam: J. a Ravensteyn, 1659; D. de Meara, *Pathologia haereditaria generalis, sive de morbis haereditariis*, c. 3: Fernelianae opinionis confutatio, Amsterdam: G. Schagen, 1666.

7   A. v. Haller, *Elementa physiologiae corporis humani*, t. 5, p. 468, Lausanne: Grasset, 1763. With regard to Haller's *Bibliothecae*, P. Diepgen, 'Albrecht Haller und die Geschichte der Medizin', *Historische Studien und Skizzen zur Natur und Heilwissenschaft, Festgabe Georg Sticker zum siebzigsten Geburtstage dargeboten*, p. 102, Berlin: J. Springer, 1930, writes: 'Er sieht auch in den ältesten Quellen noch etwas durchaus Gegenwärtiges, mit dem er sich wie mit der modernen Literatur auseinandersetzt.' Diepgen rightly points out the broader view Haller took of medical history as a whole.

8   G. Rosen, 'Levels of integration in medical historiography: a review', *J. Hist. Med.* 1949, 4, 460–7 (see p. 465).

9   G. W. F. Hegel, *Wissenschaft der Logik* II, 3 in *Sämtliche Werke*, vol. 5, p. 236, ed. H. Glockner, 20 vols., Stuttgart: F. Frommann, 1927–30.

10 *Vorlesungen über die Philosophie der Geschichte*, Einleitung, b, dd, ibid., vol. 11, p. 33.

11 O. Temkin, 'German concepts of ontogeny and history around 1800', *Bull. Hist. Med.* 1950, 24, 227–46 (see p. 245).

12 P. Geyl, *Debates with historians*, p. 14, New York: Meridian Books, 1958.

13 O. Temkin and C. L. Temkin, 'Wunderlich *versus* Haeser: a controversy over medical history', *Bull. Hist. Med.* 1958, 32, 97–104 (see p. 101).

14 Ibid., p. 102.

15 O. Temkin, 'Wunderlich, Schelling and the history of medicine', *Gesnerus* 1966, 23, 188. On the general theme of German medical historiography of

the period see E. Heischkel, 'Die deutsche Medizingeschichtsschreibung in der ersten Hälfte des 19. Jahrhunderts', *Klin. Wschr.* 1933, 12, 714–17.

16 J. E. Dezeimeris, *Lettres sur l'histoire de la médecine*, pp. 200ff, Paris: chez l'auteur, 1838.

17 Ibid., p. 200.

18 Ibid., pp. 85f.

19 W. Stark, *The sociology of knowledge*, p. 213 (heading), Glencoe, Illinois: The Free Press, 1958; 'Intrinsic and extrinsic study of the history of ideas.' The fact that Dezeimeris stressed the difference between internal and external history does not imply that he invented it.

20 E. Bouchut, *Histoire de la médecine et des doctrines médicales*, p. iv, Paris: Germer Baillière, 1864.

21 Ibid., p. 7.

22 G. Genil-Perrin, *Histoire des origines et de l'évolution de l'idée de dégénérescence en médecine*, Paris: A. Le Clerc, 1913.

23 These statements need qualifications. The political, cultural, and philosophical background of medical history was by no means neglected by medical historians at least as far back as K. Sprengel. Moreover, the generation of J. Pagel and K. Sudhoff, and that of C. Daremberg before them, was engaged in much historical work that had little bearing upon medical problems of its own days. My remarks are aimed at the historiography of ideas only.

24 H. E. Sigerist, 'William Harveys Stellung in der europäischen Geistesgeschichte', *Arch. Kulturg.* 1928, 19, 158–68. (English translation in *Henry E. Sigerist, On the history of medicine*, pp. 184–92, ed. F. Marti-Ibañez, New York: MD Publications, 1960.

25 J. G. Curtis, *Harvey's views on the use of the circulation of the blood*, New York: Columbia University Press, 1915.

26 H. Wölfflin, *Principles of art history, the problem of the development of style in later art*, transl. M. D. Hottinger, Dover Publications, n.d.
Edith Heischkel-Artelt, 'The concept of baroque medicine in the development of medical historiography', Ithaca: 26.VIII.–2.IX.1962, *Actes du Dixième Congrès International d'Histoire des Sciences*, 2, 913–16, has challenged the concept of baroque medicine altogether.

27 As outstanding examples related to medicine I mention: R. Klibansky, E. Panofsky, F. Saxl, *Saturn and melancholy: studies in the history of natural philosophy, religion and art*, New York: Basic Books, 1964, and W. S. Heckscher, *Rembrandt's anatomy of Dr. Nicolaas Tulp*, Washington Square: New York University Press, 1958.

28 B. A. Morel, *Traité des dégénérescences physiques, intellectuelles et morales de l'espèce humaine et des causes qui produisent ces variétés maladives*, Paris: Baillière, 1857.

29 Apart from the work by Genil-Perrin (note 22, above), see E. A. Ackerknecht, *A short history of psychiatry*, ch. 7, pp. 47ff, transl. S. Wolff, New York–London: Hafner Publishing Company, 1959; P. Burgener, *Die Einflüsse des zeitgenössischen Denkens in Morel's Begriff der 'dégénérescence'*,

Zürich: Juris, 1964 (Zürcher medizingeschichtliche Abhandlungen, neue Reihe, No. 16); W. Leibbrand und A. Wettley, *Der Wahnsinn, Geschichte der abendländischen Psychopathologie*, pp. 524ff, Freiburg-Munich: K. Alber, 1961 (Orbis academicus); A. Wettley, 'Entartung und Erbsünde, der Einfluss des medizinischen Entartungbegriffs auf den literarischen Naturalismus', *Hochland* Munich 1959, 51, 348–58; A. Wettley, 'Zur Problemgeschichte der "dégénérescence"', *Sudhoffs Arch. Gesch. Med. Naturw.* 1959, 43, 193–212.

30 K. W. Swart, *The sense of decadence in nineteenth century France*, The Hague: Nijhoff, 1964, and A. E. Carter, *The idea of decadence in French literature, 1830–1900*, University of Toronto Press, 1958, to which cf. C. E. Rosenberg's review in *Bull. Hist. Med.* 1961, 35, 483–4. Swart, p. 115, cites evidence for Baudelaire's having considered society decadent rather than the art dealing with it.

31 Morel, op. cit. (note 28, above), p. 78: 'Nous devons prouver, quelle que soit la difficulté de la situation, que la médecine, bien loin d'être frappée d'impuissance comme le prétendent quelques-uns de ses détracteurs, peut encore, malgré la prédominance des cas incurables, devenir pour la société un précieux moyen de salut. Elle seule peut bien apprécier la nature des causes qui produisent les dégénérescences dans l'espèce humaine, à elle seule appartient l'indication positive des remèdes à employer. Sa prétention n'est pas de se poser comme une force médicatrice exclusive; elle convie à cette œuvre de régénération ceux auxquels sont confiés le bien-être et les destinées des populations, et qui possèdent les moyens de réaliser les projets d'amélioration que la science médicale soumet à leur examen.' p. 691: '...[la société] doit faire de la *prophylaxie préservatrice* en essayant de modifier les conditions intellectuelles, physiques et morales de ceux qui, à des titres divers, ont été séparés du reste des hommes; elle doit, avant de les renvoyer dans le milieu social, les armer pour ainsi dire contre eux-mêmes afin d'atténuer le nombre des récidives.' The book concludes with the words (p. 693): 'Amélioration intellectuelle, physique et morale de l'homme, ou, si l'on préfère, sa Régénération.' Morel (p. 693) refers to a treatise on physical and moral hygiene where the principles of the use of regenerative conditions will be set out in detail. See also p. 586. The appeal to administrative authority is clear from these words (p. 77): 'Si donc les causes de tant de misères peuvent céder en grande partie devant l'action favorable que seule l'autorité administrative peut exercer d'une manière utile, nous sommes en droit de réclamer son intervention.'

32 E. H. Ackerknecht, *Rudolf Virchow: doctor, statesman, anthropologist*, p. 205, Madison: University of Wisconsin Press, 1953, asks whether Virchow, the anthropologist, in attributing deviations from a parent race to a pathological process, was succumbing 'to the same trend that in his time made the new "degeneration" concept of the psychiatrist-anthropologist Morel...so universally popular?' Wettley, 'Zur Problemsgeschichte der "dégénérescence"', op. cit (above, note 29), p. 198 refers to pathology but

leaves the question of a common ground open, whereas Leibbrand and Wettley, op. cit. (above, note 29), deny a relationship in view of Morel's 'new' departure. While it is true that Morel developed the notion of degeneracy from a theological point of view, characteristic for him and for his friends (see Burgener, op. cit., above, note 29), it was not his theology that impressed those after him. The old idea of degeneration neither originated with him nor was it bound to the particular form he gave to it, interesting and important though the latter was. See also below, note 49. I find that the article 'Dégénérescence' in the *Dictionnaire encyclopédique des sciences médicales*, ed. A. Dechambre, vol. 26, pp. 212–54, Paris: G. Masson-P. Asselin, 1882, actually treats the anthropological aspect (E. Dally) as well as the anatomical-pathological (Ch. Robin), with a common introduction for both on pp. 212f. G. Hertel, *Der Begriff der Degeneration bei Virchow*, Diss. Munich, 1959, became available to me only after the completion of the present article.

33 A. O. Lovejoy, *The great chain of being*, pp. 3–23, New York: Harper, 1960 [reprint]; Lovejoy, 'Reflections on the history of ideas', *J. Hist. Ideas* 1940, 1, 3–23; 'The historiography of ideas', reprinted in A. O. Lovejoy, *Essays in the history of ideas*, pp. 1–13, Baltimore: The Johns Hopkins Press, 1948. For G. Boas see above, note 1, and 'The history of philosophy', in Y. H. Krikorian (ed.), *Naturalism and the human spirit*, pp. 133–53, New York: Columbia University Press, 1944.

34 W. Pagel, *William Harvey's biological ideas: selected aspects and historical background*, New York: Hafner, 1967. This book gives a very comprehensive panorama of influences that made themselves felt in Harvey's time. W. Pagel's *Das medizinische Weltbild des Paracelsus*, Wiesbaden: F. Steiner, 1962, should also be mentioned here.

35 Lovejoy, 'Reflections on the history of ideas', op. cit. (above, note 33), pp. 16ff.

36 A. R. Feinstein, *Clinical judgment*, p. 1, Baltimore: Williams and Wilkins, 1967.

37 Pagel, op. cit., 1967 (above, note 34), p. 209, discusses this as part of the general problem of what makes a genius of former times arrive at his discovery.

38 This is the thesis propounded by C. Hill, 'William Harvey and the idea of monarchy', *Past and Present*, 1964, 27, 54–72, and rejected by G. Whitteridge, 'William Harvey, a royalist and no parliamentarian', ibid. 1965, 30, 104–9. Commenting on this controversy, continued in later issues of *Past and Present*, C. Webster, 'Harvey's De generatione: its origins and relevance to the theory of circulation', *Brit. J. Hist. Sci.* 1967, 3, 262–74, has pointed out (p. 274 n. 64) that if *De generatione* was composed in 1638 (as Webster argues with good reason), the political explanation would hardly be tenable.

39 E. Hirschfeld, 'Virchow', *Kyklos* (Leipzig) 1929, 2, 106–16.

40 E. H. Ackerknecht, 'A plea for a "behaviorist" approach in writing the history of medicine', *J. Hist. Med.* 1967, 22, 211–14.

41   M. Neuburger, *Die Lehre von der Heilkraft der Natur im Wandel der Zeiten*, Stuttgart: F. Enke, 1926.

42   E. H. Ackerknecht, 'Aspects of the history of therapeutics', *Bull. Hist. Med.* 1962, 36, 389–419 (see pp. 412 ff).

43   L. Febvre, *Combats pour l'histoire*, seconde édition, pp. 206–20 ('Histoire et psychologie') and pp. 221–38 ('La sensibilité et l'histoire'), Paris: A. Colin, 1965.

44   H. R. Trevor-Roper, *Religion, the reformation, and social change*, pp. 99ff, 146ff, 172, 192, London: Macmillan, 1967. In this connection see also G. Rosen, *Madness in society: chapters in the historical sociology of mental illness*, especially the introduction, pp. 1–18: 'Psychopathology in the social process', London: Routledge & Kegan Paul, 1968.

45   R. K. Merton, 'Singletons and multiples in scientific discovery: a chapter in the sociology of science', *Proc. Amer. Phil. Soc.* 1961, 105, 470–86.

46   I have, therefore, left out of historical consideration 'ideas' as inspirations or working hypotheses, a use common with Claude Bernard.

47   G. Rosen, 'The philosophy of ideology and the emergence of modern medicine in France', *Bull. Hist. Med.* 1946, 20, 328–39.

48   E. H. Ackerknecht, *Medicine at the Paris Hospital 1794–1848*, p. 69, Baltimore: The Johns Hopkins Press, 1967.

49   The article by Dr Bertulus, 'Considérations sur les causes de la dégénération physique et morale du peuple des grandes villes, et sur les moyens d'y remédier', *Gazette médicale de Paris* 1847, pp. 799–803 and 819–24, which appeared ten years before Morel's book, is significant; cf. above, note 31 and the respective text.

50   R. H. Shryock, 'The interplay of social and internal factors in modern medicine: an historical analysis', reprinted in R. H. Shryock, *Medicine in America, historical essays*, pp. 307–32, Baltimore: The Johns Hopkins Press, 1966; cf. also O. Temkin, 'Scientific medicine and historical research', *Perspect. Biol. Med.* 1959, 3, 70–85.

51   Shryock, op. cit. (above, note 50), pp. 321f and O. Temkin, 'The role of surgery in the rise of modern medical thought', *Bull. Hist. Med.* 1951, 25, 248–59.

52   Lovejoy, 'Reflections on the history of ideas', op. cit. (above, note 33), p. 17, has discussed the problem of historical relativism as posed by K. Mannheim's sociological philosophy. See also Maurice Mandelbaum, *The problem of historical knowledge* [reprinted with a new preface in] Harper Torch books, 1967.

53   E. H. Ackerknecht, 'Recurrent themes in medical thought', *Scient. Mon.* (N.Y.) 1949, 69, 80–3.

54   S. Buchanan, *The doctrine of signatures, a defense of theory in medicine*, p. x, London: Kegan Paul, Trench, Trubner, 1938. The content of this book might be paraphrased as 'the idea of medicine'.

55   B. Lusk, *Concepts of medicine*, Oxford: Pergamon Press, 1961; G. Canguilhem, *La formation du concept de réflexe au XVIIe et XVIIIe siècles*, Paris: Presses universitaires de France, 1955; E. Berghoff, *Entwicklungs-*

geschichte des Krankheitsbegriffes, 2nd ed., Vienna: Maudrich, 1947; N. Dain, *Concepts of insanity in the United States, 1789–1865*, New Brunswick, N.J.: Rutgers University Press, 1964.

56 C. McC. Brooks and P. F. Cranefield (eds.), *The historical development of physiological thought*, New York: Hafner, 1959.

57 L. G. Stevenson, *The meaning of poison*, Lawrence: The University of Kansas Press, 1959 (Logan Clendening lectures on the history and philosophy of medicine, seventh series). Other titles that might be mentioned are W. Riese, *La pensée causale en médecine*, Paris: Presses universitaires de France, 1950, and *La pensée morale en médecine*, ibid., 1954.

58 *Current work in the history of medicine* 1967, 55, 215 (no. 413).

59 For instance, see Neuburger, *Die Lehre von der Heilkraft der Natur im Wandel der Zeiten* (above, note 40). Formerly, the term 'Auschauungen' was very popular in the German literature.

60 I have dealt with this question rather imperfectly in 'An historical analysis of the concept of infection', in *Studies in intellectual history*, pp. 123–47, Baltimore: The Johns Hopkins Press, 1953 (a book by several authors sponsored by the Johns Hopkins History of Ideas Club in honour of A. O. Lovejoy).

61 R. Virchow, *The freedom of science in the modern state*, 2nd ed., p. 31, London: J. Murray, 1878.

62 M. M. Katz *et al.* (eds.), [Proceedings of a conference held in Washington, D.C., November 1965 on] *The role and methodology of classification in psychiatry and psychopathology*, p. 24, U.S. Department of Health, Education and Welfare, Public Health Service, National Institute of Mental Health, Chevy Chase, Md. [1968].

63 All this is closely connected with a general, philosophical, interest in 'meaning', for which see G. H. R. Parkinson (ed.), *The Theory of Meaning*, Oxford University Press, 1968.

2 The Medical Profession, Medical Practice and the History of Medicine

CHARLES E. ROSENBERG

At least once every four months, at a luncheon table or cocktail party, someone asks how the history of medicine differs from the history of science; it is one of those inevitable conversation-making academic questions. The answer is equally predictable. Medicine, like science, is a body of knowledge and a community of men. But unlike science, it is an organic social function. Medicine is as old as the tendency of the human mechanism to dysfunction. People become sick and demand care: individuals with specialized knowledge and often a specialized function visit them, diagnose their ills, treat them. This is the root, the defining function of the physician. The specific body of knowledge he brings with him to the sickroom may vary; his prescriptions may rely on incantation or antibiotics. Yet the primary situation remains. Whether the patient lies on a pallet of skins or an adjustable hospital bed, he must be seen and his complaints assuaged. These aspects of the physician's world are always the same.

This distinction is no more than a truism. Yet anyone even passingly familiar with the literature of medical history will agree that it fails to reflect this basic fact. The greater portion of medico-historical writings relates to the physician's intellectual equipment—not to his function as healer. Thus, for example, as recently as 1967 a prominent medical historian felt it necessary to appeal for a 'behaviourist' history of medicine, the study that is of what physicians did, not what an elite said they should have done. At almost the same time, another eminent medical historian called programmatically for the study of 'People, Disease, and Emotion'.[1]

There do exist, of course, a great many books and articles on medical men and medical institutions. Most studies of the physician tend however towards the episodic and anecdotal, emphasizing the atypical, even the quaint and quack at the expense of systematic consideration of patient care. The majority of institutional studies, moreover, tend to be construed in the narrowest of internal terms: histories of hospitals, of associations, of societies based on a one-dimensional narrative of overt incident supplemented by arbitrary biographical compilation.

All this is not terribly surprising. For most of these criticisms apply equally well to history generally—and to intellectual history particularly; much intellectual history tends also to lack feeling for social context and the structural configuration of ideas. The bulk of our medico-historical literature is, moreover, not written even by the unsystematic if usually assiduous professional historian, but by physicians in their spare time. And with such limitations in time—and thus almost necessarily in depth—it is hardly surprising that one misses so often a sense of context and proportion.

When undertaking historical research, moreover, practising physicians and scientists often face a handicap greater even than lack of time. The historical orientation of most contemporary physician-historians reflects the values of our medical schools: medicine as science, the centrality of discovery and priority; it is hardly surprising that they see the essential history of their profession as a naggingly slow, if ultimately comforting accumulation of verifiable knowledge and deserved status.

A new emphasis seems necessary, one which concerns itself more directly with the physician as healer and as member of a profession.* Three general areas of research are, I think, implied by this emphasis. One is a study of the provision of medical care and the physician-patient relationship: who treated whom for what and how. Secondly, this emphasis implies a more sensitive and detailed analysis of relationships between physician and physician, of the profession's internal institutional life. Third, and least obvious, is the connection which these approaches underline between the

* It is certainly no part of my intention to discourage the study of medical history as the elaboration of verifiable knowledge, of particular disciplines and meaningful techniques. I hope only to suggest what seems a disproportionate lack of interest in the social aspects of medicine. Such programmatic demands are hardly original with the present author; yet the paucity of answers to calls for a social interpretation of medical history would seem only to underline the strength of institutional resistance against the approach.

physician's social exigencies and the formal ideas with which he explains his patients' ills and justifies modes of therapy. I shall try to discuss each of these contexts in turn, with the preliminary *caveat* that their interconnections are so numerous and organic that some overlapping is inevitable.

II

The logical place to begin any study of medical practice is the creation of an adequately-balanced picture of medical care. With the exception of casual and in some ways gratuitous generalization, there has been little systematic historical investigation of the provision of medical care in the post-Enlightenment West, almost no recognition indeed of the need for such studies.

To some extent, this is an artifact of the sources. Until comparatively recent times, most medical practice has been in the hands of informal, rural, semi-educated practitioners and such men and women leave few tracks in the archival sands. Thus the history of medical practice has tended to be the chronicle of a self-conscious and comparatively articulate urban elite. The greater availability of their written records only increases—seems almost to make inevitable—the predilection of medical historians for the discoverer, for representatives of medical high-culture. And perhaps this is all for the best; perhaps the ideas of members of London's Royal College of Physicians are intrinsically significant, the affairs of—let us say—Dorsetshire apothecaries and their patients eternally trivial. Yet one does conceive a radically different view of English medical history when one makes the appropriate correction for scale and perspective, realizing that the Royal College played an extremely modest role in the provision of medical care and one little if any greater in controlling access to the profession.[2]

Certainly, it must be conceded, the study of medical practice represents far greater methodological difficulties than do most traditional subjects. Yet data do exist. By the late eighteenth and nineteenth centuries, hospital records, manuscript diaries and account books, travel accounts, fee bills, records of malpractice suits, insurance examiner's manuals, medical journals and transactions become available; even advertisements in the general and medical press can provide much insight into the nature of practice and the character of its practitioners.* Vade-mecums and collections of prescriptions as well as surviving pharmacy records shed additional light on prevailing modes of treatment. Memoirs, diaries, even devotional manuals illuminate lay attitudes towards sickness, health, death, the nature and emotional content of specific ills, towards the sick role generally—and thus help explain something of the encounter likely to have taken place between patient and physician in the sickroom. (Such values shape, for example, so basic an aspect of medical care as the decision to call a physician.†)

It must be emphasized, however, that an understanding of medical care in the past cannot be gained through an uncritical acceptance of the facile generalizations offered by contemporary polemicists. (So often the source of medico-historical summations or practice.) Thus, for example, in my own work on American medicine, I was originally misled by the frequency of hand-wringing mid-nineteenth-century attacks on the average American physician and depressing analyses of the reasons for his declining status.[3] When I read somewhat more widely in comparative sources, it soon became clear that American medical practice was not really unlike that of many European countries: except that in Germany, France, or Russia, the existence and necessity of a 'second-class' medical profession for 'second-class' or geographically isolated patients was explicitly acknowledged. Nineteenth-century Americans were simply unwilling to acknowledge and formalize status distinctions. All practitioners reached for and assumed the same title, although, speaking functionally, the provision of medical care was not radically different from that prevailing in much of Europe: an elite of urban physicians treated the wealthy and educated, less elaborately trained practitioners saw to the health needs of the poor.‡

* Though some of these materials are used relatively routinely by medical historians, it is often with a viewpoint constricted by their discipline's intellectualistic canon of significance—a process likened in a well-known metaphor to shining the beam of a searchlight into the murk of the past. Great areas outside the beam's focus lie in darkness. This is, I think, no unjust description of the way in which most medical historians have utilized nineteenth-century medical journals.

† Lay expectations provide in general, of course, a significant parameter in determining the physician's role.

‡ The applicability of this generalization varies from country to country and is, on the whole, decreasingly accurate as the nineteenth century progressed. The general contrast between Europe and the United States seems clear enough however. I should like to thank Professor Owsei Temkin for his kindness in warning of the danger in overstating this generalization.

The relevance of extra-medical values is clear enough; yet the true situation has been obscured by too literalistic a reading of jeremiads deploring the 'American physicians'' failings. In this case, acceptance of medical reform rhetoric without investigation of existing medical care patterns would have obscured a most significant structural development within the profession—the gradual emergence of an articulate European-oriented elite (the authors, of course, of these morally-outraged pamphlets and editorials). One can, moreover, now deal with a question previously unperceived: how do such rhetorical conventions influence future development within the profession? For once established, such value-embracing rhetorical formulae become inevitably a component of the system itself.*

There is still another factor which should be considered in evaluating the doctor-patient relationship in its most comprehensive sense. This is disease. In any culture at any particular moment in time, the pattern of disease incidence is a determinant of physician–patient relationships. The prevalence of acute, infectious disease in a society unable to prevent or assuage such ills implies, for example, physician–patient interactions quite different in quality from those prevailing in the mid-1960's. Disease incidence has another effect, moreover, creating paradigmatic models which shape ideas of disease and disease causation. Aetiological and therapeutic theory—and by implication the treatment of all patients—reflects, that is, the influence of particularly common ills. Thus, for example, the prevalence of malaria in classical Greece must have lent plausibility to the doctrine of critical days. Or, to cite another example, paresis, which in the second half of the nineteenth century offered a suitably mechanistic somatic model into which all mental disease could be fitted.

III

Thus far we have been discussing primarily the relationship between physician and patient. There is, of course, another and in some ways distinct area of professional life: education, access to practice, ethical

---

* Thus one possible explanation for the thoroughness and remarkable uniformity of the revolution in American medical education and licensing in the first decades of the twentieth century. It was impossible seriously to entertain the idea of an explicitly and avowedly second-class practitioner.

relationships, the conduct of institutions—the internal life of the profession.

There is, to be sure, a tradition of the historical study of such problems, a tradition supplemented by a vigorous new interest within medical sociology. It seems equally undeniable, however, that most historical treatments of such intra-professional problems have been in essence chronicles, chronicles written by men assuming medical 'progress' as an absolute value and honestly dismayed at the seeming weakness and deficiency of past institutional arrange-ments. The implicit interpretive schemes of their studies tends always to the same hortatory form: reformers arrayed against inertia, traditionalism, even iniquity. Aside from the assumption that a 'forward-looking' scientifically-oriented—and thus moral—elite constitutes the dynamic element in any social or institutional change, comparatively little is available by way of interpretation. (And even this interpretation remains largely implicit; there is little of the intellectually-arresting complexity of reality in so schematic and morally polarized a design.)

This rather narrowly defined form has produced some useful, even admirable works. Yet existing institutional studies have, it would be fair to say, failed on the whole to exploit the potential of their subjects. Many indeed, especially those of the 'centennial' sort, are so thin and lacking in critical framework as to be of almost no use to succeeding scholars. And this failure in the literature is dis-appointing to general as well as medical historians; for if seen in broad social terms, the institution and its history can provide a kind of sampling device, a limited and controlled context in which to evaluate the impact and dimensions of social change. General societal factors—attitudinal and economic primarily—external to a particular institution are inevitably significant elements in shaping its inner history.

Thus, for example, the physician's status—and by implication the prerogatives granted him by society in terms of controlling access to practice—are related generally to social structure and to the strength of assurance granted any occupational status. Let me sug-gest an illustrative example. The proper perspective, it might well be argued, in which to interpret the reform of American medical education in the first decades of this century is that of a general movement towards the rationalization and control of an increasingly complex, technologically-oriented and highly-structured society.[4] In medicine a more and more sophisticated—and efficacious—basis in science became at once the occasion and justification for a sweeping reform in medical education and the creation of an unprecedentedly firm control of access to practice. The Carnegie wealth which paid for the Flexner Report and which continued—with the help of the Rockefeller Foundation—to help underwrite medical reform was equally a product of the new economic and industrial order. None of the ideas for medical reform were novel; they had been the clichés of a European-oriented elite since the late 1870's and 1880's —but it was not until conditions outside the profession itself had become propitious that these conceptions of reform could become a programme for action.

Specific aspects of institutional development of course also reflect changes in medical thought and practice. And the institution, whether it be hospital, society, or licensing agency, is more likely than the independent practitioner to have preserved adequate records. (Records often of things done; not simply formal admonitions as to that which should be done.) Hospital and asylum archives are, for example, a significant source of data for studies of therapeutics and aetiological thought.[5] Hospital records often indicate admission diagnoses and courses of treatment, thus providing valuable data in regard to both disease incidence and the practice of clinical medicine. Records of drug purchases may also document trends in therapeutics; even architectural conceptions reflect both medical and social thought. Changes in organization—the creation of special services, of out-patient facilities, of bacteriology laboratories and X-ray units—also reflect and in their turn promote intellectual change. Similarly, valuable insights can often be gained from the artifacts of medical education; examination papers, theses, student publications, bulletins and circulars all shed light on the educational process and thus into the total context of ideas and experience in which a medical generation grew to professional maturity.

Or to suggest another class of historically significant yet comparatively neglected institutional materials: the archives and publications of local medical societies may provide valuable insights into the dissemination of a discrete idea or technique, into prevailing modes of therapeutics, into the actual apportionment of professional status and the relationship between knowledge and status within and without the profession. The present author, for example, was interested some time ago in constructing a case study of medical practice at one time and place; I chose New York City a century ago and it soon became apparent that the city's medical profession was dominated socially and intellectually by a somewhat disparate yet essentially cohesive elite. Yet how were the holders of real power within the medical community to be identified in more than impressionistic terms? For without such definition, it would be impossible to make precise statements in regard to the relationship between status and specialization, between institutional power and intellectual achievement. As I soon discovered, it was only through institutional records and institutional connections—membership in an exclusive medical society and possession of attending and consulting appointments at the city's several hospitals—that I was able to outline an elite group and then evaluate such factors as their pattern of education, interest in specialties and the like.[6]

IV

Perhaps most complex—and in this sense alluring—are the connections between the physician's social function and his medical thought. One can hardly mistake the manner in which the formal explanations of the healer in primitive cultures reflects the necessities of his role in the patient–physician nexus. Yet this contextual point of view is utilized comparatively little by students of these aspects of medical thought in the post-Enlightenment West.

Let me try to clarify this point with a more specific example. Ludwig Edelstein's influence on contemporary understanding of medical thought in classical antiquity seems clearly related to his social and contextual point of view, one somewhat atypical among the classical philologists of his generation. It seems undeniable that Edelstein's characteristic insight was at once historical and sociological; the historian must, his writings on classical medicine suggest, gain some understanding of the physician's social role—into the nature of the modal physician–patient relationship—before gaining an adequate understanding of the intellectual tools with which the physician rationalized this encounter.[7]

The problem is timeless. A physician is called to see a patient anxious and often in discomfort. The demands of his role imply the reassurance of the patient and himself; both must maintain confidence in the reality of his skills. Hence the need to elaborate some aetiological and therapeutic scheme to explain and thus control the disquieting reality of sickness. (The almost universal elaboration of the healer role by cultures diverse in time and place indicates a functional recognition of the patient's need for care and reassurance; the creation of such a role would seem to be a part of society's response to the inevitably recurring demands of the sick.)

We are all 'primitives' in our unwillingness to tolerate the random; we all demand explanation, control, power over the disquietingly irrational incidence of disease. This need for explanation and hence control has been a central element in aetiological thought from Imhotep to the present.

This, despite its philosophical connections, was clearly the social function of the humoral theory.* It helped that is to rationalize and thus legitimize the physician's role. The humoral physiology and pathology provided a dynamic system in which health and disease could be explained as the consequence of a complex physiological state, one in which equilibrium meant health, disequilibrium illness. The humoral balance was, of course, the resultant of an interaction between basic constitution, climate, and regimen—food, sleep, exercise. All these factors might through individual imprudence or unfortunate circumstances become unbalanced and produce disease. Health was never a stable good, but always a state of becoming; and the physician's task was to fill in the appropriate elements in the ever-varying health equation; the system itself was so circular and open-ended that he might never be at a loss in explaining either the occurrence of a disease or continued health. Could any hypothetical scheme more implacably justify the physician's role?

Thus the persistence of these ancient ideas through at least the mid-nineteenth century. It was not traditionalism alone, but the continued relevance of these explanations which made physicians continue to embrace aspects of the humoral theory—if only in the

---

* The origin of the humoral theory and the precise interaction between physicians and philosophers is, of course, still unclear. It may be argued, however, that even if physicians simply borrowed the central elements of their humoral physiology and pathology from others, that the needs which drove them to embrace such formal rationalistic schemes and the function of their belief can only be explained in terms of the social exigencies of their role as physicians.

30

attenuated form of temperament and constitution. (While the various haemato-pathologies so fashionable in mid-nineteenth century served in many ways the same schematic function, the physician was never at a loss to explain how 'disorders of nutrition' might occur, how they might be prevented even in those of inadequate hereditary endowment.)

V

Though the previous pages have at least referred to a great number of separable issues, there is one theme which has implicitly asserted itself in a number of different contexts and which I should now like to discuss more explicitly. This is the interdependence of ideas and institutions. It is indeed almost impossible in the history of medicine to disentangle factors purely institutional from those largely intellectual. And most studies which proceed in the assumption that this can be done are destined for at most a partial success; the best medical history is to some degree always a historical sociology of medical knowledge.

The distribution of ideas is very much a part of the relationship between power, prestige, and status. The tracing of particular ideas or techniques represents indeed one of our most valuable means of access to the inner structure of the profession; they can, if the metaphor be excused, serve as discrete 'tagged' elements in the system; where and when they are recovered indicates a great deal about the physiology and anatomy of the system into which they were originally introduced.*

Such an analysis of the dissemination of particular ideas might well, for example, provide insight into the changed structural relationships which have accompanied the development of medicine in

* The ways in which these ideas or techniques may be changed in the process of transmission from elite to non-elite or from metropolis to rural area—the form in which tagged elements are retrieved, to expand our metaphor—also tells us a good deal about their relationship. One might indeed even define these structural relationships in terms of the changes wrought in ideas as they passed from one sector of the profession to another.

The present author, for example, is at work on a study of the introduction and diffusion of the germ theory in the United States. In the course of this investigation, changes in the social and spatial relationship between elite and general practitioners, between teaching and practice, between the metropolis, the region, and the town have manifested themselves as central aspects of a study which had—originally—been projected in narrower and more intellectualistic terms.

this past century.[8] The 'scientification' of medical research has created new disciplines and sub-disciplines, the members of which —though holders of the medical degree—look for status and define their aspirations in terms of their disciplinary peers, not in terms of medicine as a social function. They care little, that is, for the rewards traditionally granted clinical skills, but seek rather an identity as biochemists, let us say, or cytogeneticists. What then is the relationship between these new academics and their colleagues in practice? How are new patterns in the allocation of status effecting patterns of research and ultimately medical care? How, on the other hand, are social attitudes and patterns of medical care effecting trends in research? These are real questions and have been asked with increasing urgency for at least several decades now; yet they are historical questions as well, their roots clearly discernible in the nineteenth century. Here is a significant problem for the medical historian— but one on the whole undefined, let alone studied in detail. Almost every discrete and consequential innovation from the mid-eighteenth century to the present represents a potential case study in the diffusion of knowledge and—as we have argued—necessarily in the social structure of the profession assimilating the new idea.* It is difficult, on the other hand, to think of more than a handful of such opportunities utilized.

To complete such studies, one must necessarily cast a wide net among available sources, including not only the literary products of an articulate elite, but a sample of the profession approximating as closely as possible its social and geographic structure. Clearly, however, the lower one descends in the order of status and knowledge, the sketchier the evidence available, the more one must extrapolate, and the greater the weight necessarily placed on individual bits of evidence. It would be unreasonable to ask that history be as complex and tentative as reality; yet it is the historian's task to approach this end as best he can.

---

* And it seems little more than a truism to emphasize that the structural aspects of the professions, in particular cultures, mirror and affirm basic social values. An understanding of medical care—like that of any other social function—offers insight into social values and attitudes generally. What is the value placed upon innovation and the innovator? What is the difference between the medical treatment accorded the rich and the poor? Are these differences acknowledged or unacknowledged?

VI

There is, I think, a final unifying theme in this somewhat dyspeptic catalogue of medico-historical ills. It rests, as I have argued, in the failure of medical historians habitually to utilize in their construction of research designs a structural, contextual view of the society in which their protagonists act and think. There are, it must be conceded, areas within the canon of medical history in which our general criticisms fail to apply: primitive medicine, for example, or as we have suggested, medicine in classical antiquity. Yet consideration of these exceptions only emphasizes the general relevance of the observations made on preceding pages. The reasons for the atypically contextual interpretation of medicine in these cultures are, I think, both apparent and revealing. One, of course, is that its very alienness makes us see the culture—whether it be the Mano or Azande or Periclean Athens—as organic, as necessarily interrelated in values, institutions, and attitudes.[9] Medicine as a cultural artifact must then partake of and relate to these general social characteristics. And, it must be confessed, the historian of medicine in such cultures is not overwhelmed by the abundance of discrete events, practice, ideas and institutions which make up the changing intellectual texture of medicine in the nineteenth- and twentieth-century West. With no path towards the truth, the structure of the literature need not trace this uplifting saga of insight and discovery. Much of the contemporary literature in these fields is, moreover, not written by practising physicians; classicists and cultural anthropologists have come to dominate these fields. The lack of an autonomous 'modern science' as a component of medical thought in these areas has made the formal intellectual aspect of medicine transparently clear in its relationship to the demands of practice. In the West today—it might be argued—the exigencies of practice assume a secondary, if not subterranean, role in the shaping of formal medical thought.

VII

The discussion has thus far had to do with the content of medical history, with broadening, deepening, and balancing the body of knowledge making up the discipline. There is still another, and I

33

think more than negligible, argument for the vitalization of a profession-centred literature within the history of medicine. This is pedagogic.

Much of the contemporary interest in medical history evinced by some medical educators relates to the possibility of its serving a meaningful role in the social education of the student-physician.[10] Medical history from this point of view may help provide insight and perspective into the social and clinical aspects of medicine, perhaps help the medical student see his profession in its relationship to the patient and to society as well as a science pure and applied. What could more accurately answer the purpose than a medical school history programme based on a consideration of the ways in which social needs and dimensions effect the physician's role; what might be more likely to attract the interest of the critically minded student? How could one, finally, even from the narrow disciplinary viewpoint of medical history more successfully recruit energetic and imaginative young practitioners into the field?

NOTES AND REFERENCES

1 E. H. Ackerknecht, 'A plea for a "behaviorist" approach in writing the history of medicine', *J. Hist. Med.* 1967, 22, 211–14; George Rosen, 'People, disease, and emotion: some newer problems for research in medical history', *Bull. Hist. Med.* 1967, 41, 5–23. Henry Sigerist and Bernhard Stern have, of course, made analogous programmatic statements in the past.

2 For a revision of older views, cf. R. S. Roberts, 'The personnel and practice of medicine in Tudor and Stuart England. Part I. The provinces'. *Med. Hist.* 1962, 6, 363–82; 'The personnel and practice of medicine in Tudor and Stuart England. Part II. London', ibid. 1964, 8, 217–34; S. W. F. Holloway, 'The Apothecaries' Act, 1815: a reinterpretation. Part I: the origins of the Act', ibid. 1966, 10, 107–29; 'Part II: The consequences of the Act', ibid. 1966, 10, 221–36. For some American parallels, cf. Barnes Riznik, 'The professional lives of early nineteenth-century New England doctors', *J. Hist. Med.* 1964, 19, 1–16.

3 For the present author's earlier views, cf. C. Rosenberg, 'The American medical profession: mid-nineteenth century', *Mid-America* 1962, 44, 163–71.

4 There is no definitive account of the movement for reform in American medical education at the beginning of this century. Important material

may be found, however, in the following: A. Flexner, *Medical education in the United States and Canada. A report to the Carnegie Foundation for the Advancement of Teaching*, New York: The Foundation, 1910; J. G. Burrow, *AMA. Voice of American medicine*, Baltimore: The Johns Hopkins University Press, 1963; *I remember. The autobiography of Abraham Flexner*, New York: Simon and Schuster, 1940; S. Flexner and J. T. Flexner, *William Henry Welch and the heroic age of American medicine*, New York: Viking Press, 1941.

5 Such case records and other hospital records exist from the mid-eighteenth century. These have, however, been little used. The compilation of a guide to such archival materials would certainly increase the likelihood of their being consulted in the future.

6 C. Rosenberg, 'The practice of medicine in New York a century ago', *Bull. Hist. Med.* 1967, 41, 223–53.

7 Edelstein's major papers in this area have been recently collected: *Ancient Medicine. Selected papers of Ludwig Edelstein*, ed. Owsei Temkin and C. Lilian Temkin, Baltimore: The Johns Hopkins Press, 1967; Fridolf Kudlien, 'In memoriam Ludwig Edelstein, 1902–1965: Edelstein as medical historian', *J. Hist. Med.* 1966, 21, 173–8; O. Temkin, 'Greek medicine as science and craft', *Isis* 1953, 44, 213–25.

8 Systematic historical studies of the diffusion of innovation are almost non-existent. For two systematic monographs, based on contemporary research in the diffusion of agricultural and therapeutic innovation, see B. Barber, *Drugs and society*, New York: R. Sage, 1967; E. Rogers, *Diffusion of innovation*, New York: The Free Press, 1962.

9 A similar point might be made in regard to medicine in contemporary China. Cf. Ralph C. Croizier, *Traditional medicine in modern China: science, nationalism, and the tensions of cultural change*, Cambridge: Harvard University Press, 1968.

10 For a sampling of contemporary positions on the appropriate place for medical history in the medical school, see J. B. Blake (ed.), *Education in the history of medicine: report of a Macy Conference. Sponsored by the Josiah Macy, Jr. Foundation in cooperation with the National Library of Medicine. Bethesda, Maryland, June 22–24, 1966*, New York and London: Hafner, 1968.

3 The Use of Literary and Documentary Evidence in the History of Medicine

R. S. ROBERTS

It would be wrong to suggest that there is any simple 'new way' to use literary and documentary evidence. The prime need for care, accuracy and impartiality has not changed; and it is not always true, unfortunately, that contemporary historians of medicine are any better in this regard than their predecessors. Similarly it would be wrong to suggest that there is any obvious 'new way' of acquiring evidence of this sort. Hitherto unknown documents and forgotten or lost works are sometimes brought to light; but no matter how enlightening these may be on particular topics, it is not likely that such acquisitions will significantly change the overall pattern of the history of medicine.

This, however, does not mean that there is no improvement to be achieved in technique or knowledge. Evidence that has long been known can often be used to yield new insights in many ways. For the truth is that evidence has usually been regarded as if it is immutable or fixed in significance, whereas in fact each generation is interested in slightly different facets of the 'evidence'. Each generation has a slightly different attitude to the problem of history which is modified by *previous* attitudes as much as by *new* evidence; professional historians, and even their students, accept this fact and it is almost a truism that 'each generation rewrites history in its own image'.

Amongst medical historians, however, such an attitude is not fully accepted in practice. Surprisingly for a new discipline, medical history still has an old-fashioned appearance; and much of what is written today is based on assumptions and attitudes that flourished among 'universal' and Whig historians a hundred years ago. For the purposes of illustration of this point, it can be said that there are three main ways in which evidence assembled in the past has 'fossilized' the writing of much medical history today.

Firstly, there is a great amount of literary evidence, mainly in the form of manuscripts, pamphlets and books written over the centuries which describe disease; such works often give valuable case-histories or eyewitness descriptions of epidemics, but their value for the reconstruction of the history of disease is tempered by the fact, often ignored, that they were written with certain traditional or philosophical assumptions. The task of medical historians is to discover those assumptions *before* the so-called facts derived from the evidence are put to use.

Secondly, there is a great amount of medical evidence, mainly in the form of articles and books, written by medical practitioners over the last hundred years or so. Such works give valuable, scientific descriptions of the causes and progress of disease, but their value in the reconstruction of the history of disease is nevertheless tempered by the fact that diseases are not immutable in history. The relationship between host and invading organism is rarely simple or static, and is certainly far more complicated than was realized by the first generation of proponents of a 'scientific' germ theory of disease. Consequently, it does not necessarily follow that modern descriptions of a disease will exactly fit the course of that disease throughout history.

Thirdly, there is a great amount of evidence, mainly in the form of books written by medical practitioners over the last century, which describe the history of the medical profession. The general tone of these works was largely defined in the nineteenth century when a facile view of progress was dominant. Consequently in the history of medicine every event, whether great like the Renaissance or small like the founding of a medical corporation, is treated as an integral part of a continuous process of improvement in which the contemporary situation is seen as the inevitable, and perfect result.

If evidence has become fossilized in this sense, that it has been made to fit certain preconceived patterns, then it must follow that the form of medical history itself, to some extent at least, is predetermined and rigid; and in the following elaboration of the three groupings of evidence it will be shown that sympathetic use can lead to better results and that there is in fact evidence of other sorts, not essentially medical, which could often be called in to help overcome the preconceptions and rigidity of analysis so often prevalent.

37

II

LITERARY EVIDENCE

This term is somewhat arbitrary in that 'literary' is here used in distinction to the 'scientific' writings that are subsumed under the second main type of evidence. Literary evidence in its widest sense can, of course, include the *literature* of any period. Therefore there may be value in perusing Shakespeare's plays, for example, for references to medicine which throw light on the ideas, practice and personnel of medicine in sixteenth-century England; and this has often been done.[1] Where except in literature would one find evidence for unpleasant, but medically important, environmental facts such as the ubiquity of infestation by human fleas?[2] Where, except in the memoirs of a Boswell or a Hickey, would one find the intimate details of prophylaxis against, and treatment of, venereal disease?[3] Nevertheless, for the medical historian the usefulness of this sort of evidence is limited. Shakespeare's frequent references to syphilis tell us virtually nothing of the aetiology of the disease, and give no clues about the supposed American origin of it; it is the student of literary forms and ideas who finds these references to syphilis vitally important as evidence of the repressed fears of the author, of the incipient fear of his age that pleasure was now to be bought only at cost. It is puritanism (or libertinism in Boswell and Hickey's case) that is illuminated rather than syphilis or gonorrhoea.

It is in a narrower sense, however, that 'literary' is used here, to mean the pre-scientific medical writings, manuscript or printed, of medical men through the ages. These are the main source of our knowledge of disease in the past and form the basis of most histories of medicine. Typical of works written upon this sort of basis are the standard histories of epidemics by Corradi,[4] Hecker,[5] Hirsch[6] and Creighton.[7] Of these works, Creighton's is undoubtedly the best known in the English-speaking world and may therefore be used as an example to illustrate the 'fossilization' of evidence that has been postulated above.

Creighton's massive two volumes on the history of epidemics in Britain have never been superseded, and the editors of the recent second edition are probably correct in their claim that footnote references to his work are more frequent today than ever before.[8]

38

Most readers realize, of course, that Creighton's explanations of epidemics are wrong in that he resolutely rejected the germ theory of disease. Nevertheless many who use Creighton today proceed upon the assumption that his erroneous theories on the causation of disease can simply be separated out from his work, leaving a solid basis of indisputable fact to which the correct scientific explanations can then be given. What is not realized is that the 'facts' themselves have in the first place emerged from a process of selection, whether conscious or not, designed to prove Creighton's theories.

Before Creighton's 'standard' work can therefore be used medical historians must do as demanded in the introduction, and discover the theoretical presuppositions which underlie the whole. In Creighton's case this is not merely that he believed in the localist-miasmatic theory of disease causation; the important point is that he was a Malthusian whose firm belief in the *de novo* origin of disease could not be reconciled with the rudimentary germ theory of causation at a time when mutation of viruses, for example, was not even postulated. Creighton in his history, therefore, was always on the look-out for sudden eruptions of 'new' diseases, preferably highly localized, to give point to his dislike of an admittedly crude germ theory which seemed to imply not only that diseases were uniform but also that they might be ubiquitous.

A typical example of Creighton's procedure is his treatment of the sweating sickness which caused many deaths in Tudor England. After much inconsistent argument about the route and exact date of the introduction of the first epidemic in 1485, the main thesis which Creighton advances is that this was a disease which affected only Englishmen and that it erupted only five times (1485, 1508, 1517, 1528 and 1551). Such a thorough-going example of 'localist' disease has naturally become something of a puzzle to medical historians. To replace Creighton's wrong explanation, however, is not easy in view of the singular nature of the 'facts' of the disease. Consequently attempts have been made to solve the problem in the only logical way available, namely to ascribe the five outbreaks to food poisoning,[9] in exactly the same way that eighteenth- and nineteenth-century physicians explained outbreaks of influenza and encephalomyelitis as the result of poisoning by radish seeds (Raphania) or by Swabian sausage (so-called botulism, properly allantiasis).[10]

When such explanations are scrutinised, it is quickly seen that

39

they must fail for lack of evidence.[11] That, however, is not the most important aspect of the matter. For the basic point to be made is that the 'facts', on which rests the whole description of the outbreaks, and the consequent explanations, have been established by a highly selective means in the first instance in order to prove the singular 'localist' disease! A careful examination of Creighton's sources will show that he omitted reference to the works of several observant contemporaries of the 'sweat'. Paradin, Fernel and Jordanus, for example, all described 'sweating' fevers which swept not only England but also the rest of Britain, the Low Countries, Germany and France on several occasions in the 1520's; furthermore there is scattered evidence for other outbreaks outside England in 1543, 1545–46 and 1551, and for other outbreaks in England in 1545 and 1558.[11] The careful reader of Creighton's footnotes will in fact see allusions to some of these awkward facts which he seems to have determined not to fit into his main description lest it invalidate his 'localist' exposition.[12] The most awkward facts of all, however, are completely omitted and it is difficult to avoid the conclusion that Creighton deliberately suppressed them; the numerous and irrefutable instances of the 'sweat' in Ireland, especially in 1491–92 for example, are nowhere referred to by Creighton despite the fact that he used the famous 'Tables of Pestilences' of the 1851 Census which tabulated all the references to the 'sweat' in the various Irish Chronicles.[13]

Lest this seems too harsh a judgement, it need only be remembered that Creighton also consistently misused the evidence relating to the early history of smallpox in the sixteenth century in order to minimize both the incidence and the severity of smallpox before the seventeenth century. The purpose of this was to emphasize the rapid but entirely natural rise and fall of disease, which proved that the later decline of smallpox was not due to any supposed virtue of vaccination! Thus famous epidemics of smallpox such as that of 1561–62 are completely omitted from Creighton's narrative, despite the well-known fact that Queen Elizabeth herself suffered such a severe attack that many at Court contemplated the need to appoint a successor![14]

Creighton's notorious dislike for Jenner is of course well known. Consequently when Razzell a few years ago based part of his argument on Creighton's 'facts' concerning variolation and vaccination, it was hardly surprising that there was a swift repudiation by medical writers.[15] This episode, however, provides a doubly interesting illustration of the need for a 'new way' in medical history: firstly it is only in the present collection of essays that attention has at last been given to Razzell's more general but related arguments on population growth;[16] secondly, it is surprising to note that this sort of medical criticism is not generally brought to bear on Creighton's 'facts' and arguments on the pre-Jennerian history of smallpox, or indeed on the history of other diseases.

The general conclusion that emerges from this examination then, is that all 'literary' works must be studied carefully *within* the traditional framework in which their facts are presented. Even purported eyewitness accounts must be scrutinized; when medical writers of Tudor times, for example, describe rats, moles and snakes leaving their holes before plague struck, it must be remembered that in fact they are repeating Avicenna, almost verbatim![17]

III

MEDICAL EVIDENCE

As explained in the introduction, this term is taken to mean scientific writings of medical men over the last century in distinction to that of their predecessors who have been discussed under the heading of 'literary'. The scientific demonstration of the causes of diseases has, of course, made it much easier for the medical historian to unravel the problems of historic epidemics. Armed with modern knowledge, one can read Rhaze's differentiation of smallpox from measles, with appreciation of his accurate observation and succinct description but with complete disregard for his explanations of the causes. Nevertheless it has been made clear from the dangers inherent in the 'facts' of the older writers that even this innocent procedure has its dangers.

There is, however, a positive 'new way' of approaching medical evidence. Briefly this is to appreciate the danger that modern scientific knowledge may often appear so comprehensive in its explanation of disease that its application to medical history becomes too rigid. The historiography of plague is a good case in point.

The work on the third pandemic, notably in India, has been comprehensively summarised by Hirst and Pollitzer;[18] consequently historians of plague rarely go beyond these authorities for their explanations of the ways in which the historic outbreaks of plague occurred. This procedure suffers from none of the defects that are inherent in reliance on 'literary' evidence or Creighton's facts; but this must not be allowed to obscure the existence of two, complementary, weaknesses in total reliance on medical evidence.

The first point noticed by a *historian* is that the incidence of bubonic plague cases in the studies of the Indian Plague Commission is very different from that found in London, Pamplona, or Venice, for example, in the sixteenth and seventeenth centuries. Modern experience '...confirmed through ample observations in various plague areas [is] that...the plague cases appearing...in individual houses usually remain single.'[19] In Pamplona in 1599, however, only twenty-two out of three hundred and forty-four deaths were solitary cases.[20] Similarly in Crediton in 1546–47 and Chesterfield in 1586–87 fifty per cent of the deaths occurred in a mere eight and fifteen per cent of the families, respectively.[21] Deaths in Croydon in 1665 were even more localized,[22] and the result of such multiple incidence was often the death of whole families, both in small villages[23] and great cities.[24]

These facts will, it is feared, be neglected as long as total reliance is given to the standard medical works on the subject. Only when these facts have been exhaustively studied can their significance, if any, be evaluated. This is not the place to offer hypotheses or explanations, but it does need to be pointed out that the few medical historians who have taken cognizance of the detailed evidence of historic outbreaks of plague have tended to come to one conclusion: that bubonic plague was largely spread by *Pulex irritans*, and not the fleas of rats![25] One detailed study has, admittedly, come to the conventional conclusion on the mode of transmission,[26] but it is remarkable that the questions raised have largely been ignored. Only one writer, apparently, has called for investigation and this too seems to have been ignored.[27]

The second, complementary, weakness due to reliance upon standard medical works, is that there develops a similar neglect by the medical historian of more recent *medical* work. A medical historian may perhaps be forgiven ignorance of the social historians' detailed findings of the sort indicated above; but if so it would be hoped that acquaintance with recent scientific research might suggest historical analogies, and in that way encourage a study of the incidence and mode of transmission of bubonic plague in the past. For the fact is that much scientific work has been done since the publication of the standard works by Hirst and Pollitzer in 1953–1954;[28] and whether this work stands the test of time or not, it is again surprising that its implications for medical history have not at least been given some attention. If this could be done, the facts discovered by social historians might suddenly take on a new meaning.

The value of attention to modern scientific work can, however, be even greater than this; for it can also lead back to other scientific work hitherto ignored by medical historians. Thus in the case of plague, acquaintance with Baltazard's publications may open up new lines of inquiry; the long tradition of work on plague in North Africa by Frenchmen, for example, raises the whole question of the route by which plague may have reached Europe.[29] Similarly the work of Devignat raises the problem of the disappearance of plague from Western Europe by the late seventeenth and early eighteenth centuries and also provides a framework for the better understanding of the differences between the three pandemics.[30]

In concluding this section on modern medical work it is interesting to note that medical historians have often appeared strangely reluctant to use scientific work as a basis for their work on disease in the past. Instead, there appears to have been a preference for what we have called 'literary' evidence despite its disadvantages. Yet it can hardly be disputed that modern examination of, for example, rural diets and pellagra are as sure a guide at least to deficiency diseases in the past, if only by analogy, as any selective 'literary' descriptions.[31] Similarly the whole problem of the origin of epidemic (or was it endemic?) syphilis in late fifteenth-century Europe needs to be looked at in a new way. Sudhoff's 'literary' evidence[32] should be checked not only against earlier documentary evidence but also against modern knowledge of the history and behaviour of the *Treponema pallidum* and the related treponemata.[33] In this way two distinct sorts of evidence can be used, to complement and check each other.

IV

EVIDENCE CONCERNING THE HISTORY OF THE MEDICAL
PROFESSION

The history of the education and practice of medical men, and of
the institutions to which they belong, has always fascinated members
of the profession; and much has been written particularly in the last
hundred years or so since professional regulation was introduced by
the Medical Act of 1858. The evidence on which this work is based
comes from both the categories which have been described. The
earlier evidence is 'literary' and consists of the books and pamphlets
written over the centuries by medical men, many of whom had
access to the documentary records of institutions like the Royal
College of Physicians of London. The later evidence is 'medical' in
the sense that modern scientific knowledge has been used to show
the significance of the work of men such as Harvey.

The value of this work, however, has often been marred by the
ways in which the evidence has been used. By and large, the history
written has been fitted into a rigid (though attractive) framework of
progress. Instead of fitting the evidence into its contemporary background, most historians of the profession have interpreted it only
in the light of nineteenth- and twentieth-century standards of medical
ethics and knowledge. The consequent perversion of our understanding of the past has lasted till today. The rigid insistence on
orderly progress, for example, has led to the almost universally poor
opinion of Anglo-Saxon medicine as evidenced by the early Leech
Books. These works, it is argued, are nothing but a jumble of
barbarous folk remedies and superstitious ideas, whereas later texts
such as the *Peri Didaxeon* are much superior in their use of rational
medicine.[34] In fact, however, a careful comparison of the early
Leech Books with both classical texts and the later English texts
show clearly that the Leech Books not only owed much to Greek and
Roman authorities but also were superior in some respects to the
later texts.[35]

Similarly the fact that English surgeons of the late fourteenth and
of the fifteenth centuries were highly skilled, well-read and interested in chemistry[36] is usually obscured by the uncritical acceptance
of the Renaissance as the beginning of progress. Yet again the 'pro-

gressiveness' of Renaissance medicine is largely unquestioned, and consequently there is little consideration of the fact that much of the popularity of Galen in England, for example, was often highly selective.

The whole question of the nature of medical practice and knowledge in the period of the Renaissance has in fact been bedevilled by *a priori* assumptions. Nowhere is this clearer than in the way in which the history of institutions like the Royal College of Physicians of London has been presented. For nearly two hundred years surgeons and apothecaries in London fought a continual battle against the privileges of this monopolistic body; ultimately they won in 1704 on the clear decision of the House of Lords that it was not in the public interest so to limit the practice of medicine. Yet this undoubted fact has never been made the basis for a new perspective. Still the Licensing Act of 1512 and the Charter of the College in 1518 are presented as milestones in the development of modern medical organization. The pleas of surgeons in their books, the testimony of witnesses in law cases, the attitude of public bodies,[37] all suffer from neglect because 'establishment' history of the physicians is uncritically accepted.

Even events which have always been something of a puzzle are presented in this way, despite the abundance of documentary evidence that has long lain unconsulted. The most glaring example of this is the London Pharmacopoeia of 1618: the obvious questions of why it was published when it was, and why there were two editions within the year have been interpreted solely within a framework of planned medical progress. No attempt has been made to look at evidence of the attitude of the Grocers Company from whom the new Apothecaries Company had separated; little consideration has been given to evidence of the constitutional and economic structure of the City of London within which the Apothecaries, Grocers and Physicians operated; no search has ever been made of the legal evidence of cases in the courts where their demarcation disputes were decided. In short, medical history all too often is treated as an abstraction from the social-economic context within which medical men and their patients lived. The consequent limitations of much of the writing on the profession and practice of medicine can only be compared with an attempt to survey contemporary medical practice in Britain which consistently ignored the existence of the National Health Service!

45

This sort of fossilization of evidence has also had the undesirable effect that whole areas of medical history have been neglected. The pervasive belief in orderly progress has often destroyed interest in periods when nothing striking appears to have been achieved. Thus the forty-three years between the Apothecaries' Act of 1815 and the Medical Act of 1858 have been almost totally ignored despite their crucial significance in the evolution of the medical profession; the Apothecaries' Act was the first step in the reform of the profession, so it appears to be tacitly assumed, and the Medical Act was the natural complement. That the leaders of the medical profession resisted, rather than planned, reform during these forty-three years is a human failing resolutely ignored; consequently the fact that the Apothecaries' Act was not reformist in intention or effect was not realized until a sociologist, and not a medical historian, took the trouble to study the legal cases brought under that Act.[38]

V

THE 'NEW WAY' OF USING EVIDENCE

The conclusion that emerges from the survey of our three types of rigidity is that there must be much greater flexibility in the use made of evidence by medical historians. It is no longer appropriate to rely on any one sort of evidence or any one sort of approach. Unfortunately much writing of medical history has become 'fossilized' and recent descriptions of the 'sweat', of the plague or of the medical corporations are largely reworkings of the standard evidence with nothing really fresh to say. The new and exciting history that is being written today is only marginally medical history, but its successes can be taken as a measure of what can be done. As this essay has hitherto been largely negative, it would be useful at this point to illustrate with positive examples the ways in which evidence can be used.

It has been shown that the history of the medical profession and the medical corporations in the sixteenth and seventeenth centuries has been written in narrow, exclusively medical terms, but there is ample evidence which is relevant and yet has never been fully utilized. The study of the records of the City of London, for example, would show that the dominating consideration for the Royal College of Physicians in the Tudor period was not medical progress, but the related problems of monopoly of practice and the constitutional tradition of freedom enjoyed by citizens of the City. The Acts of Parliament of 1540, when viewed against this background, take on a new meaning; the searching of the apothecaries, the right of the physicians to practise surgery, the union of the surgeons with the Barber-Surgeons, are all matters which are municipal rather than medical in origin and intention. Similarly, consideration of the cases brought in the Court of Exchequer thereafter, would illustrate the difficulties of enforcing the monopolies of surgery and medicine.[37] It can then be seen why the surgeons had a strong economic interest in Galen and Paracelsus. The texts of Galen translated by surgeons were essentially those which related to medical treatment by internal as well as external means; it was not Galen's knowledge but his concept of unified treatment by a *medicus*, or general practitioner, rather than by both physician and surgeon, that appealed to the surgeons.[39] In the actual details of treatment, innovation came largely from the very same surgeons who were translating Galen in order to exploit his authority; for they, and not apothecaries or physicians, led the field in experimenting with new chemical remedies.[40]

A study of Port Books which give the statistics of imports for this period would also confirm this view that experiment in pharmaceutical preparations lay in the field of chemicals rather than of Galenicals or exotics. For it is surprising that, almost a century after the opening up of the new oceanic trade routes, the only 'new' drugs imported regularly into England were guaiacum, china root and sarsaparilla, all remedies for syphilis.[41] Further study of the Port Books for the seventeenth century, on the other hand, would demonstrate a rapidly changing situation in which the import of exotic drugs was increasing year by year;[41] and it is against this medical background rather than any supposed battle over the use of chemicals, that the first British Pharmacopoeia should be studied.

Nevertheless it needs to be emphasized that medical considerations of this sort were not necessarily the most important in medical history; and any detailed consideration of the 1618 Pharmacopoeia and its two editions of that year must rather take account of the municipal situation in London. For a study of the records of the Corporation of London and of the Grocers on the one hand, and of the Court of Star Chamber and Chancery on the other, would show

47

that the difference in the contents of the two issues of the Pharma-copoeia were not due to any rivalry of therapeutic theories, but were the result of complicated legal battles amongst the traders of the City of London.[42]

Almost the whole history of the medical profession, its practice and its institutions, in fact, will be brought to life only when there is adequate research into the social and economic context of which medicine was but a part. With this theoretical generalization nobody presumably would disagree; but to translate this into practice has proved remarkably difficult for medical historians in this country and basically it is a question of methodology: records not medical in character must be studied in order to appreciate and evaluate those which are. What the limits to such an approach are, is not easy to define. The most unlikely sources can illuminate a medical problem: the history of the regulation of midwives in the sixteenth and seven-teenth centuries, for example, has taken a new meaning for the present author by a study of the attitude of the Church in England towards childbirth and baptism in relation to the religious changes from Catholicism to Protestantism and back to Catholicism again, and then finally to Protestantism.

This sort of approach to evidence is not limited to the social aspects of the history of medicine, although of course not every problem can be handled in exactly the same way. Some aspects of the history of medicine such as new discoveries in anatomy are not likely to be illuminated by the sort of 'external' evidence that has just been described; Harvey's experiments and discoveries, for example, are 'internal' in that they are to be understood as part of a continuing tradition of interest *within* medicine. Nevertheless even this sort of scientific history should not be studied in isolation, and a consideration of evidence illustrating the development of philo-sophy can often supply a framework of reference similar in nature to the social framework necessary for the medical profession and its practice. In the case of the discovery of the circulation of the blood the significance of Harvey's methodology and success can be fully appreciated only when due weight is given both to his conservative attitude and to the potentiality of Aristotelianism at Padua.[43]

Similarly the history of disease can be extended by attention to evidence usually neglected. The standard histories of disease in Britain, for example, whether of the 'literary' or 'medical' variety, have relatively little to say about the years after the 'last' outbreak of 'sweat' in 1551. Economic historians, however, have paid attention to this period because it appears to have been a time of considerable crisis. Hoskins noticed the number of harvest failures and the high mortality, especially in 1557–58, and he found that parochial registers of burials and wills proved, indicate a death-rate four times higher than usual; indeed there was a contemporary assessment, ignored in the standard works, that one-third of the population was carried off in these years by epidemics of influenza.[44] Another contemporary opinion, again usually ignored, was that these epidemics were further outbreaks of the 'sweat'.[45] Work of other social and economic historians, using other evidence, tends to confirm the drastic extent of this epidemic crisis. Fisher in comparing wage-rates and prices of food in Elizabethan England came to the conclusion that the strange divergence of these indices can only be explained by an extremely high mortality in these years.[46] Local histories and parish registers similarly confirm the importance of these years, which in fact seem to have been a complicated famine-epidemic crisis in which plague and typhus were as important as influenza or the 'new sickness'.[47]

The importance of such work is not merely that it may correct former knowledge. Far more important than correction, or even amplification, is the awareness that more can be discovered about the pattern of disease than former medical historians ever realized. Registers of baptism, burial and marriage can be used to yield a vast amount of information, as French and British historical demographers have shown. Thus Drake and Howson in their limited studies have already indicated that the pattern of disease was very different from what is usually assumed. In the period when plague is thought of as the main killer, for example, burials rose much higher in winter months than in summer in the years of exceptionally high mortality. The reasons for this may vary from region to region; in the West Riding it was probably trade depression but in north-west England it was more likely to have been poor harvests. In either case, however, it is interesting to note the importance claimed in these preliminary studies for high food prices and the mobility of the population.[48] Similarly for the eighteenth century, detailed local studies have been made by historical demographers and economic and social historians;[49] and these contain considerable

49

material on disease and death rates which has not so far been utilized by medical historians.

Indeed it is with some envy that the medical historian in Britain today looks at this sort of evidence which lies to hand but which was assembled by historical demographers. The latter's use of traditional 'literary' evidence has been combined with a study of the parish records, and by virtue of techniques like 'family reconstitution' exciting new insights are being obtained.[50] Furthermore the foundation of the Cambridge Group for the History of Population and Social Structure has made possible the development of co-ordinated detailed research, locality by locality.[51]

VI

This, it seems, is one of the 'new ways' that medical history should take. The implication of much of the argument above has been the need to break down the barriers between literary and medical evidence, to encourage interest in neglected sources like parish records, and to promote local studies in depth. It is not only the history of disease that awaits reconstruction. In most British Record Offices there are the inventories, wills, medical licences, and prescription books left by medical men since Tudor times; in the Public Record Office there are similar records of legal cases, bankruptcies, apprenticeships, imports of drugs, all awaiting systematic use. In 1962 the present writer twice made a plea for detailed local work to be done on these records,[52] but little has been achieved so far. Consequently there is an almost complete absence in Britain of that sort of local 'case-study' which is available for many areas of Germany and France. Clearly, a county-by-county, town-by-town medical history of Britain, with national and international comparative studies in order to avoid antiquarianism and with the incorporation of the few existing, widely-dispersed writings, is needed. If, for example, there was a detailed study of London apothecaries in the seventeenth century of the sort that Doucet has done for Nantes,[53] then many of the legends of British medical history would fall away. For it could more easily be seen that the apothecaries of London in the 1630s were not struggling for freedom to practise medicine; on the contrary those who did devote themselves to medicine were deprived of seniority in the Society in order that power remained in the hands of 'true' apothecaries whose interest was in the free sale of drugs. Similarly it would be seen that the emergence in the eighteenth century of the apothecary as a general practitioner was more often than not a verbal illusion, behind which surgeons, often home from naval and military service, successfully appropriated the trade of the apothecary and the practice of the physicians.[53]

Generalizations of the sort discussed above, whether about the social history of the profession or the course of historic epidemics, can be validated, however, only when there are numerous case-studies which provide the factual proof and the means of comparison; and in Britain these studies are not likely to be made until there is some academic centre to plan and coordinate research. Furthermore such a centre, on the model of the Cambridge Group for the History of Population as part of a department of the history of medicine and in contact with related academic disciplines, is all the more necessary because the 'new way' in using evidence outlined above postulates considerable interdisciplinary activity. As another contributor points out,[54] it is dangerous for an economic historian to venture into the field of virology; but if the available evidence of the different sorts is to be used properly, then historians must somewhere be able to learn the essentials of epidemiology just as medical men need instruction in historical methodology. Furthermore they must have somewhere to meet, to cooperate and to achieve that cross-fertilization of ideas that a protean subject like medical history demands. Only then will the 'new way' of using evidence be realized.

REFERENCES

1 See for example, P. M. Yearsley, *Doctors in Elizabethan drama*, London, Bale & Danielsson, 1933;
   R. R. Simpson, *Shakespeare and medicine*, London: E. & S. Livingstone, 1959;
   P. G. Brewster, 'Physician and surgeon as depicted in 16th and 17th century English literature', *Osiris* 1962, 14, 13–32.
2 G. Gascoigne [d. 1577], 'Gascoygnes good night' in J. W. Cunliffe (ed.), *George Gascoigne: the poesies*, Cambridge: University Press, 1907 (vol. 1 of J. W. Cunliffe (ed.), *The complete works of George Gascoigne*, 2 vols.) in 'Flowers', pp. 35–95, see p. 59.

3   F. A. Pottle (ed.), *Boswell's London journal 1762–1763...*, pp. 49–50, 155–8, 173, 227, 237, 255, 262, London: Heinemann, 1950;
    C. Ryskamp and F. A. Pottle (eds.), *Boswell: the ominous years 1774–1776*, pp. 326–7, London: Heinemann, 1963;
    P. Quennell (ed.), *Memoirs of William Hickey*, p. 171, London: Hutchinson, 1960.

4   A. Corradi, 'Annali delle epidemie occorse in Italia dalle prime memorie, fino al 1850...con varie note e dichiarazoni', *Mem. Soc. med.-chir. Bologna*, 1865–92, vol. 6, fasc. 3–9; vol. 8 [postumo], Bologna: Gamberini and Parmeggiani, 1894.

5   J. F. C. Hecker, *The epidemics of the Middle Ages*, transl. B. G. Babington, London: Sydenham Soc., 1844.

6   A. Hirsch, *Handbook of geographical and historical pathology*, transl. (from 2nd German ed.) C. Creighton, 3 vols., London: New Sydenham Soc., 1883–6.

7   C. Creighton, *A history of epidemics in Britain from A.D. 664 to the extinction of the plague*, 2 vols., Cambridge University Press, 1891–4.

8   D. E. C. Eversley, 'Epidemiology as social history' in C. Creighton, *A history of epidemics in Britain from A.D. 664 to the extinction of the plague*, with additional material by D. E. C. Eversley, E. A. Underwood and L. Ovenall, 2 vols., 2nd ed., I, 4 [Introduction], London: F. Cass, 1965.

9   For example, see A. Patrick, 'A consideration of the nature of the English sweating sickness', *Med. Hist.* 1965, 9, 272–9.

10 F. G. Crookshank, 'The history of epidemic encephalomyelitis in relation to influenza', *Proc. R. Soc. Med.* (*Sect. Hist. Med.*), 1918–19, 12, 1–21 [reprinted in F. G. Crookshank (ed.), *Influenza: essays*, pp. 81–101, London: W. Heinemann, 1922];
    Sir A. S. MacNalty, 'Encephalitis lethargica', *Br. med. J.* 1926, i, 1073–6, and idem., *Epidemic diseases of the central nervous system*, London: Faber and Gwyer, 1927 [Milroy Lecture], *passim*.

11 See R. S. Roberts, 'A consideration of the nature of the English sweating sickness', *Med. Hist.* 1965, 9, 385–9.

12 See Creighton, op. cit. (above, note 7), vol. I, pp. 245, 264 (footnote I), 280, 400 (footnote 2).

13 *The census of Ireland for the year 1851. Part V. Tables of deaths*, 2 vols., vol. I, Sect. I, 'Table of cosmical phenomena, epizootics, epiphitics, famines and pestilences in Ireland', pp. 41–333; and Sect. II, 'Analysis of the foregoing table...', pp. 334–64, Dublin: A. Thom, 1856 [*Accounts and papers* (Ireland), 1856 (2087–1), XXIX, 261; 1856 (2087–11), XXX, 1].

14 J. Caius, 'Annalium Collegii medicorum Londini Liber, Anno 1555 institutus, Johanne Caïo praesidente & authore' [1518–72], p. 55, in E. S. Roberts (ed.), *The works of John Caius, M.D....*, Cambridge University Press, 1912;
    J. A. Froude, *History of England from the fall of Wolsey to the death of Queen Elizabeth*, 12 vols., vol. 7, p. 429, London: Longmans, Green, 1862–70;

J. E. Neale, *Queen Elizabeth I*, p. 123, London: Penguin Books, 1960.

15 P. E. Razzell, 'Edward Jenner: the history of a medical myth', *Med. Hist.*
1965, 9, 216–23; 'Comment by Professor A. W. Downie, M.D., F.R.S.',
ibid., pp. 223–5; 'Mr. Razzell's reply', ibid., pp. 226–9; N. Schuster,
'Edward Jenner: a medical myth', ibid., pp. 381–3; D. Baxby, 'Inoculation and vaccination: smallpox, cowpox and vaccinia', ibid., pp. 383–5.

16 P. E. Razzell, 'Population change in eighteenth century England: a reinterpretation', *Econ. Hist. Rev.* 1965, 18 (2nd ser.), 312–22; idem.,
'Population growth and economic change in eighteenth- and early nineteenth-century England and Scotland' in E. L. Jones and G. E. Mingay
(eds.), *Land, labour and population in the Industrial Revolution, essays presented to J. D. Chalmers*, pp. 260–81, London: E. Arnold, 1967; and T.
McKeown, 'Medical issues in historical demography', below, ch. 4,
pp. 57–74.

17 Cf. Avicenna, [*Canon medicinae*, libri I–IV], 2 vols., vol. 2, lib. quart., fen.
I, tract. 4, cap. 3, p. 69: Venice: Juntae, 1608; and descriptions in G.
Skeyne, *Ane breve descriptioun of the pest...*, Edinburgh: R. Lekprevik,
1568; and T. Lodge, *A treatise of the plague...*, for E. White and N. L[ing],
1603.

18 L. F. Hirst, *The conquest of plague: a study of the evolution of epidemiology*,
Oxford: Clarendon Press, 1953;
R. Pollitzer, *Plague*, Geneva: W.H.O., 1954.

19 Pollitzer (1954), op. cit. (above, note 18), p. 485. See also Hirst, op. cit.
(above, note 18), pp. 146, 236.

20 J. Viñes Ibarrola, *Una epidemia de peste bubónica en el siglo XVI...*, p. 46,
Pamplona: Editorial Aramburu, 1947.

21 W. G. Hoskins, 'Epidemics in English history', *The Listener* 1964, 72,
1044–6, see p. 1045;
W. E. Godfrey, 'The plague in Chesterfield, 1586–7', *Journal of the Derby-
shire Archaeological and Natural History Society* 1954, 74, 32–42, see
p. 38.

22 A. G. E. Jones, 'The Great Plague in Croydon', *Notes and Queries* 1956,
201 (N.S. 3), 332–4;
C. A. F. Meekings (ed.), *Surrey Hearth Tax 1664*, Surrey Record Society
17, 1940, see p. xciii.

23 A. Gooder (compiler), *Plague and enclosure: a Warwickshire village in the
seventeenth century (Clifton-upon-Dunsmore)*, Coventry and North Warwickshire History Pamphlets: No. 2, 1965 [University of Birmingham and
the Coventry Branch of the Historical Association], pp. 45, see p. 6.

24 T. Vincent, *Gods terrible voice in the city...*, p. 31, London: G. Calvert,
1667.

25 E. Rodenwaldt, 'Pest in Venedig 1575–1577. Ein Beitrag zur Frage der
Infektkette bei den Pestepidemien West-Europas', *Sber. heidelb. Akad.
Wiss.* (*Mathematische-Naturwissenschaftliche Klasse*) 1952, pp. 119–381,
see '4. Die Infektkette der Pest bei ihren Westeuropäischen Epidemien',
pp. 336–77 [2. Abhandlung, pp. 263, see pp. 218–59];

G. Lavier, 'Étude épidémiologique de la célèbre peste de Marseille en 1720', *Bull. Soc. Path. exot.* 1953, **46**, 728–40;

P. Diosi, 'Étude épidémiologique de la célèbre épidémie de peste enregistrée en 1709 en Transylvanie', *Maroc Méd.* 1961, **40**, 1090–2; idem, 'Cserei Mihaly a bubopestis terjedesi modjarol' ['Michael Cserei: the epidemiology of pestilential bubo'], *Orvosi Szemle* 1961, **7**, 222–4; idem, 'Bemerkungen eines Zeitgenossen über die Verbreitungsart der Pest in Burzenlande im Jahre 1786', *Centaurus* 1963–64, **9**, 38–44; idem, 'Aufzeichnungen eines Augenzeugen über die Pestepidemie der Jahre 1718–1720 in Siebenbürgen', *Janus* 1964, **51**, 221–5.

26   E. Woehlkens, *Pest und Ruhr im 16. und 17. Jahrhundert*, Hanover: Niedersächsischer Heimatbund, 1954.

27   G. Rath, 'Von Ratten, Flöhen und dem Erlöschen der Pest in Europa', *Z. ärztl. Fortbild.* [West Germany] 1961, **50**, 10–12; but see the present author's forthcoming study, 'A reconsideration of the history of plague', which is in preparation.

28   See the publications of M. Baltazard and his many collaborators which have been summarized in 'La peste: état actuel de la question', *Acta med. iran.* 1961, **4**, 1–19; M. Baltazard *et al.*, 'Séance especiale consacré à la mémoire de Georges Blanc. Étude de l'épidémiologie de la peste dans le Kurdistan iranien', *Bull. Soc. Path. exot.* 1963, **56**, 1101–246.

29   G. Blanc, 'Une opinion non conformiste sur le mode de transmission de la peste', *Revue Hyg. Méd. soc.* 1956, **4**, 535–62; G. Grenoilleau, 'Notes sur la peste en Algérie', *Bull. mens. Off. int. Hyg. publ.* 1946, **38**, 419–31 [English translation, ibid., pp. 432–44].

30   R. Devignat, 'Réflexions sur la conservation du virus de la peste à travers les âges', *Bull. Séanc. Acad. r. Sci. colon. (outre Mer)* 1964, **4**, 942–3; for a discussion of, and references to, other work of this author, see R. S. Roberts, 'The place of plague in English history', *Proc. R. Soc. Med. (Sect. Hist. Med.)* 1966, **59**, 101–5.

31   R. S. Roberts, 'Epidemics and social history: an essay review', *Med. Hist.* 1968, **12**, 305–16, see p. 316.

32   K. Sudhoff and C. Singer, *The earliest printed literature on syphilis: being tractates from the years 1495–1498*, Florence: R. Lier, 1925.

33   See notably, C. J. Hackett, 'On the origin of the human treponematoses (pinta, yaws, endemic syphilis and venereal syphilis)', *Bull. Wld. Hlth. Org.* 1963, **29**, 7–41; and the work of E. H. Hudson, summarized in 'Treponematosis and African slavery', *Br. J. vener. Dis.* 1964, **40**, 43–52 and in *J. Hist. Med.* 1969, **24**, 86.

34   J. F. Payne, *English medicine in the Anglo-Saxon times*, Oxford: Clarendon Press, 1904; and also, J. H. G. Gratton and C. Singer, *Anglo-Saxon medicine and magic illustrated especially from the semi-pagan text 'Lacnunga'*, London: Oxford University Press, 1952.

35   C. H. Talbot, *Medicine in medieval England*, pp. 18–23, London: Oldbourne, 1967.

36   Ibid., pp. 195–6; C. H. Talbot and E. H. Hammond, *The medical prac-*

titioners in medieval England : a biographical register, sub nomine Bradmore, Morstede and Weseham in 'General Index', London: Wellcome Historical Medical Library, 1965.

37 R. S. Roberts, 'The personnel and practice of medicine in Tudor and Stuart England, Part II. London', *Med. Hist.* 1964, 8, 217–34; idem, 'The Royal College of Physicians of London in the sixteenth and seventeenth centuries', *History of Science* 1966, 5, 87–100.

38 S. W. F. Holloway, 'The Apothecaries' Act, 1815: a reinterpretation', *Med. Hist.* 1966, 10, 107–29, 221–36.

39 *The questyonary of cyrurgyens...with the fourth Boke of the Terapentyke* [*sic*], *or Methode curatyfe of Claude Galyen...*, transl. R. Copland, sig. Ai^v–Aii, London: R. Wyer for H. Dabbe & R. Banckes [1542]; *Certaine workes of Galens called Methodus medendi, with...an Epitome of the third booke of Galen, of naturall faculties...*, transl. T. Gale, sig. Hvii, pp. 23–33 [London: H. Denham?, 1566]; C. Baker (ed.), *Guydos questions newly corrected. Whereunto is added the thirde and fourth booke of Galen...*, transl. R. Copland, London: T. East, 1579; see also, J. Hall, *A most excellent and learned worke of chirurgerie called Chirurgia parva Lanfranci...*, sigs. *iv^v, Ai^v–ii, London: T. Marshe, 1565.

40 P. H. Kocher, 'Paracelsan medicine in England: the first thirty years (*c.* 1570–1600)', *J. Hist. Med.* 1947, 2, 451–80; A. G. Debus, *The English Paracelsians*, pp. 56–7, 69–70, London: Oldbourne, 1965.

41 See the statistics in R. S. Roberts, 'The early history of the import of drugs into Britain', in F. N. L. Poynter (ed.), *The evolution of pharmacy in Britain*, pp. 165–85, see pp. 173–83, London: Pitman, 1965.

42, See the present author's forthcoming study 'The origin of the British pharmacopoeia: medical rivalries, City government and the two editions of the London Pharmacopoeia of 1618', to be published by the British Society for the History of Pharmacy.

43 See, for example, J. H. Randall, Jr., *The career of philosophy, from the Middle Ages to the Enlightenment*, New York and London: Columbia University Press, 1962.

44 Hoskins, 1964, op. cit. (above, note 21), p. 1045.

45 J. Jones, *A dial for all agues : conteininge the names in Greeke, Latten, and Englyshe...*, sig. Ii^v, London: W. Seres, 1566.

46 F. J. Fisher, 'Influenza and inflation in Tudor England', *Econ. Hist. Rev.* 1965, 18 (2nd ser.), 120–9.

47 M. Drake, 'An elementary exercise in parish register demography', *Econ. Hist. Rev.*, 1961–62, 14 (2nd ser.), 427–45, see especially references to plague in footnotes 6–7 on pp. 431–2; W. G. Howson, 'Plague, poverty and population in parts of North-West England, 1580–1720', *Transactions of the Historic Society of Lancashire and Cheshire* 1961 [for the year 1960], 112, 29–55.

48 Drake (1961–62), op. cit. (above, note 47), pp. 435–7; Howson (1961), op. cit. (above, note 47), 'V. The wanderers', pp. 49–55.

49 See, for example, J. D. Chambers, *The Vale of Trent, 1670–1700: a regional*

study of economic change, Econ. Hist. Rev. Supplement 3 [1957]; idem, 'Population change in a provincial town: Nottingham 1700–1800' in L. S. Pressnell (ed.), *Studies in the Industrial Revolution presented to T. S. Ashton*, pp. 97–124, London: Athlone Press, 1960.

50   See, for example, D. E. C. Eversley, 'A survey of population in an area of Worcestershire from 1660–1850 on the basis of parish records', *Population Studies* 1956–57, 10, 253–79; E. A. Wrigley, 'Family limitation in pre-industrial England', *Econ. Hist. Rev.* 1966, 19 (2nd ser.), 82–109.

51   See E. A. Wrigley (ed.), *An introduction to English historical demography from the sixteenth to the nineteenth century*, London: Weidenfeld & Nicolson, 1966;

P. Laslett, *The world we have lost*, London: Methuen, 1965.

52   R. S. Roberts, 'The apothecary in the 17th century', *Pharm. J.* 1962, 189, 505–9, see p. 508; idem, 'The personnel and practice of medicine in Tudor and Stuart England, Part I. The provinces', *Med. Hist.* 1962, 6, 363–82, see p. 376; cf. the similar plea by F. Roberts, 'The effects of epidemics on population and social life', *Proc. R. Soc. Med. (Sect. Hist. Med.)* 1955, 48, 785–9.

53   J. Doucet, *Les apothicaires nantais sous l'ancien régime*, Thèse de Rennes (Faculté de Médecine et Pharmacie), pp. 300ff, Fontenay-le-Comte: P. & O. Lussaud, 1959; this is one of many French *thèses* dealing with local pharmaceutical history which emanate mostly from the Universities of Strasbourg and Nancy; R. S. Roberts, 1962, op. cit. (above, note 52), pp. 375–6; idem, 1964, op. cit. (above, note 37), p. 228.

54. See T. McKeown, below, ch. 4, p. 68.

4 Medical Issues in Historical Demography

THOMAS McKEOWN

For the demographer and economic historian all movements of population are important and deserve, so far as possible, to be explained; but for the student of social and medical history the modern rise of population is a unique event whose interpretation is not only of the greatest historical interest but is also essential to an understanding of some of the most formidable contemporary problems.

The distinction between the earlier recurrent changes of population and the modern rise is of particular significance in the eighteenth century. The methods as well as the aims of enquiry are different according to whether the increase in numbers is regarded as analogous to that in previous periods (given particular but not necessarily unique significance because of its coincidence with the Agricultural and Industrial Revolutions), or whether it is considered as the beginning of the modern expansion whose dimensions and continuity distinguish it from all previous changes.

If eighteenth-century growth is no more than the most remarkable of many movements of population, it is permissible to argue by analogy and to invoke the same kinds of explanations as are accepted for earlier periods. This treatment has been adopted by some economic historians, for example when a decline of mortality has been attributed to cyclic changes in the behaviour of infectious diseases or even of a single disease.[1] But if the eighteenth century saw the beginning of the modern rise of population such explanations are clearly inadequate, for as the event was unprecedented so too, it seems reasonable to believe, must be the explanation for it.

There is no serious doubt that in Britain the modern rise of population did begin during the eighteenth century. It was certainly well established before registration of births and deaths (1838) and even at the time of the first census (1801) the increase in numbers was much greater than that which occurred in earlier periods. For the purpose of interpreting the modern rise of population it is unnecessary, and probably impossible, to state precisely when it started. It is sufficient to know that whatever the explanation in the early years of the eighteenth century, at some time before its end the first phase of the unique expansion had begun.

II

METHODS OF INVESTIGATION

For interpretation of this expansion there is no more important decision than the choice of methods by which it is to be investigated. I should like to make four suggestions concerning them.

(a) Data for the eighteenth century are not available, and are unlikely to become available, which put the major issues beyond dispute.

(b) It is therefore desirable to begin by examining post-registration data and to consider the uncertainties in the eighteenth century in the light of conclusions concerning the later period.

(c) Some of the most important questions which arise are medical in character.

(d) In the pre-registration period, the issue which has preoccupied many economic historians—the relative importance of changes in birth rate and death rate—is less significant than the question what disturbed either rate.

(a) Eighteenth-century data

The inadequacy of eighteenth-century sources is notorious, but this has not deterred investigators from advancing explanations that would be hard to sustain on twentieth-century evidence. Some have been prepared to write confidently about specific causes of death in a period when the death rate is unknown, and even to attribute the remarkable growth of population before registration to the behaviour of a single disease. In fact the data are so unreliable that it is all too easy for the investigator to persuade himself that he has found evidence to support any hypothesis which appeals to him: an increase in fertility,[2,3] a decrease in mortality;[4] the appearance of the potato,[5] the disappearance of plague;[1] the effectiveness of variolation,[6] the ineffectiveness of all medical measures.[4]

The lack of evidence which makes it difficult to sustain an hypothesis makes it almost equally difficult to refute it. When, for example, it is asserted that the rise of population in the eighteenth century was due to the introduction of inoculation against smallpox,[6] even a virologist cannot be expected to produce historical or other evidence which proves conclusively that it was not.[7] He can state only that such an interpretation seems most improbable in the light of his knowledge of the disease and its behaviour in a later period for which data are more tangible. It therefore adds nothing to the acceptability of an hypothesis that convincing evidence cannot be mounted against it from contemporary sources, and we must rely largely on later information and the judgement of those whose experience enables them to give an informed opinion.

But while recognizing the limitations of existing data, some demographers and economic historians have high hopes from new material which may become available, for example, by investigation of parish registers and of selected population groups such as peers. In assessing what can be expected from such sources one can only express a personal opinion, that the evidence which can be assembled for the eighteenth century is very unlikely of itself to answer the main questions, and conclusions will still be largely influenced by prior hypotheses. This somewhat pessimistic judgement is based not only on the obvious limitations of contemporary sources, but on recognition of the difficulties presented by the major issues. On the last point it is salutary to be reminded that in countries such as Ceylon, where a rapid expansion of population has occurred within the past few decades, there are considerable differences of opinion between informed observers about the relative contribution of malaria control, other medical measures and a rising standard of living, particularly nutrition.[8,9]

(b) Post-registration data

If conclusions concerning the eighteenth century must be largely influenced by prior hypotheses, it is clearly important to decide on what evidence they are to be based. The best evidence, I suggest, is from the time when there is sufficient information to support an interpretation; and the minimum requirements are data concerning birth rate, death rate and cause of death. The birth rate and death rate are needed to assess the contribution of an increase of the one or a decrease of the other to population growth, the issue which has had so much attention in eighteenth-century studies; and cause of death is essential for appraisal of the influences which contributed to the decline of mortality. In England and Wales these minimal data are available from 1838.

The problem of extrapolating from the later to the earlier period is in some respects less difficult than it appears to be. For example, if in the light of knowledge of the diseases which declined after 1838 it is concluded that specific measures of preventing or treating disease in the individual made no significant contribution to the reduction of the death rate during the nineteenth century,[10] it seems reasonable to conclude that such measures are very unlikely to have been effective a hundred years earlier. Since the introduction of improved sanitation coincided with the decline of the bowel infections in the 1870's[10] we can be fairly confident that this was not a significant influence during the eighteenth century. And if a reminder is needed that mortality from a single infection may fluctuate apparently without medical or other intervention, in a period when more important influences are changing the whole pattern of disease, it is provided by experience of scarlet fever in the nineteenth and twentieth centuries.

The failure to make full use of nineteenth-century evidence before turning to the uncertainties of the earlier period, although regrettable, is understandable. Historians have been particularly interested in the association between population growth and the beginning of the Industrial Revolution, one of the important issues in economic history, and they have been less concerned with the nineteenth century when the relationship seemed more obvious and therefore less challenging. But whether the focus of interest is the eighteenth century, or interpretation of the modern rise of population as a whole, the most promising approach to an understanding of the first phase of population growth is through investigation in the years immediately after registration, when the data are sufficient to raise discussion above the level of speculation.

(c) *Medical issues*

Both before and after registration some of the most important questions raised by investigation of population growth are medical in character. They include the following.

The reason for the reduction of mortality from tuberculosis. Mortality from this disease was declining rapidly from the time of registration of cause of death and this appears to have been responsible for nearly half of the total reduction of mortality (from all causes) between that time and the end of the nineteenth century. No treatment was effective, and the main issue is the relative importance of a change in the character of the disease and of improvement in the environment.[10]

Reliability of certification of cause of death. There must be uncertainty concerning the acceptability of diagnoses, not only before the discovery of the bacterial origin of infectious disease, but throughout the nineteenth century because of the limitations of methods of investigation. It is particularly important to decide whether the reduction of mortality from tuberculosis can be attributed substantially to changes in diagnostic practice, resulting in a transfer of deaths from this to other causes.

Interpretation of the behaviour of mortality from infections in the absence of intervention by medical or other measures. Although this matter should present no great difficulty to biologists who recognize the unstable relationship of organism and host, the attention given to it in the literature shows that it has been a source of misunderstanding by some economic historians. The significance attributed to the disappearance of plague[1] is an example of the failure to distinguish between the changing pattern of infectious disease and the type of explanation which must be sought for the beginning of the unprecedented modern rise of population.

The effects on fertility of advancement or postponement of age of marriage. This is largely a matter for the demographer but there is one issue on which judgement is influenced by acquaintance with contemporary medical evidence. No one familiar with this evidence could, I believe, be in any doubt that infant mortality due to infectious disease rises sharply with increasing birth rank. There could be no better indication of the treacherous character of early data when viewed without reference to later medical evidence than the conclusion by a distinguished demographer that this association is not supported by a study of bourgeois families in Geneva between the sixteenth and nineteenth centuries.[11]

The effectiveness of inoculation against smallpox. It is significant that the claim that this measure contributed substantially to control of the disease, and even to the total decline of mortality and rise of population in the eighteenth century, has not been advanced by medical writers but has been disputed by some of the best informed among them.[7,12] This matter will be referred to later and is mentioned here only as an example of a medical question which has perhaps been given undue prominence.

These are among the medical issues which arise in investigation of the most important problem in historical demography, the explanation of the modern rise of population. It seems remarkable that so far they have had little attention from medical historians, but interpretation of the decline of mortality has not been a theme of medical history in the way that interpretation of population growth has been a theme of economic history. Medical writers have been interested in the behaviour of individual infectious diseases and a considerable literature is concerned with possible reasons for the decline of mortality from smallpox, typhus, scarlet fever, typhoid and other infections. But there have been few attempts to assess the contribution of medical and other influences to the trend of mortality as a whole, or the relation between mortality and growth of population. And in so far as such questions have been considered, there has been an unfortunate tendency to confuse very different measures—environmental, preventive, therapeutic—under the large umbrella of scientific medicine.

(d) The relative importance of birth and death rate

One of the consequences of the focus of interest on the eighteenth century has been the disproportionate attention given to the birth rate–death rate controversy; when neither rate is known the way is open to interpretations which are as difficult to support conclusively as they are finally to refute. However interesting this discussion may be to economic historians, in relation to investigation of the reasons for the modern rise of population it is of secondary importance compared to the question what disturbed either rate. For if the first phase of the modern rise cannot be attributed to medical measures or to fortuitous change in the infections—and this is the conclusion which emerges from examination of post-registration evidence (discussed below)—the deduction is inescapable that the standard of living rose in the eighteenth century, whether its most significant effect was an increase in the birth rate or a decrease in the death rate. This is not to suggest that discussion need stop at this point; on the contrary it leads to a more realistic appraisal of the features of the environment which were ameliorated and their likely effect on births and deaths.

Adopting the procedure suggested above I shall now consider in turn the possible reasons for the rise of population after and before registration.

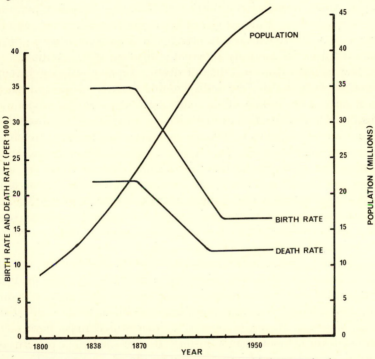

FIG. I. Data from national statistics concerning birth rate, death rate and population in England and Wales.

III

POPULATION GROWTH AFTER REGISTRATION OF BIRTHS AND DEATHS

The figure summarises the data concerning birth rate, death rate and population in England and Wales from the times when national statistics put them beyond serious doubt. It shows that an excess of births over deaths was established before registration and has continued until the present time. The birth rate remained high until 1880 when it began to fall; mortality was fairly constant until about the same time when it too began to decline. The growth of population from 1838 was clearly due to the margin of births over deaths established before and maintained after registration, and to the decline of mortality from the eighth decade which compensated to some extent for a declining birth rate. The main task is to account for the reduction of mortality in the late nineteenth century, and in the light of the conclusions to investigate the margin between birth rate and death rate already apparent at the time of registration.

The national data on cause of death, available only for Britain from so early a date, are indispensable for examination of these problems. The decline of mortality between 1840 and 1900 was restricted to the infections and McKeown and Record[10] showed that five diseases or groups of diseases were responsible for it: tuberculosis for a little less than a half; typhus, typhoid and continued fever for about a fifth; scarlet fever for a fifth; cholera, dysentery and diarrhoea for nearly a tenth; and smallpox for a twentieth. Investigation of reasons for the changes in each disease or disease group, and if possible formulation of a general hypothesis based on the conclusions, is one of the most important tasks confronting medical historians. It has not yet had the attention it deserves.

McKeown and Record[10] suggested that the possibilities for each disease can be considered under three headings: specific medical measures of preventing or treating disease in the individual; a 'spontaneous' decline of mortality not attributable to medical effort or environmental change, analogous to that which must have contributed throughout man's history to the changing pattern of infectious disease; and improvement in the environment. The last comprises a wide range of influences but at the outset it is convenient to group them under the same heading.

Of the diseases which declined, only smallpox was influenced significantly by specific medical measures and even if the whole of its decline is attributed to vaccination it can account for only a small part of the total reduction of mortality. Scarlet fever is the outstanding example of an infective organism whose virulence changed over quite a short period, apparently independently of medical or other intervention, and its decline can be attributed confidently to the second heading ('spontaneous' change).

Since the reduction of mortality from bowel infections began in the eighth decade when sanitary reform began to make its impact on water supplies and sewage disposal, there is also no serious doubt that it was due mainly to improved sanitation. In the case of typhus (which is not identified from typhoid in national statistics before 1871) this explanation may not be adequate, but for the two groups as a whole (typhus, typhoid and continued fever; and cholera, dysentery and diarrhoea) it seems acceptable.

The chief difficulty, already referred to, is in explaining the early, rapid and continuous decline of mortality from tuberculosis. It occurred from the time of registration (and almost certainly preceded it), at least several decades before the reduction of mortality from the other main causes. The decline was not due to treatment, which did not become really effective until after the Second World War, and McKeown and Record[10] concluded that it was due mainly to a rising standard of living, particularly of nutrition. Their reasons for not accepting as more probable 'spontaneous' change in the disease, the explanation favoured by some epidemiologists, were (a) because so large a reduction of mortality would be unlikely to occur in this way in a population already exposed to the disease for several centuries, and (b) because substantial movements of population from country to town were too late to explain a large decrease in the fourth decade (if it is assumed that the rural population of Britain had not long been exposed to the disease). Nevertheless it is impossible to be confident about so complex an issue, one of the most important in medical history, which fully merits further study.

In summary of the conclusions in respect of each of the main diseases (or groups) it was suggested that in order of relative importance the influences responsible for the reduction of mortality in the second half of the nineteenth century were: (a) a rising standard of living, of which the most significant feature was possibly improved diet (responsible mainly for the decline of tuberculosis and, less certainly and to a lesser extent, of typhus); (b) hygienic changes, particularly improved water supplies and sewage disposal, introduced by sanitary reformers (responsible for the decline of the typhoid and cholera groups); and (c) a favourable trend in the relationship between infectious agent and human host (which accounted for the decline of mortality from scarlet fever and may have contributed to that from tuberculosis, typhus and cholera). The influence of specific prevention or treatment of disease in the individual was restricted to smallpox and made little contribution to the total reduction of the death rate.

Is it possible to be confident, if not in detail at least about the main lines of this interpretation? There are three reasons for believing that specific medical measures contributed little: the reduction of mortality was due to the decline of infectious diseases; smallpox was the only infection on which medical measures then had an applicable effect; and only about a twentieth of the total reduction of mortality between 1838 and 1900 was due to the decline of smallpox.

It is not possible to be equally confident about the relative importance of environmental influences (a rising standard of living and the more specific hygienic measures) and spontaneous decline of infections. But there is reason to believe that an advance in the standard of living, generally agreed to have occurred by the mid-century, contributed substantially to the reduction of mortality from tuberculosis, and that sanitary measures were mainly responsible for the decline of mortality from the bowel infections which coincided with improvements in water supply and sewage disposal. Hence while it is impossible to assess precisely the contribution of spontaneous change in the infectious diseases, the evidence that other important influences were at work, and the improbability of a fortuitous explanation for so large a reduction of mortality, appear to justify the main lines of the interpretation. In this communication no attempt will be made to extend it beyond 1900, although elsewhere[13] I have suggested that for the whole period from 1838 until the present day the order in time of the main influences is also the probable order of their importance: a rising standard of living, at least from 1840; improved sanitation from about 1870; and prevention and treatment of disease in the individual, with the exception of vaccination against smallpox from the second quarter of the twentieth century.

66

IV

POPULATION GROWTH BEFORE REGISTRATION

In investigation of reasons for the growth of population in the eighteenth century there are three main causes, or more accurately, classes of causes, to be considered: medical measures of preventing or treating disease in the individual, leading to a decline of mortality; a spontaneous reduction of mortality; and improvements in the environment, whether leading to an increase of the birth rate or decrease of the death rate. It is possible to think of other influences on population growth, for example a reduction of the birth rate such as occurred in France or a spontaneous increase in fertility, but none likely to have contributed significantly to the rise of population in eighteenth-century Britain. In the discussion which follows no assumptions will be made about the levels or trends of birth rate or death rate, and an interpretation will be sought mainly in the light of conclusions from the nineteenth century.

Medical measures

If it is accepted that with one interesting but not large exception (vaccination), prevention or treatment of disease in the individual was ineffective in reducing mortality in the late nineteenth century, it would seem to follow that they can have had no significant influence on the trend a century earlier. Indeed there is good reason to believe that some kinds of medical intervention were harmful, for example expansion of hospital care with the attendant risks of the spread of infection. However a little to the surprise of most medical writers the suggestion that inoculation against smallpox made a substantial impact on mortality in the eighteenth century[6] makes it necessary to enquire whether this procedure was a remarkable early exception.

It is unnecessary to review the history and methods of inoculation in Britain which have been discussed extensively in recent years, and it will suffice to note that it was a crude procedure which no one would dare to use today, introduced without knowledge of its mode of action or attendant risks. The difficulties of resolving medical issues by reliance on eighteenth-century evidence are nowhere more apparent than in the wide differences of opinion concerning the frequency of inoculation and its effectiveness in preventing smallpox. It is said that the procedure was common[6] and that it was uncommon;[14] that it afforded substantial protection[6] and that it is likely to have contributed to the spread of the disease.[14] The frequency of inoculation is perhaps a matter for general discussion, but in the absence of firm evidence, assessment of its probable effectiveness should be based on laboratory, clinical and epidemiological experience of the disease. Yet an economic historian has not hesitated to debate this issue with a distinguished virologist.[15]

The conclusion of those who know the disease is that mortality in the eighteenth century was not significantly reduced by inoculation; it is in accord with extensive recent experience of immunization. After nearly a hundred years of investigation there are a number of vaccines which offer substantial protection against some infectious diseases. Had they been available and used efficiently in the eighteenth century, even in the absence of other influences it is probable that they would have led to a reduction of mortality from the specific infections and one or two, for example measles vaccine, might have had a temporary effect on total mortality. But it is most unlikely that any of them would have had an effect so large and prolonged as to explain the increase of population in the eighteenth century. This conclusion rests on judgement, not of the effectiveness of vaccines, but of the probable contribution of any single infection to total mortality over a considerable period. Hence even if very large assumptions are made about the frequency and effectiveness of inoculation, it cannot account for the rise of population which had occurred before the time of registration, when other influences associated with a rising standard of living were certainly present.

A spontaneous decline of mortality

It is convenient, but somewhat misleading, to describe a decline of mortality as spontaneous if it was not influenced by medical or other measures such as improvements in the environment. The relationship between an infective organism and its host is clearly not independent of the environment in which they are placed; nevertheless a distinction should be made between the changes which presumably occurred throughout man's evolution, leading sometimes to an increase and sometimes to a decrease in mortality, and those which have been associated with the reduction of mortality during the past two centuries. For the latter there must be a more specific explanation.

In the post-registration period it was possible to consider the significance of spontaneous change in the character of the individual diseases which contributed to the total decline of mortality. This procedure cannot be used before 1838 when cause of death is unknown, and we must rely on a judgement of probabilities, assisted by knowledge of the nineteenth century.

The following are among the few undisputed facts relevant to assessment of spontaneous change. A decline of mortality, if it occurred before registration, would have been due to a reduction of infectious causes of death. The relationship between organism and host is variable, but the rate of change is very different for different organisms. Without effective medical or other intervention, over any considerable period some deaths from infections must have increased, some decreased and others remained fairly constant. There is therefore no reason to question that one or more infections may have declined spontaneously in the eighteenth century as did scarlet fever in the nineteenth and other diseases, undoubtedly, in previous centuries.

If it is accepted that medical measures had no significant effect on national mortality trends before registration, without knowledge of cause of death we must ask for how long the rise of population could reasonably be attributed to spontaneous change. While no precise answer can be given it seems hardly credible that this alone can explain the unprecedented increase before registration. Even if some reduction in mortality in the early years of the eighteenth century is analogous to that which occurred in previous centuries, before its end the modern rise of population had begun. Its extent, continuity and coincidence with the Agricultural and Industrial Revolutions were all unique, and it cannot be explained by a decline of mortality which was independent of medical or other measures. We are therefore left with the third interpretation, that the rise of population was associated with the profound changes in way of life which occurred in the late eighteenth and early nineteenth centuries.

Against this background it will be convenient to refer briefly to the proposal that eighteenth-century population growth can be explained by the disappearance of plague.[1] As in the case of small-pox, the data are quite unreliable, and it needs faith as well as discernment to find regularity in a cycle of mortality whose wavelength was several centuries. On medical grounds it is also difficult to accept that prolonged changes in mortality (from all causes) and population growth can be attributed to the behaviour of a single disease.

But even if plague had the significance suggested, reasons for its decline must be sought under the three headings listed above. It was certainly not due to prevention or treatment of the disease in the individual. If it occurred spontaneously it may have contributed to population growth in the early eighteenth century but cannot be accepted as the main reason for the first phase of the modern increase. And if plague declined because of environmental improvement, the explanation is consistent with the interpretation which follows.

Improvement in the environment

The conclusion that a rising standard of living was the most important reason for the reduction of mortality after registration was suggested by examination of the diseases which declined, and was consistent with the fairly uniform opinion of economic historians that by this time conditions had improved. The fact that for several decades after cause of death was first registered, the most notable feature was a decline of mortality from tuberculosis made it possible to go further, and to suggest that the most plausible explanation for its decline was a better diet. This explanation was consistent with what is known about the behaviour of the disease and the consequences of higher employment rates and better wages.

Before registration the grounds for emphasizing improvements in the environment as the probable explanation for a rising population are inevitably somewhat weaker. The conclusion is reached after exclusion of the alternatives (medical measures and fortuitous change) and cannot be supported by examination of individual causes of death. Moreover some economic historians do not agree that on balance living conditions improved in the late eighteenth and early nineteenth centuries and they have reservations about the interpretation on this account.

In a review of the position McKeown and Brown[16] concluded as follows: 'It would probably be unwise for medical writers to attempt to go beyond a general conclusion. It is that in the light of an assessment of the evidence after registration, it seems most reasonable to attribute the rise of population which had occurred before that time to improvement in the environment. For the purposes of a general interpretation it is not necessary, and indeed it may never be possible, to specify the nature of the improvement, or to state a time from which it can confidently be said to have begun. But the fact that the population had trebled in a relatively short period before 1851 leaves little doubt that it was well established before the date when economic historians are agreed that the standard of living had risen.'

There are now reasons for thinking that this conclusion was unnecessarily cautious. Data referred to by Hutchinson[17] in his Presidential Address to the British Association in 1966 suggest that the explanation for the rising standard of living should be sought in the striking advances in British agriculture. He quotes Ernle:[18] 'In 1811 [the population of England and Wales] had grown to 10 150 615. On these figures the population had doubled itself in 125 years and even if no allowance is made for an improved standard of living, it is probable that England during the same period had doubled her production of food.' Hutchinson states that by the end of the Napoleonic Wars production had outstripped consumption, and it was not until the 1870's that imported food supplies from North America began to make a significant contribution.

This emphasis on the importance of food supplies is not only consistent with the explanation suggested for the decline of mortality in the years after registration; it is also in keeping with more general conclusions concerning the basic requirements for human health.[19] There are four requirements—food, oxygen, warmth (or more accurately, avoidance of excessive heat loss) and water—but only the first has been so deficient as to have a profound impact on human health, numbers and evolution. The position was correctly assessed by Malthus ('The tendency of all animated life is to increase beyond the nourishment prepared for it') and until the eighteenth century any improvements in food supplies were rapidly offset by increasing numbers. The agricultural advances to which Hutchinson and Ernle[17,18] refer were able to support a vastly increased population, which was further expanded by the reduction of mortality consequent upon sanitary reform. But in time, and on an evolutionary scale fairly short time, these advances would again have been overtaken by increasing numbers if the decline of the birth rate from 1870 had not brought population growth under control. Not sufficient control, in Hutchinson's view, to meet the needs of a technically advanced society, but at least enough to maintain a change in health unique in human history.

V

This interpretation of the modern rise and eventual control of population in Britain puts the emphasis on three influences: improved food supplies from 1770 or earlier; removal of adverse influences in the physical environment by sanitary measures from 1870; and limitation of numbers by a declining birth rate from about the same time. It is not suggested that these advances began precisely in the years mentioned. The improvements in agriculture —enclosure, manuring, wintering of stocks, introduction of root crops, etc.—occurred over a period; there may well have been some advances in hygienic practice, as there undoubtedly were in hygienic teaching, during the eighteenth century; and both French statistics and English literature indicate that contraceptive measures were not used for the first time in the 1870's. Furthermore there were periods in man's history when other influences may have been temporarily more important than food in restricting numbers, at least of special groups; for example in England for many centuries royal and aristocratic families were presumably adequately, if unhygienically, fed, and their risk of death from violence was probably much greater than from malnutrition. Nevertheless in respect of the population as a whole over any considerable period the Malthusian thesis seems unassailable; and while the three influences—improved diet, sanitation and birth control—were not perhaps unique in kind, they were in the scientific, educational and political circumstances which led to their introduction and continuity in the eighteenth and nineteenth centuries.

VI

This interpretation of population growth rests largely on judgement of medical issues: the effectiveness of treatment during the eighteenth and nineteenth centuries; the reasons for the decline of mortality from intestinal infections, scarlet fever and, above all, tuberculosis; the value of inoculation against smallpox; and the likelihood of a sustained reduction of total mortality as a result of 'spontaneous' change in a number of infectious diseases or of a single disease such as plague. These issues are brought into focus by investigation of the modern rise of population, a subject which has had the attention of economic historians and demographers, but not, so far to any extent, of medical writers. Medical historians have largely ignored this theme, or have restricted enquiry to individual infections. Yet behind the problem of population growth lies what is among the most important questions in medical history, the reasons for the transformation of man's health during the past two centuries.

REFERENCES

1 K. F. Helleiner, 'The vital revolution reconsidered', *Canad. J. Econ. pol. Sci.* 1957, **23**, 1–9.
2 H. J. Habakkuk, 'English population in the eighteenth century', *Econ. Hist. Rev.* (2nd ser.), 1953, **6**, 117–33.
3 J. T. Krause, 'Changes in English fertility and mortality, 1781–1850', *Econ. Hist. Rev.* (2nd ser.) 1958, **11**, 52–70.
4 T. McKeown and R. G. Brown, 'Medical evidence related to English population changes in the eighteenth century', *Popul. Stud.* 1955, **9**, 119–41.
5 W. L. Langer, 'Europe's initial population explosion', *Am. Hist. Rev.* 1963, **69**, 1–17.
6 P. E. Razzell, 'Population change in eighteenth century England. A reinterpretation', *Econ. Hist. Rev.* (2nd ser.) 1965, **18**, 312–32.
7 N. Schuster, Letter to the Editor, *Med. Hist.* 1965, **9**, 381–3.
8 *Lancet*, Leading article, 1968, **1**, 899–900.
9 H. Frederiksen, Letter to the Editor, *Lancet* 1968, **2**, 346–7.
10 T. McKeown and R. G. Record, 'Reasons for the decline of mortality in England and Wales during the nineteenth century', *Popul. Stud.* 1962, **16**, 94–122.
11 L. Henry, *Anciennes familles genevoises*, Paris: P.V.F., 1956.
12 A. W. Downie, Comment on P. E. Razzell, 'Edward Jenner: the history of a medical myth', *Med. Hist.* 1965, **9**, 223–5.
13 T. McKeown, 'Medicine and world population', *J. chron. Dis.* 1965, **18**, 1067–77.

14   C. W. Dixon, *Smallpox*, pp. 195–6, 239–48, London: J. and A. Churchill Ltd, 1962.
15   P. E. Razzell, Reply to A. W. Downie, *Med. Hist.* 1965, 9, 226–9.
16   T. McKeown and R. G. Brown, 'An interpretation of the rise of population in England and Wales', *Economic History Congress*, Munich, 1965.
17   J. Hutchinson, 'Land and human populations', *Listener*, 1 September 1966, pp. 303–11.
18   R. E. P. Ernle, *English farming past and present*, London: Longmans, Green, 1919, pp. 266.
19   T. McKeown, 'The seed-bag and the urn', *Proc. R. Soc. Med.* (*Sect. Hist. Med.*) 1967, 60, 575–9.

5 The Medico-Historical Significance of Young and Developing Countries, illustrated by Australian Experience

BRYAN GANDEVIA

Mere curiosity acts as the initial stimulus to the study of the history of medicine in a community young in years and small in numbers. The development of a national self-consciousness, of which it forms one aspect, gives some impetus to the study, and a pride in local traditions, institutions and practice may thus be encouraged. In Australia, the first phase began tentatively about half a century after its foundation[1] but more definitely only after a century.[2] The second phase was well developed within another sixty or seventy years, as a check list of the literature on the subject up to 1957 reveals,[3] and considerable progress has been made in the past decade. In the circumstances, it is inevitable, and probably desirable, that this work should be carried out by amateur historians; it is equally inevitable that there should at first be a bias towards relatively finite and definable subjects, such as biography and the history of individual diseases and institutions. None the less, in recent years there is evidence of a more professional, a more scientific and a more mature approach to the history of Australian medicine, manifest in the standards of historical research and presentation, and in a broader approach to more complex subjects. The influences which are effecting this change are not far to seek. On the one hand, history itself is now written more in terms of social change than as the biographies of leaders, and it concerns itself more with movements and trends than with dates and events. Locally, on the other hand, Australian history has become not only an acceptable subject for scholarly study but also one which has created such widespread interest as to promote a rapidly increasing literature and the growth of numerous historical societies.

75

II

CAN AUSTRALIAN MEDICAL HISTORY CONTRIBUTE?

At this time, it is therefore appropriate to examine whether the study of the history of medicine in Australia can contribute to a fuller understanding of the evolution of medicine in general. Indeed, in this paper the hypothesis is advanced that the study of medical history in a localized area is a valid scientific technique in historical research which is of universal significance. Whilst the illustrations in this essay will be drawn from Australia, as the writer's special interest, the principles involved are applicable to other countries with entirely different backgrounds. In Singapore, for example, where traditional medicine from three cultures is practised side by side with Western medicine, there is obvious scope for study of the modification of the one by the other over even comparatively recent years; the historian might go so far as to borrow an approach from the epidemiologist and institute a prospective study of the interaction between these several medical 'cultures' in order to throw light on questions of the transference, assimilation and decay of medical procedures in earlier times and other civilizations, and under the influence of different religions and socio-economic backgrounds. Here too there is a unique opportunity for the evaluation not merely of ancient therapeutic methods but also of the social contribution of traditional patterns of medical practice. One might see, over the past century or so, how each had coped with the changing environment as a modern city grew from a village on a tropical island; one might even watch the adaptations as entrepôt trading gives way to industry and technology as the basis of the national economy. But these observations are occurring in advance of the argument.

To appreciate how medical history may profit as a discipline from the study of local medicine, it is necessary first to examine some fundamental principles governing the evolution of medicine. In the light of the rationalistic, or at least naturalistic, philosophy of his era and his culture, it is not remarkable that Hippocrates should have discounted the supernatural in aetiology; a more fundamental or more positive contribution lay in his recognition of the influence of the environment on man's physical and mental attributes and on the characters of his diseases. It is, of course, mere coincidence that he should describe not only the common view of the Australian environment but also the Australian's popular image of himself:[4]

But where the land is bare, waterless, rough, oppressed by winter's storms and burnt by the sun, there you will see men who are hard, lean, well-articulated, well-braced, and hairy; such natures will be found energetic, vigilant, stubborn and independent in character and in temper, wild rather than tame, of more than average sharpness and intelligence in the arts, and in war of more than average courage.

The history of medicine is one facet of the story of man's adaptation to his environment. Complex interactions between man and the physical, cultural, religious and socio-economic components of his environment determine not only the medical problems encountered but also the manner of medical practice. The adoption of this view of the evolution of medicine is necessary if one is to accept that the detailed medical history of an isolated continent over a century or two is worth studying for any wider purpose than the furtherance of national pride and the establishment of local tradition. The medical influence of some aspects of man's physical, mental and social environment can sometimes be studied by more or less experimental methods in which, by design, most of the variables are specifically controlled. It is rare for this direct approach to be available to the historian, but he can adopt another approach from modern epidemiology, whereby a comparison is made between two communities which differ only in those characteristics the influence of which it is desired to study. The people who came to Australia were European, predominantly British, and they brought with them the same European social organization, the same physical and mental attributes, the same religion, and the same concepts and knowledge of science and medicine. With these essential similarities and with continuing, indeed growing, contact with the old world, it is not surprising that the general trend of medical evolution was more or less the same in Australia as in Europe; until scientific research became established, we cannot look to Australia as the source of any radical influence on Western medicine. In the presence of these basic similarities, it is the differences which are significant for their effects on medicine and its practice. We have the same stock, the same medicine, transported to a different environment and thus

77

confronted with different problems. Both medically and administra-
tively, new patterns of reaction in medical practice emerge.

Before considering some of these differences and their medico-
historical significance, it may be pertinent to look at some of the
other factors which make Australian medicine peculiarly appropriate for a study of this kind. The first is a chance matter of time.
Australia was first colonized in the last decade or so of the eighteenth
century, a period not so remote that the medical concepts and
philosophy of the time are wholly strange to the modern student.
More particularly, however, this offers a short 'control' period before
the sweeping changes of the nineteenth century; the development of
Australia is contemporaneous with the most radical and important
developments in medicine since perhaps the era of Hippocrates. In a
microcosm, as it were, it is possible to study the introduction and
acceptance of these advances in more detail, and at times to see the
difficulties or consequences of them with greater clarity, than is
possible in larger or less isolated communities. Secondly, the isolation
of the continent is valuable in that events such as the introduction of
a disease or the news of great events (for example, vaccination,
anaesthesia or 'Listerism') can often be dated with great precision;
diffusion of disease or of news often proceeded from one or two isolated points, identifiable in space and time, and was uninfluenced
by other contacts with the outside world.

Thirdly, as will be illustrated below, Australia offers a wide range
of physical environments differing from those previously familiar
to the colonists, and there were also several different forms of social
organization, at different periods and places; the age and sex distribution of the population was also unusual. Changes in the sociological environment, rapid and striking on occasion, occur in such
a way as to permit comparisons; these changes resulted sometimes
from legislation but more often from a gradually developing control
over the physical environment.

Finally, documentation is tolerably good, although the sources
are many and varied,[5] and some reliance must be placed on evidence
from lay sources;[6] in the absence of a more appropriate forum, and
sometimes in spite of one, considerable space in the lay press was
devoted to medical controversies. Local medical journals[7] and
societies[8] have maintained some continuity of existence from about
1850, and the detailed records of some of the societies are extant.

78

The local publication of pamphlets and books in some profusion commenced about the same time; although no comprehensive bibliography has been published, some valuable collections of medical Australiana exist[9] and are belatedly being systematically expanded.[10] References to Australian medical problems were also frequent in the British medical press.[11] Separate 'states', enthusiastically accepting their responsibilities as independence evolved, conducted many inquiries and Royal Commissions on matters of medico-social significance. Unfortunately there are all too few medical autobiographies, diaries and letters from the nineteenth century; it may be that some are still hidden with family skeletons in European cupboards!

III

The remainder of this paper is devoted to an indication of some of the altered medical problems produced among the Europeans after their introduction to an environment which, although different, was at least of more or less virgin purity from the medical point of view. The settlers brought their own diseases and their own medicine with them: only the physical and social environments, themselves interrelated, were changed. The story of the aborigines' adaptation to the alterations in their environment is equally fascinating and instructive, albeit as yet less successful; although relevant as illustrating the principles involved, it is too complex for consideration here, and the interested reader is referred to the bibliography of Pedersen and Moodie[12] and to relevant sections of the *Australian Encyclopaedia*.[13] Suffice it to say that the impact of the European invasion was felt not only medically, in terms of new diseases, but also psychologically and socially in the destruction of age-old concepts and beliefs. By contrast, the aborigines had no demonstrable effect on European morbidity (excluding some understandable trauma), presumably because of their small numbers (an estimated 300 000 were scattered over the continent in 1788) and nomadic existence.

IV

SOME BASIC ENVIRONMENTAL INFLUENCES

Next to its isolation from the old world, the outstanding feature of Australia to its early settlers was its vastness; even today, in proportion to its population, this significantly influences medical practice. Its area is nearly 3 000 000 square miles, approximately the same size as the United States of America, and many times the size of the islands from which the first migrants came. Today, with only three people per square mile, it remains the most sparsely populated of all civilized countries. A century ago, a quarter of the population lived in the State capital cities, but now the proportion is more than half; there is thus the historically important contrast of rapidly developing urban communities in association with relatively gradual changes in rural population density.

The physical environment varies widely from a relatively fertile coastal strip with reasonable rainfall to an arid central desert and a tropical jungle to the north. Large rivers and lakes are few; over a third of the continent receives less than 10 inches of rain each year. Water supply (whether for human beings, agriculture or stock), droughts and bushfires remain consistently recurring problems over much of the country, while other environmental problems, largely related to health, delayed the effective settlement of the more tropical regions. The weather generally was hotter, and the hours of sunshine longer, than the inhabitants had previously known. They were also closer to their environment; even the more permanent homes of the pastoralist, the farmer, and the shepherd were for many years much the same—a slab, or 'wattle and daub', hut with a bark or shingle roof and earth floor.

Certain physical and social consequences of this altered environment, not without medical significance, were the subject of comment by travellers within half a century of the first settlement. The colonists were observed to eat more, drink more, smoke more, exercise more and wash more often; their voices and accents had changed, they wore locally made hats specifically designed to keep off the sun, they were independent and egalitarian, and their rather wild children were of excellent physique.

The social organization offers remarkable contrasts and changes.

The first settlements, at Sydney and Hobart, were penal settlements, whilst Melbourne and Adelaide were founded some years later largely by private enterprise, the first through local initiative and the second as a planned programme of colonization organized in Britain. Within three-quarters of a century, these settlements had become politically independent states, with universal franchise and secret ballots, subject to the authority of the British Crown only in certain fields. By contrast with this apparently rapid progression to conventional social organization and administration, the gold rushes, occurring more or less successively in several states between 1850 and 1900, produced wholly unplanned communities with dramatic suddenness in areas capriciously determined by nature, rather than thoughtfully selected by man, as township sites. At the same time, tiny isolated communities, based perhaps on a station homestead, with seasonal fluctuations in population (depending, for example, on sheep-shearing demands) strove to make themselves as independent as possible, perhaps days or weeks by horse or bullock dray from centres approximating civilization.

The age and sex distribution of the population differed greatly from the European norm for about a hundred years. Its growth in the first few decades after 1788 was almost entirely dependent on the transportation of convicts and of the persons necessary for their administration and for the preservation of law and order. Gradually 'free' emigration was accepted and encouraged, so that about three-quarters of a 175 per cent increase in the population (to about 190 000) during the fourth decade of the nineteenth century may be attributed to this source. After the gold rush of the 1850's, emigration slowed, and natural increase became the dominant factor, almost exclusively so by the turn of the century. Prior to about 1830, the normal relationship which exists between population and economic growth did not obtain; as a result, problems of starvation and unemployment recurred, with their various socio-medical consequences. Whilst the population increase in the middle years of the century allowed the development of secondary industries, the limited labour requirements for primary pastoral industries, on which the country's economic status depended, inevitably aggravated the drift of population towards the towns. This was particularly marked towards the end of the nineteenth century, severely straining urban resources, so that, in some degree, the earlier problems of feeding and employing the population returned. It would, of course, be possible to extend this brief summary of population growth into the twentieth century, and especially into the post-World War II period of assisted migration and population increase, but enough has been said to indicate the patterns of population growth which formed the background to medical practice in the new continent. Indeed, the country has a unique experience in the assimilation of migrants, who have still their own particular problems in adjusting to the local environment.

The sex constitution of the population was also grossly abnormal by European standards over most of the nineteenth century. Males outnumbered females by three to one in 1830, and the gold rushes produced a predominantly male migration. None the less, the masculinity ratio fell to 1.4 : 1 by 1860, and by 1880–1900 the socio-medical consequences of the preponderance of males were becoming less apparent as the ratio fell to about 1.1 : 1. At least wives were not offered for sale in the street, as one was in 1811.

Periods of intensive migration and of high natural increase inevitably produce a relatively youthful age distribution in the population, and this state, for one or other reason, obtained in Australia for a century or so after its foundation. Half the population in 1881 was under the age of 21 years, while in Victoria in 1855–60, people aged 20–44 years formed nearly 60 per cent of the population. Between 1850 and 1880, the proportion over 50 years of age (again taking Victoria as an example) increased from about 3 per cent to 10 per cent; since 1910, it has risen to around 15 per cent. Where youth predominates, fertility is high; the increase in life expectancy lowers fertility rates as the age structure of the population changes. Thus, the concern over the declining birth rate manifest at the turn of the nineteenth century is not altogether surprising,[14] although the other factors discussed in relation to this trend ('direct reversal of the ordinary courses of morality', enhanced 'cerebral development', increased awareness of birth-control measures, separation of husbands and wives due to Australian conditions of life, a marriage rate rendered acceptable only by 'the mischances of ante-nuptial intercourse') are of considerable medico-social significance.[15]

An awareness of the relevance of all the environmental factors outlined above—as well as others—is inherent in the disciplines of demography, epidemiology, geographical pathology, sociology, public health, economics and even politics. It is hoped that it is not inappropriate to draw the attention of the medical historian, whose discipline incorporates a measure of understanding of all these facets of human society, to a country where extremes, wide ranges, and rapid changes in these factors may be studied more or less in controlled fashion, more or less in isolation, in an intellectual, philosophical and medico-scientific environment common to the communities of the new and old worlds.

Against the preceding background, it now becomes possible to formulate more precise questions to be asked if Australian medical history is to provide information of value to the study of the history of medicine generally. In what ways did the distinctive features of the local physical and social environment influence the pattern of disease as it presented itself to the medical practitioner? In what ways did these same features, and the consequent disease pattern, influence the overall conduct of medical practice? Can any distinctive features in Australian medical practice be related specifically to environmental factors? In some instances, provisional answers may be checked against the results of change in the environmental factors, as, for example, in the influence of a changing age constitution of the population on the morbidity due to the acute infectious diseases. In other instances, the environmental circumstances remain unchanged but the means of coping with the same problem changes with increasing technical resources—the influence of isolation and distance on medical practice remains, but the doctor on a horse, or even in a car, has given way to the wireless and the aeroplane.

It is, of course, not the purpose of this essay to provide answers to these questions, even if these were available in definitive historical studies deliberately undertaken to answer them. Even less is it possible to point to studies where this approach to Australian medical history has been chosen specifically to illuminate the general history of medicine, as it could and should be. All that can be done is to draw attention to areas where Australian experience, for one environmental reason or another, has differed sufficiently from the European norm to offer some contrast. It will not be possible in this review to do more than accept the obvious hypothesis that the difference is due to the defined environmental factor, but, in evaluating this methodological approach as a research technique, it

83

deserves to be noted that often the emerging hypothesis can be stated in a form which can be tested; as indicated above, this possibility arises from the frequency with which the environment has changed in a definable way, or with which the methods of dealing with the situation have changed. In either event, comparative evaluations at different points in time may confirm or deny the hypothesis. The conclusions may sometimes be given added weight by comparisons over the same time interval with, for example, British or other experience, where, perhaps, the environment may have remained unchanged, or even altered in the reverse direction.

V

ENVIRONMENT AND DISEASE

As an early illustration of how environmental factors may sometimes be isolated and identified, we may look briefly at the mortality on the convict ships. Multiple causes were certainly operative—the introduction of infection by convicts brought from hulks harbouring various diseases, pre-existing malnutrition and scurvy, inadequate ventilation and exercise, overcrowding, trauma of various kinds and shipwreck. On the First Fleet, there was a tolerable mortality of about 6 per cent amongst the convicts, and only 1 per cent amongst the other personnel. The difference is statistically significant, and the mere fact of transportation, with its immediately related hazards, is thus excluded as an inevitable factor in the mortality. For a variety of reasons, mortality on some ships of the Second Fleet reached 25 to 30 per cent; after an almost inevitable decline on these appalling figures, there was a further peak in 1814. Largely as a result of a medical report prepared by a former convict, William Redfern,[16] more emphasis was placed on shipboard hygiene, and more responsibility and authority was given to the surgeons on the transports. The measures adopted had an immediately favourable effect on mortality but subsequently there was a steady rise until about 1840. During this period, the hygiene, medical supervision and diet on the transports remained relatively constant and reasonably satisfactory, and obviously diseased individuals were supposedly rejected before departure. Fig. 1 shows the mortality over the whole period of transportation, together with the numbers of convicts transported and an index of the space allotted to them (the ships' tonnage divided by the numbers of convicts embarked). The graph indicates that in the earlier years mortality bore little or no relation to the numbers transported or the space available to them, but between 1820 and 1840 there is a clear correlation between the rising mortality, on the one hand, and, on the other, the numbers transported and the 'space factor'.[17] The duration of the voyage tended to fall, emphasizing the conclusion that transportation *per se* was not responsible for the mortality. It is thus justifiable to relate the rising mortality of this particular period solely to over-crowding and its concomitant evils, engendered basically by the administrative stress of transporting larger numbers. In individual ships, of course, other factors played a part. Even lower mortality rates were recorded in the last transports, where possibly the shorter voyage to Perth and other factors were contributory.

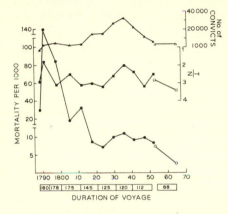

F IG. 1. Mortality (lower line) on convict transports, 1788–1865. The upper line shows the number of convicts embarked and the intermediate line the space-factor (T/N: tonnage divided by number of convicts). The average duration of the voyages in days is shown in the lower panel. Closed circles relate to Sydney or Hobart and open circles to Perth as the ports of disembarkation. Reproduced by permission from *Med. J. Australia* 1967, 2, 941 (17).

There are two points to be made from this elementary analysis. Firstly, the data exist to allow examination of several environmental factors separately in a specific situation which is directly relevant to the medical history of life at sea at this period. Secondly, attention may be directed to the use of an environmental index (the 'space factor') to explain some of the mortality; the more customary approach is to use the mortality data simply as an indication of the combined effects of environment and medical care. An analogous approach using other environmental indices in other fields might prove equally rewarding in effecting some distinction.

A similar method, more elegantly and elaborately developed, has

85

been used by Gordon[18] in relating morbidity and mortality in the convict settlement at Moreton Bay, Queensland, to changes in social conditions and living standards. It is, as he observes, a study in human ecology, based on the migration of Northern Europeans 'to a subtropical climate with preconceived ideas garnered from living in a temperate climate'. Both mortality and morbidity were higher amongst the convicts than amongst the accompanying soldiers. The major problems of the settlement were dysentery, fever (probably malaria), malnutrition and violence; ophthalmia was common and infant mortality high. Allowing for differences in the characteristics of the local fevers, the problems were essentially similar in all the early settlements, from Melville Island and Port Essington[19] in the north to Hobart and Port Arthur[20] in the south, and including the first settlement in Sydney. In the tropical areas, the index of the settlers' adjustment was a change in the peaks of morbidity and mortality from the summer to the winter months; Queensland was to become 'the first (and for a long time the only) instance of successful colonisation of a tropical and subtropical land by a population almost entirely white'.[21]

Perhaps the best illustration of failure of adaptation to the environment is the high prevalence of scurvy common to all the settlements, in spite of the accumulated knowledge derived from the experience of the British navy over the preceding century. During 'the hungry years' (1788–92)[22] when the first settlement was nearly starved out of existence, a search for native antiscorbutics was conducted by the surgeons with only partial success. Scurvy was to occur in all the remote areas of Australia throughout the protracted pioneering phase; a major contribution towards its control was made by Chinese migrants in search of gold who ultimately turned to growing vegetables. Even in Hobart, with a familiar climatic pattern and reasonable soil, the settlers took about two years to banish the scurvy by local vegetable production.[23] The presence of other hypovitaminoses may be inferred from clinical descriptions and the relatively standardized diet (rations of meat, flour, tea, sugar and tobacco) of a high proportion of the work force for much of the nineteenth century.

Certain types of violence and trauma were specific to the penal settlements, or rather to the convict population. Apart from judicial hanging, death commonly occurred after attempted escapes, either from starvation or disease, or at the hands of aborigines; the Australian bush is harsh and unfriendly, and more remote from China than many of the early convicts thought. Some instances of cannibalism occurred amongst groups of escapees. In the harsher penal establishments, occasional murders were committed for the sake of the trip to a centre of settlement for trial, in spite of its inevitably fatal outcome. 'Flagellatio' was inevitably an outstanding cause of morbidity; over 9000 lashes with a double cat-o'-nine-tails were administered in 1823 to a population of about 230 convicts at Macquarie Harbour; about 6000 convicts yearly received an average of 45 lashes in the 1830's. These macabre causes of disease and death obviously reflect a particular social environment, but mortality from violence amongst the general population remained higher than in the United Kingdom throughout the nineteenth century for reasons largely connected with the physical environment. Accidental death—commonly from horse-riding in difficult country, or from drowning—was exceedingly common, with an overall mortality rate higher than that attributable today to the motor car.[24] Children and alcoholics were prone to get lost in the bush, and to die of thirst or heatstroke; on the goldfields, even after these had ceased to be active, falling down a disused shaft was a recognized hazard. As one might expect, the mortality from violence predominantly affected males, producing a reversal of the sex ratio by comparison with European experience in late childhood and early adult life.

Inland, or 'outback', Australia posed medical problems based essentially on isolation and distance.[6,25] Their significance is obvious in relation to accident, acute disease, childbirth—many dramatic or tragic accounts, clinical, biographical, fictional and poetic, of such events are extant—but perhaps less apparent with regard to malnutrition and insanity. Whilst true isolation, at most in small groups, limited the spread of infectious and intestinal disorders, overcrowded conditions in a one- or two-roomed hut meant the certain spread of any introduced contagion. Whole families might be affected at one time, remote from help, by influenza or more serious infections; outbreaks of respiratory infection were expected with the seasonal arrival of the shearers. Before properties were fenced, the lonely and indolent occupation of shepherd harboured many social misfits and ex-convicts, amongst whom suicide, insanity, alcoholism or simply 'queerness' were common. Labourers' wages were usually paid partly in rations (with a margin of profit allowable to the employer); rations included liquor to obviate the necessity for the employee to walk thirty miles or more for a 'spree'. Townships grew up haphazardly, with little or no regard to town-planning, sanitation or water-supply; typhoid fever in country towns was a recurring problem until the present century. Generally speaking, mortality and morbidity were lower in the remote areas, in spite of the special hazards.

Just as isolation basically determined the medical problems of the outback, so overcrowding in makeshift camps on unsuitable sites dominated goldfields medicine.[6,25] Typhoid fever and dysentery were rife, rheumatism was disabling in the southern winters, and ophthalmia or sandy-blight (some of which was trachoma) was ubiquitous. Accidents, which carried a mortality as high as 50 per cent in those requiring admission to a hospital, were an everyday occurrence. Water, required for extracting the gold, was often scarce,[26] and that for drinking was not as a rule effectively designated; pollution was inevitable. Fortunately, a severe enough shortage would restrict both mining operations and the population. 'Grog', often scandalously adulterated or concocted, was easier to obtain, at a price, than fresh meat or vegetables. Although reasonably law-abiding, or at least conforming to certain unwritten codes of 'diggerdom' or mateship (later to become a part of the national character which asserted itself in the 'diggers' of two world wars), instances of violence were not uncommon.

In spite of the social and economic disturbance produced by the gold itself, by the influx of 'new chums' into almost uninhabited country, and by the diversion—or desertion—of the population from their usual avocations, wholesale famine and distress were avoided. Assimilation of the multitude proceeded remarkably smoothly towards a period of prosperity and stability immediately following the exhaustion of the superficial alluvial gold. However, the increase in population, the relative youth of the migrants, the increasing number of eligible females and the emergence of major towns were all to have their effects on the epidemiology of disease.

VI

DISEASE IN A NEW ENVIRONMENT

A changing pattern of morbidity and mortality is, of course, a striking feature of many diseases during the past century or so. Interest in Australian experience is again centred on differences in the pattern of change by comparison with long-established European societies, and occasionally on interstate differences. These differences may be due to variations in the population structure from that of a 'standard population', differences in the physical or socio-economic environment, or changes in some intrinsic property of the disease itself or its causal agent. Investigation of these questions is as much a matter of epidemiological science as of history, and for this reason, the history of the infectious fevers, intestinal disease and tuberculosis in Australia has been studied in detail;[27] the collations of historical and statistical data by Cumpston deserve special mention.[28]

Perhaps rubella best illustrates not only the scientific significance of historical and geographical epidemiology but also the major local influences on the epidemiology of the infectious diseases, namely, isolation and the size, density and age distribution of the population at risk. Large epidemics occurred in 1898, 1924–25 and 1938–41, and can be correlated with immediately following epidemics of deaf-mutism.[29] Isolation and a population inadequate to maintain the virus are the factors necessary to determine epidemicity and to ensure a high proportion of non-immune females in the child-bearing age. It is only in a country fulfilling these conditions that the classical observations of Swan and of Gregg on the relationship of congenital abnormalities to maternal rubella could be made. The epidemic character of deaf-mutism was noted in Australia as far back as 1911; fluctuations were not apparent in British figures until about 1936. In the circumstances, it is not necessary to postulate a special Australian variant of rubella as responsible for congenital disorders, although this was done at one time.

The epidemiological behaviour of measles in Australia was similar, but is more readily identifiable over a longer time because of its episodic effects on mortality. Intervening periods when deaths, and the disease, were absent led to deaths in later epidemics amongst older age groups than might be expected in a conventional situation. Thus, analysis of the age distribution of deaths in measles epidemics of the second half of the nineteenth century provided support for an otherwise unsubstantiated, secondhand, report of an epidemic in the 1830's. Further research revealed proof, in an extensive medical correspondence in the contemporary lay press.[30] It then became possible to trace the probable source (a crowded ship from England), and the spread of the disease from Sydney to Hobart and New Zealand. Australian measles epidemics showed some relationship to high periods of mortality in England, and also some evidence of interstate transfer, a finding consistent with reintroduction and subsequent local spread.

In spite of the intensive gold migration between 1850 and 1856, when diphtheria was already present in England, no transfer to Australia occurred until 1858, the year in which this disease suddenly became more prevalent and more fatal in Britain. Once introduced, epidemics in the several states were usually independent of one another and of epidemics abroad. Their occurrence was influenced to some extent by the birth rate and the proportion of the population in the most susceptible age group (0–5 years). Fatality rates in successive epidemics tended to decrease gradually over the years. Scarlet fever, first introduced in 1833 at a time of recrudescence in Britain, also behaved in an independent fashion subsequently. Its epidemics could not be correlated with demographic factors, nor with other diseases now known to be streptococcal (although puerperal fever was also first recorded in 1833); extreme fluctuations in mortality were observed until the world-wide decline in severity of the disease about the turn of the century. It seems reasonable to conclude that the character of diphtheria and scarlet fever changed, the former probably only once, the latter perhaps many times. In addition to a large passenger list, a particularly hardy organism was apparently required to survive the traumatic experience of emigration, an observation possibly relevant to human experience.

The epidemiology of pulmonary tuberculosis was distinctive.[31] Although one of Captain Cook's seamen died of consumption and was buried in Australia, the disease was rare until about the middle of the nineteenth century. Through most of this early period—indeed one sees vestiges of the tradition today—Australia was a resort for the phthisical,[32] recommended by London consultants to the affluent and by the military surgeons to Indian army officers; no doubt their example was followed by many assisted emigrants. A disproportionate number of deaths from phthisis occurred amongst migrants, and gave support to a belief in the immunity of the colonial-born, a belief which at first allowed the rising mortality from tuberculosis to be viewed with equanimity. A large 'infective pool' awaited the additional numbers of non-immune children born in the gold-rush era as they reached the susceptible periods of late adolescence and early adult life between 1865 and 1890; it awaited increased aggregation of the population in towns and cities, and it awaited the development of industry and factories. The result, for which there is unequivocal clinical as well as statistical evidence, was an epidemic of 'galloping consumption', of rapidly progressive disease in young people. After about 1880 the peak mortality gradually shifted from the 20–35 years age group to the older age groups, a change towards the European norm occurring as the age constitution of the population also approached European standards. One wonders whether the same evolutionary pattern of tuberculosis may not have occurred in Europe a hundred years before, in less dramatic fashion over a longer period of time. In any case, the awareness of phthisis as a common but declining problem was probably responsible for the early recognition of 'miner's phthisis' as a cause of excess mortality after the introduction of the machine rock drill; the survey of Bendigo miners by Summons in 1906 is a landmark of some importance in the history of pneumoconiosis.[33]

Whilst it is not possible to compare Australian and overseas morbidity data, changes in the pattern of psychiatric disorder over a century deserve mention to illustrate what perhaps were primarily effects of a changing social environment. Patients with acute psychosis were more disturbed, violent and aggressive in the nineteenth century than later; acute mania and melancholia, and the affective psychoses generally, became less frequent causes for detention, even after allowance for diagnostic fashions.[34] Schizophrenic manifestations altered, with a decline in the katatonic form, and alcoholism gradually fell from a position of primary importance, whether as an aggravating or causal factor. Brothers[35] places these observations in their social context: a century ago, the patients tended to be 'illiterate, heavy-drinking, virile and adventurous

91

types living under conditions which were much cruder, rougher and tougher than today, and it is perhaps not to be wondered at that they reacted more aggressively in their psychotic state'. 'Our fevered past' fostered restlessness and irresponsibility, as at the time it excited wildness and pleasure-seeking; combined with physical hardship and isolation, psychological maladjustment and other forms of escape were predictable sequelae. As might also be anticipated, the admissions of migrants to asylums were disproportionately high in comparison with those of people born in Australia. Amongst organic disorders, general paralysis of the insane declined, while senile dementia became more common, largely as a function of the ageing of the population.

VII

MEDICAL PRACTICE, PRACTITIONERS AND PATIENTS IN A NEW ENVIRONMENT

The evolution of medical practice itself, the status of the medical practitioner and the relationships between the profession, its patients and the government show certain distinctive features over the period of Australian history.[17] Although of considerable significance to current medico-political controversies and attitudes, these questions have received surprisingly little attention from medical historians or sociologists. Certain general observations are offered with the object of indicating some appropriate fields for further study.

In the formative years, the medical service was essentially a state-salaried one, and hospital treatment could not be other than sponsored by the government, even if financed in part by the somewhat dubious method of encouraging the rum traffic.[36] Private practice in Sydney was not established for about thirty years after the foundation of the colony.[16] Gradually, the numbers of ex-convicts and 'free' settlers or emigrants seeking medical aid rose; they predominated, of course, in the non-penal settlements, such as Port Phillip (Melbourne). The government declined to accept, as a principle, responsibility for indigent paupers, although in practice it had to do so for variable periods in the several states. There was a progressive change, accelerated by the cessation of transportation of convicts, away from direct government control and responsibility,

and towards the conventional British pattern of hospital organization and of private and public medical practice. Instead, government
encouragement and finance were given to voluntary charitable and
benevolent institutions.[37] It seems curious that, in such a wholly
different environment, posing special problems of medical practice,
an exact copy of the British system was evolved. In a country which
sought and obtained radical political reform, which introduced
universal franchise, which forced the release of Crown land to the
small selector, and which came to lean heavily on the government
to solve any sort of sectional problem, one might have anticipated
a more comprehensive social, or at least medical, programme. Perhaps, as has been suggested in regard to lunacy administration,[38]
the public was repelled by any arrangement resembling the English
Poor Law system. Perhaps, too, the colonists were satisfied by the
generally better living conditions and standards than obtained from
whence they came, and with the resultant indirect benefits to health.
In due course, they organized friendly societies which were to
become a powerful medico-political force in the twentieth century.

Outside the larger towns, medical practice during the nineteenth
century was, as a rule, both unremunerative and arduous.[6] Doctors,
or practitioners of medicine, were not in short supply in relation to
the size of the population; population density was low, and long
distances had to be negotiated on horseback; the expenses of practice were necessarily high. The inhabitants were for the most part
in the prime of life; they were subject only to occasional epidemics
of acute disease, accidents, alcoholism and malnutrition. Their
isolation had taught them to be self-reliant, and they had their own
medical aids and household guides. Paradoxically, the very conditions which produced a tradition of independence and comprehensive care in Australian general practice led to the necessity for
subsidizing medical practice by other occupational activities. This
phase passed as the population became older and its distribution
relatively fixed towards the turn of the century.

The social status of the doctor in Australia was always high,
especially in the nineteenth century, by comparison with his British
colleagues. One early factor, which greatly enhanced the medical
image, was the obviously beneficial effect of good medical care on
mortality and morbidity in convict and emigrant ships. Doctors were
amongst the better-educated members of society, and more of their

93

number ventured into the rural areas than from other professions. They were a homogeneous (if not always harmonious) group, with little intraprofessional gradient, as between physicians and surgeons, for example. Most practitioners were both, and, largely because of the shortage of midwives,[39] obstetricians as well. The first specialists tended to be obstetricians and gynaecologists,[40] perhaps reflecting the local practitioners' considerable experience, and ophthalmologists,[41] reflecting a colonial medical need as well as technical advances. The comparative absence of specialization delayed the relative decline—in the public eye—in the status of the general practitioner which has accompanied increasing specialization in modern times.

What of the patients, who should perhaps occupy a central position in any study of environmental adaptation? To the best of my knowledge, there has been no deliberate historical study of the changing attitudes of patients, over the past century or two, to their diseases and to their doctors. The attitudes of governments to medical practice reflect the attitudes of all patients, on average, to all doctors; they do not reflect the attitude of patients to *their* doctor, which may have changed less. Probably the most useful index of patients' attitudes are the attitudes expressed in the lay press by editors, journalists and correspondents. In fact, one cannot fail to be impressed by the immense tolerance and respect shown by the newspapers of a century ago to 'the faculty', in spite of its public controversies, which could scarcely engender confidence, over fundamental matters of diagnosis and treatment in common conditions. Today it is not quite the same, and surely it is worth defining the differences and seeking for their causes.

The medicine practised, the conditions of its practice and the position accorded its practitioners are ultimately related to the attitudes of society to health and disease, whatever the state of medical science, and whatever the physical environment. No opportunity should be lost to examine any aspect of these problems, and the restricted Australian scene, well-delineated and relatively simple in structure, is particularly suited to such study.

VIII

The thesis advanced in this paper is that the medical history of a newly established, developing country, whatever its cultural background, can be viewed as a deliberate experiment in history; what it lacks in antiquity is offset by a gain in documentation and detail. As such, it becomes a peculiarly appropriate method of analysing the complex interactions which occur in the course of man's adaptation to his environment. The present era of social and technological change, with its medical implications, could, and should, give a sense of immediacy and purpose to these studies.

ACKNOWLEDGEMENTS

The references have been selected with the object of facilitating further study, or of illustrating a method of approach, rather than to substantiate any particular statement in the text; a review of this kind is indebted to many authors not listed individually. My thanks are due to Dr B. D. Foote, Biomedical Librarian, University of New South Wales, and my secretary, Miss Jennifer Kearney, for particular assistance in the present survey, but my debt in fact extends to many colleagues and librarians over the years.

REFERENCES

1 D. J. Thomas, 'Valedictory address of the President', *Australian med. J.* 1865, **10**, 40–51, 70–82.
2 G. T. Hankins, 'The history of medicine from the early times to the year 1833', *Australasian med. Gaz.* 1893, **10**, 194–202.
3 B. Gandevia, *An annotated bibliography of the history of medicine in Australia*, Sydney: Australasian Medical Publishing Co., 1957.
4 Hippocrates, 'Airs, waters and places', transl. W. H. S. Jones, vol. 1, p. 137, Loeb Classical Library, London: William Heinemann, 1923.
5 D. Gordon, 'How to use historical sources in Australian medical history', *Med. J. Australia* 1967, **2**, 933–7.
6 B. Gandevia, 'Land, labour and gold: the medical problems of Australia in the nineteenth century', *Med. J. Australia* 1960, **1**, 753–62.
7 B. Gandevia, 'A review of Victoria's early medical journals', *Med. J. Australia* 1952, **2**, 184–8; R. R. Winton, 'Australian medical journals: their history and current locations', *Bull. Post-Grad. Committee Med., Univ. Syd.* 1969, **24**, 259–61.

8   A. Tovell and B. Gandevia, 'Early Australian medical associations', *Med. J. Australia* 1962, 1, 756–9, and ibid., 1962, 2, 397–8.

9   B. Gandevia and A. Tovell, 'The first Australian medical libraries', *Med. J. Australia* 1964, 2, 314–20.

10 A seminar on 'The problems of Australian medical libraries in relation to historical collections and research', held under the auspices of the Post-Graduate Medical Foundation, was published in full in a special issue of *Bull. Post-Grad. Committee Med., Univ. Syd.* 1969, 24, 244–309. In a series of papers, the history, resources and policies of the major medical libraries are reviewed; a list of separate publications on the history of medicine in Australia is appended. *A collection of medical books and pamphlets of Australian interest from the library of Bryan Gandevia*, issued in roneoed typescript form by the Biomedical Library, University of New South Wales in 1967 (supplement, 1968), lists about 600 separate publications.

11 A. Tovell and B. Gandevia, *References to Australia in British medical journals prior to 1880*, Museum of Medical History, Medical Society of Victoria, Melbourne, 1961.

12 E. B. Pedersen and P. M. Moodie, *The health of Australian aborigines: an annotated bibliography with classification by subject matter and locality*, School of Public Health and Tropical Medicine, University of Sydney, Sydney, 1966.

13 *The Australian Encyclopaedia*, ed. A. H. Chisholm, 10 vols., Sydney: Angus and Robertson, 1958. See also J. B. Cleland, 'The ecology of the aboriginal in South and Central Australia' in B. C. Cotton (ed.), *Aboriginal man in South and Central Australia*, Adelaide: Govt. Printer, 1966.

14 T. A. Coghlan, *Childbirth in New South Wales: a study in statistics*, Sydney: Govt Printer, 1899.

15 T. A. Coghlan, *The decline in the birth-rate of New South Wales and other phenomena of child-birth: an essay in statistics*, Sydney: Govt. Printer, 1903. See also A. T. Gover, 'The pattern of population change in Australia', *J. & Proc. Roy. Aust. Hist. Soc.* 1946, 32, 295–340.

16 E. Ford, 'The life and work of William Redfern', *Bull. Post-Grad. Committee Med., Univ. Syd.* 1953, 9, 1–36.

17 B. Gandevia, 'Medical history in its Australian environment', *Med. J. Australia* 1967, 2, 941–6. See also D. R. McNeil, 'Medical care aboard Australia-bound convict ships', *Bull. Hist. Med.* 1952, 26, 117–40.

18 D. Gordon, 'Sickness and death at the Moreton Bay convict settlement', *Med. J. Australia* 1963, 2, 473–80.

19 A. M. McIntosh, 'Early settlement in Northern Australia', *Med. J. Australia* 1958, 1, 409–15, 441–9.

20 J. B. Cleland, 'Morbidity and mortality in the convict settlement at Port Arthur, Tasmania, from 1830–1835', *Med. J. Australia* 1932, 2, 347–50.

21 R. Cilento and C. Lack, *Triumph in the tropics: an historical sketch of Queensland*, Brisbane: Smith & Paterson, 1959. For a general review, relating especially to population, migration and the aborigines, see A. P.

Elkin, 'Man in Australia', in *A century of scientific progress: the centenary volume of the Royal Society of New South Wales*, Sydney: Royal Society of New South Wales, n.d. [1968]. For the history of the early settlements, see papers listed in op. cit. (above, note 3).

22 L. Davey, M. Macpherson and F. W. Clements, 'The hungry years: 1788–1792', *Historical Studies* 1947, 3, 187–92.

23 A. W. Hume, *Hobart General Hospital: its early history*, Hobart, n.d. [c. 1920].

24 H. O. Lancaster, 'The mortality from violence in Australia, 1863 to 1960', *Med. J. Australia* 1964, 1, 388–93.

25 F. McCallum, 'Bionomics of Australian history', *Health* 1926, 4, 45–53. This review is particularly pertinent to the general theme of the present essay, but, as with op. cit. (above, note 6) and other relevant papers listed in op. cit. (above, note 3), no comprehensive analysis of rural and gold-field medicine has been attempted; these topics require further study to establish the validity of the generalisations offered here. The special problems of truly remote areas led to particular solutions, such as the Flying Doctor Service and the Australian Inland Mission, with its wire-less medical advisory service. See C. Fenton, *Flying Doctor*, 3rd ed., Melbourne: Georgian House, 1949; J. Bilton, *The Royal Flying Doctor Service of Australia: its origin, growth and development*, Royal Flying Doctor Service Federal Council, Sydney, 1961; W. S. McPheat, *John Flynn: apostle to the inland*, London: Hodder and Stoughton, 1963.

26 M. C. Harris, 'Water: tragedy and triumph on the Western Australian goldfields', *Early Days (J. & Proc. West. Aust. Hist. Soc.)* 1947, 9, 18–26. Different water supply problems were encountered elsewhere.

27 H. O. Lancaster, *Bibliography of vital statistics in Australia and New Zealand*, Sydney: Australasian Medical Publishing Co., 1964.

28 J. H. L. Cumpston, *The history of diphtheria, scarlet fever, measles and whooping cough in Australia, 1788–1925*, Melbourne: Govt Printer, 1927; J. H. L. Cumpston and F. McCallum, *The history of the intestinal infections (and typhus fever) in Australia 1788–1923*, Melbourne: Govt Printer, 1927 (Commonwealth of Australia Department of Health Service publications Nos. 37 and 36 respectively). Cumpston, whose other works are listed in op. cit. (above, note 27), summarises much relevant material in 'Public health in Australia', *Med. J. Australia* 1931, 1, 491–500, 591–7, 679–85; see also H. O. Lancaster, 'Vital statistics as human ecology', *Aust. J. Sci.* 1963, 25, 445–53.

29 H. O. Lancaster, 'Deafness as an epidemic disease in Australia', *Br. med. J.* 1951, 2, 1429–32.

30 J. W. Donovan, 'Measles in Australia and New Zealand, 1834–1835', *Med. J. Australia* 1970, 1, 5–10.

31 M. J. Holmes, 'Tuberculosis in Australia', *Med. J. Australia* 1937, 2, 813–27; J. H. L. Cumpston, 'Tuberculosis in Australia', ibid. 1931, 2, 153–63.

32 K. Bryn Thomas and B. Gandevia, 'Dr. Francis Workman, emigrant, and

the history of taking the cure for consumption in the colonies', *Med. J. Australia* 1959, **2**, 1–10.

33 W. Summons, *Report on an investigation at Bendigo into the nature, causes and means of prevention of miner's phthisis*, Melbourne: Stillwell, 1907. See also, B. Gandevia, 'Australian contributions to the study of pneumoconioses', K. F. Russell (ed.), *Proceedings of the Second Seminar on the History of Medicine, University of Melbourne*, in press [1970].

34 J. Krupinski and A. Stoller, 'Survey of institutionalized mental patients in Victoria, Australia, 1882–1959', *Med. J. Australia* 1962, **1**, 269–76, 314–21, 359–67.

35 C. R. D. Brothers, 'Archives of Victorian psychiatry', *Med. J. Australia* 1957, **1**, 341–7, 373–9.

36 M. H. Ellis, 'Governor Macquarie and the "rum" hospital', *J. & Proc. Roy. Aust. Hist. Soc.* 1946, **32**, 273–93; W. S. Campbell, 'The use and abuse of stimulants in the early days of settlement in New South Wales', ibid. 1932, **18**, 74–99.

37 See, for example, J. F. Watson, *The history of Sydney Hospital from 1811 to 1911*, Sydney: Govt Printer, 1911; K. S. Inglis, *Hospital and community: a history of the Royal Melbourne Hospital*, Melbourne: Melbourne University Press, 1958; D. Peyser, 'A study of the history of welfare work in Sydney from 1788 till about 1900', *J. & Proc. Roy. Aust. Hist. Soc.* 1939, **25**, 89–127, 169–212; A. M. McIntosh, 'The life and times of William Bland', *Bull. Post-Grad. Committee Med., Univ. Syd.* 1954, **10**, 109–52.

38 C. J. Cummins, *The administration of lunacy and idiocy in New South Wales 1788–1855*, Sydney: Department of Health (N.S.W.), 1967.

39 F. M. Forster, 'Mrs. Howlett and Dr. Jenkins: Listerism and early midwifery practice in Australia', *Med. J. Australia* 1965, **2**, 1047–54.

40 F. M. Forster, *Progress in obstetrics and gynaecology in Australia*, Sydney: John Sands, 1967.

41 D. Williams, 'Eyes, surgeons and sociality in Australasia', *Trans. Ophthalm. Soc. Aust.* 1947, **7**, 5–13; B. Gandevia, 'James Thomas Rudall, F.R.C.S. (1828–1907): his life and journal for the year 1858', *Med. J. Australia* 1954, **2**, 989–1008.

6 Diagnosis of Disease in the Past

C. J. HACKETT

The more accurate recognition of diseases from descriptions of the past and the diagnosis of pathological changes in exhumed bones and other tissues should contribute to a better understanding of the origin, spread, and thus the distribution of diseases in earlier times. Sufficient knowledge should now be available for this, and recent techniques for accurate and direct dating of ancient objects call for similar precision in diagnosis. It should not be forgotten, however, that scientific medicine started less than a century ago so that diagnosis before then depended upon clinical appearances only.

In one locality (Chowilla) in south-eastern Australia a number of skeletons have been unearthed recently. Carbon dating of one gave an age of about 5000 years. One long bone or skull among this material with diagnosable pathological changes would be of considerable value in helping to establish the pattern of disease at this particular period and perhaps in indicating some of the ways of life of the inhabitants.

It is proposed to consider in this paper first the textual and then the pathological evidence for diseases which occurred decades or centuries ago.

II

DESCRIPTIONS OF DISEASE IN THE PAST

The comprehensibility of such descriptions depends largely upon the general knowledge at the time they are recorded. Those of exceptional writers may be illumined by astute and accurate observation of natural events. Until medical knowledge was developed, however, even the best descriptions cannot be expected to be more than records of accurate observation unaided by modern techniques and can, in fact, be no better than present-day accounts by the best lay observers.

Destructive lesions especially of the face were attributed by some early nineteenth-century explorers in Australia[1] to the 'most loath-some disease' for they dreaded to say 'venereal disease' or 'syphilis'; others, however, report the high prevalence of such conditions by name. These destructions were probably due to yaws in the north or endemic syphilis in the centre and south of the continent. The former was not well described until the end of the nineteenth century and the latter was practically unknown until well into the present century. Even now, in a patient out of geographical context, yaws may be difficult to differentiate from venereal syphilis and some present-day writers do not appear to appreciate the existence of the four human treponematoses, of which pinta alone does not cause bone lesions.

In these old descriptions fact should be carefully looked for. 'The sickness followed upon the return of traders from the east', 'the infliction ceased immediately the rains started and was not seen again that year', and 'summer paralysis' are statements which might have been based upon observation and their meaning should be sought. Imprecise statements that a people was scourged by some deity may refer to epidemic outbreaks whose characterization is lacking, or to a famine.

Of the sweating sickness it has been said that whereas in plague the patient becomes sick before he dies, in this disease death occurred before the patient became sick. It appears to have been brought to England in 1485 as a new disease by French mercenaries in the army of Henry VII though they themselves were not sick. Pomeranz recalled that the sweating sickness did not affect Scotsmen, Irishmen or Frenchmen, but 'annihilated countless thousands throughout Germany'.[2] He quotes Holinshed, 'Suddenly, a deadly burning sweat so assailed their bodies and distempered their blood with a most ardent heat, that scarce one among a hundred that sickened did escape with life, for all in manner, as soon as the sweat took them, or a short time after, yielded the ghost.'[3] John Caius judged it worse than plague which '...commonly geveth iii. or iiii. often vii. sumtyme ix....sumtyme xi. and sumtyme xiiii. dayes respecte, to whome it vexeth. But that [the sweating sickness] immediately killed some in opening theire windowes, some in plaieng with children in their strete dores...'[4]

In England, until it disappeared after five epidemics in 1551, it was said to have spared the poor but 'went most among rich people'.[5] In Bavaria after the 1939-45 war infective hepatitis was seen in American troops but not in the local populace; it occurred in young individuals who had been a relatively short time in the area and affected white and coloured soldiers equally.[6] During that war the same infection broke out in Egypt amongst European but not Indian troops. Recently poliomyelitis was frequent in newly arrived European social workers in African villages, but was absent in the villagers themselves. A century ago this apparent discrimination would have been inexplicable.

Records of spectacular events in a community during the course of a disease, the cause of which had been established by laboratory methods, would be a great help in deciphering past descriptions. There is a group of people, doctors and missionaries sixty to eighty years of age, who have spent many years in what are now developing countries and who saw and perhaps understood many things that no longer occur. Thirty to forty years ago they may have often seen epidemics appear and disappear uninfluenced by immunization or chemotherapy, and they may have been impressed by dramatic incidents in community or individual health and sickness. They should be encouraged to record such occurrences in modern medical terms, in the manner of the people themselves, and as an intelligent layman might do. It may be necessary and worthwhile to assist the older members of this group, who pioneered modern medicine in the countries of their temporary adoption, by providing a medical amanuensis with a tape-recorder.

The information that would be useful is eyewitness accounts of:

(1) Onset, course and end of the outbreak of a disease and its duration, spread in a country or across a continent.

(2) Unexplained absence or presence of a disease or of disease manifestations; dramatic symptoms and persistence of symptoms or disabilities.

(3) Attack and death rates, seasonal variations, frequency of crippling, age groups attacked.

(4) Sickness among domestic or wild animals at the same time as the human illness.

(5) Concurrent non-medical events of apparent significance.

Individuals with personal experience of disease outbreaks may be expected readily to provide the information needed. The recognition of factual statements is a preliminary step in the recognition of the disease. Laymen's accounts are of particular value because of the useful, non-medical terms they employ.[7]

It is, of course, obvious that published accounts of relevant information would also be sought in medical publications[8] and in the journals of explorers of the past five or more centuries. The medical statements of ocean explorers may prove to be more factual than those of land explorers, perhaps because health and sickness were always closer to them and their crews throughout their careers, and because navigation and log-keeping exercised their powers of observation and recording.

Information of direct or indirect value in understanding the spread of disease in the past may be had from publications on the following conditions:

Tungiasis. Tunga penetrans was probably present in Africa in restricted areas in the eighteenth, and perhaps even in the seventeenth century. There was, however, apparently a reintroduction in September 1872 from Brazil by a British warship, H.M.S. *Thomas Mitchell,* from Rio de Janeiro to Ambriz in Angola.[9] By 1895 it had reached the east coast and in that year it was carried to Madagascar and three years later to Zanzibar. Soon thereafter it was conveyed to Bombay and Karachi. This spread was due to improved communications, exploration, and to troop movements. The original home of *T. penetrans* was probably tropical America between about 30°N and 30°S and the Caribbean Islands.

Relapsing fever, louse borne. Scott[10] reports that the great epidemic in West Africa started in Guinea in 1921 and spread to Dafur in western Sudan by 1926, a distance of 3000 miles in five years.

Meningococcal meningitis. The West African epidemic of the 1930's started in Mongalla Province of south-east Sudan in 1927 to 1930 and reached Sierra Leone and Gambia in 1941.[11] The spread was about latitude 14°N, south of the arid zone and north of the humid forest zone. Scott[12] states that meningococcal meningitis was first described in 1805 in Switzerland and that it reached the United States in 1893. In Ghana it occurs in the drier areas in the cool, dry season.

African trypanosomiasis. The great West African epidemic of 1912 to 1940 started in the Congo[13] and spread north-west to reach northern Nigeria in the late 1920's; thence it extended westwards to reach Sierra Leone in 1939. The disease was widely endemic before the arrival of the epidemic which may have been due to the appearance of 'a strain of trypanosome with epidemic qualities'.[14]

Other information on the spread of disease would be had in the occurrence of yellow fever among new arrivals in the Caribbean and West Africa: of plague in India and in Europe, and its introduction into California followed by the infection of indigenous rodents:[15] of cholera in the past and during the last ten years: of influenza and smallpox in the past and at present: of haemorrhagic fever at present.

There is also the relatively rapid spread of potato blight, a fungus infection, probably from the northern Andes region of South America to the eastern states of the United States (1843), thence to Belgium (end of June 1845), Holland and France (mid-July 1845), England (mid-August 1845) and to Ireland (September 1845) where the failure of the crop had such grave consequences for the Irish.[16] This provides considerable information on the speed of spread of what was at the time thought to be a new potato disease in Europe. The first report of the blue mould of tobacco plant in Europe came from England in October 1958, and in two years the disease spread across Europe to Poland, Roumania and the Transcaucasian Ukraine. This was brought about mainly by the wind transport of spores, conidia, and less importantly, by the carriage of them on man or animals.[17]

An outbreak of paralysis commenced in the Meknes region of Morocco in 1959,[18] but except for one man who had adopted the Moslem way of life, no case occurred among the Europeans, the Jews or the better-to-do Moslems. Cases were grouped at the periphery of the towns where the poorest of the Moslem population lived. The incidence was in decreasing order, in adult women, adult men and older children. During the outbreak a quarter of a million visitors came to the town, but no case among them occurred while they were there, nor as far as could be ascertained, after leaving Meknes. The cause of the paralysis was traced to adulterated vegetable oil. Outbreaks of bacterial food poisoning should be of interest for the understanding of similar occurrences in the past. Among two

hundred guests at a triple marriage feast in Timor in 1968, all
except seven fell ill within twelve to twenty-four hours and five
died. Those that were not affected complained that they arrived late
and that all the meat had been eaten.

As regards the unexpected absence or presence of diseases, some
attention might be given to those that were indigenous to the different continents when they first became known to Europeans. When
records of other and earlier explorers, for example Asian, are better
known, the dating of the information will be moved further back.
The approximate dates of continental discovery by Europeans as
far as the transmission of disease is concerned might be taken as
Africa, coastal, 1480; inland 1850–1900; America 1490; Asia 1500;
Australia 1780. A list of diseases indigenous to the continents at the
time of European discovery might be proposed:[19]

Africa. African trypanosomiasis, schistosomiasis, yellow fever,
leprosy, yaws and endemic syphilis.

America. American trypanosomiasis, pinta, bartonellosis, tungiasis.

Australia. Yaws and endemic syphilis.

Oceania. Yaws.

Asia. Dermal and visceral leishmaniasis, cholera, plague,
trachoma, leprosy, smallpox, yaws and endemic syphilis.

Similarly a list of diseases carried from one continent to another
would be useful.

To America. Schistosomiasis and perhaps yellow fever from
Africa. Leprosy and smallpox from Europe. Plague from Asia.

To Europe. Cholera, plague and smallpox from Asia. Trachoma
from Egypt, allegedly by Napoleon's troops. Perhaps leprosy
from Asia.

To Australia. Trachoma and perhaps leprosy from Asia.

To Africa. Plague from Asia.

To Oceania, Australia, Africa, and America. The common communicable diseases from Europe.

Unexplained, unexpected and perhaps dubious absences might
include: scabies from ancient Rome: syphilis in pre-Columbian
Europe, in writings and bones: bone syphilis in Addis Ababa in
recent years: tabes dorsalis and general paralysis of the insane in
Europe until their recognition as clinical entities in the second half
of the nineteenth century.

Other useful lists would be the 'new' diseases or first reported occurrences of diseases likely to produce a dramatic impact on a community; such as high mortality, widely spread paralysis, sudden death, unconsciousness, mental disturbances, or occurring especially in one section of the populace, for example, the prosperous, or the newcomers.

All this information would provide a basis of the known from which one could try to understand the unknown.

III

DISEASE IN DRY BONES

In the past the diagnosis of disease in early bones seems to have been either obvious as in septic osteomyelitis, or authoritarian as in the range of syphilitic lesions. In 1930 Pales[20] summarized admirably the difficulty in, the errors of, and the uncritical approach to the diagnosis of syphilis in dry bones. In conversation recently[21] he thought these had not changed much. In some reports of a particular dry bone of archaeological interest the only support for the diagnosis of syphilis is the author's use of such expressions as 'characteristic', 'diagnostic', 'undoubted', or 'almost certainly'. These are unconvincing to the unwilling.

Recognition of the bone lesions due mainly to communicable diseases prevalent in the past is sought. In Europe during the last two centuries the frequent bone lesions have been septic osteomyelitis and osteoperiostitis, syphilis and, less commonly, Paget's disease of bone ('osteitis deformans') and those secondary to chronic ulceration of the leg. Tuberculosis of the spine and joints might have to be differentiated and leprosy must certainly be taken into account.[22,23]

The main problem remains, as ever, the recognition of syphilitic lesions and their differentiation from other bone diseases. Syphilis should in this context be understood to include the three treponematoses that cause bone lesions; namely venereal syphilis, yaws and endemic syphilis.[24] 'Treponemal lesions' or the 'lesions of treponematoses' are rather clumsy expressions but indicate the breadth needed. At present there is no way to differentiate between these three infections in bones, if one does, indeed, regard them as individual infections by separate organisms.[25] Radiographical studies of endemic syphilis[26] and yaws[27] have been published but adequate, recent studies of the bone lesions of venereal syphilis are difficult to find.

One worker, Williams,[28] has attempted to establish diagnostic criteria for syphilitic bone lesions before tackling the problem of syphilis in pre-Columbian bones in Europe and the Americas. He examined 500 skulls labelled syphilis in European and American museums of pathology and found no differences of opinion in the various countries about what was a syphilitic skull. He estimated that lesions in over half of these skulls were not typical. He thought 'the perfectly typical syphilitic skull...a more certain criterion for diagnosis than a Wassermann reaction of four plus or an aneurysm of the aorta' (p. 784), but was not so confident of the diagnosis of syphilis in other bones. With radiography and microscopy, however, 'a high degree of probability in the diagnosis may be obtained with some long bones' (ibid.). Recent inquiry at his old department in the University of Buffalo failed to trace his notes of this study. T. M. Prudden in an article by Hyde[29] dealt at some length with the diagnosis of syphilis in archaeological bones and Weber,[30] Michaelis[31] and Wilhelm[32] were concerned with the microscopical appearances of these lesions.

The characterization of bone lesions may be attempted by their macroscopical, radiographical or microscopical appearances. The absence of cells in dry bones poses considerable problems which some workers have said rule out any expectation of microscopical criteria. Other difficulties in microscopical studies arise from chemical and structural deterioration that accompany exposure to soil and water during burial. One form of the latter has been reported by Wedl,[33] Roux,[34] Baud and Morgenthaler[35] and Werelds,[36,37] under several names: 'canaux de forage', 'Roux canals', 'Bohrgänge', etc. This is a post-mortem and microscopical tunnelling which appears in bones buried for some time, depending on the conditions of the burial. It extends longitudinally more than transversely in compact and cancellous bone tissue. It starts on the outer and inner surfaces of diaphyses and extends slowly through the calcified tissue. Osteones tend to be riddled with these changes and in the early stages the interstitial lamellae contain only a few transversely meandering tunnels. Ultimately the structure of the whole tissue is destroyed and the bone disintegrates, although this process may be measured in centuries rather than years. Roux[34] thought that these changes were due to a fungus which he named *Mycelites ossifragus*. Contact of the buried material with the soil seems to be the deciding factor in the extent and rate of the deterioration.

A study of old bones, therefore, might start with the macroscopical appearances and if they suggest criteria of a certain disease these might be sharpened by microscopy. Radiography of the whole long bones often adds little to the information derived from sagittal sections. Unless the base of the skull is missing, X-rays of calvarial changes may not be of much assistance.

Early studies in isolated communities, such as New Guinea and 25 years ago in parts of Africa, south-east Asia, Australia and some Pacific Islands, indicate that perhaps the only bone lesions present then were those of yaws. Septic conditions were rare or unknown in museum specimens and in the field. Thus it appears that the investigation needed might most usefully be based upon the diagnosis of syphilitic changes and upon their differentiation from other diseases likely to cause confusion. It would be mainly concerned with prevalent communicable diseases, for although nutritional deficiencies or congenital abnormalities may change the structure or shape of bones, they are not usually confused with these lesions.

An attempt is now being made by the writer to establish such criteria along these lines by studying bones in the museums of university departments of pathology. Bones with lesions that might be due to infections are inspected without reference to the catalogue entry and only when the features of the specimen have been fully recorded is the original diagnosis sought in the catalogue. Certain groupings of the bone lesions, and developmental sequences thereof, are becoming apparent. A major difficulty is the unsatisfactory basis of many of the catalogue diagnoses. Only 2–5 per cent of them are supported from evidence other than from the bone itself, such as clinical findings, and none by microscopical examination. The catalogue entry often consists of the name of the donor and a diagnosis and/or description, which may have been made or modified many years after the acquisition of the specimen. Some specimens have only a diagnosis and most specimens were acquired more than sixty years ago before laboratory methods of diagnosis came into general use. Wells[38] stresses the importance of distinguishing damage after death from pathological lesions.

On the basis of the label diagnosis, certain lesions are found that are diagnosed mainly or only as syphilis and others mainly or only as osteomyelitis. Closer study of the former makes the descriptions of workers of the last century more readily comprehensible.[39] The similarity of the lesions ascribed to syphilis with the pathological changes of yaws and endemic syphilis as seen radiographically, lend support to the label diagnoses. In some museums there are specimens labelled syphilis from communities such as those of Australia and of certain Pacific Islands, which during the relevant period were heavily infected with yaws; yaws infection in childhood is generally regarded as a protection from adult venereal syphilis. There are small groups of three to five specimens labelled 'syphilis' that do not fit into the other syphilitic groups of twenty to thirty specimens, and some others labelled 'periostitis' and 'osteoperiostitis' which readily fall into one of the syphilis-labelled groups. The lesions labelled syphilitic are mostly gross and readily recognizable. Until, however, the evidence is statistically satisfactory it cannot be said that the days of authoritarianism have passed.

IV

CONCLUSIONS

Knowledge of diseases in earlier times can be enhanced by improving the recognition of diseases in textual records and in pathological material from the past.

(1) *Textual.* The diagnosis of diseases, especially those of infectious origin occurring in tropical and sub-tropical countries, hazarded from past descriptions of them, may be improved by obtaining information from individuals who have personally observed them during the past half-century. This would have to be before modern therapy, prophylaxis, environment and migration influenced their course but when accurate diagnosis was possible.

(2) *Pathological.* For the more precise diagnosis of disease in ancient bones, statistically acceptable criteria are desirable and an attempt is being made to establish them. This however is difficult because the catalogue diagnoses of specimens in museums of pathology are rarely supported by evidence other than from the bone itself.

These improvements in diagnosis are needed if there is to be better understanding of the origin, spread and distribution of diseases in the past.

REFERENCES

1   C. J. Hackett, 'A critical survey of some references to syphilis and yaws among the Australian aborigines', *Med. J. Aust.* 1936, 1, 733–45.
2   H. Pomeranz, 'Medicine in the Shakespearean plays and era', *Med. Life* 1934, 41, 479–532, see p. 532.
3   Ibid.
4   J. Caius, *A boke, or counseill against the disease commonly called the sweate or sweatyng sicknesse*, fo. 8ᵛ–9ʳ, London: R. Grafton, 1552.
5   J. Renner of Bremen in C. G. Gruner, *Scriptores de sudore Anglico super-stites*, ed. H. Haeser, p. 448, '...ging meistig aver de ricken Lüe', Jena, 1847.
6   J. R. Paul, 'Epidemic hepatitis among U.S. troops in post-war Germany', *Proc. R. Soc. Med.* 1950, 43, 438–40.
7   R. S. Roberts, 'Old and new: disease in Manicaland fifty years ago, as described by an educated African, with special reference to essential thrombocytopenia', *Central African J. Med.* 1968, 14, 277–9.
8   Articles such as that by A. S. Thomson on a possible case of leprosy, for example, may be numerous: 'An account of the disease called "Ngere-ngere' by the New Zealanders (Lepra gangraenosa)' in 'On the peculiarities in figure, the disfigurations and the customs of the New Zealanders; with remarks on their diseases and on their modes of treatment', *Br. for. Med.-chir. Rev.* 1854, 13, 489–502; ibid. 1854, 14, 461–70; and ibid. 1855, 15, 520–9, see pp. 496–502.
9   R. Hoeppli, 'Early references to *Tunga penetrans* in Tropical Africa', *Acta trop.* 1963, 20, 143–53.
10 D. Scott, *Epidemic disease in Ghana 1901–1960*, pp. 121–2, London: Oxford University Press, 1965.
11 B. B. Waddy, 'The spread of cerebro-spinal meningitis across Africa', *W. Afr. med. J.* 1957, 3 (N.S.), 71–4.
12 Scott, op. cit. (above, note 10), p. 86.
13 Scott, op. cit. (above, note 10), pp. 145–7.
14 Scott, op. cit. (above, note 10), p. 147.
15 K. F. Meyer, 'The natural history of plague and psittacosis', *Publ. Hlth. Rep., Wash.* 1957, 72, 705–19.
16 P. M. A. Bourke, 'Emergence of potato blight, 1843–46', *Nature, Lond.* 1964, 203, 805–8.
17 R. W. Rayner and J. C. F. Hopkins, *Blue mould of tobacco. A review of current information*, p. 7, Kew, Surrey: Commonwealth Mycological Institute, 1962 (Miscellaneous Publication No. 16).

18   H. V. Smith and J. M. K. Spalding, 'Outbreaks of paralysis in Morocco due to *ortho*-cresyl phosphate poisoning', *Lancet* 1959, **2**, 1019–21.

19   See R. Hare, 'The antiquity of diseases caused by bacteria and viruses, a review of the problem from a bacteriologist's point of view' in D. Brothwell and A. T. Sandison (eds.), *Diseases in antiquity*, pp. 115–31, Springfield, Ill.: C. C Thomas, 1967.

20   L. Pales, *Paléopathologie et pathologie comparative*, pp. 218–25, Paris: Masson, 1930.

21   Personal communication, 1964.

22   V. Møller-Christensen, *Bone lesions in leprosy*, Copenhagen: Munksgaard, 1961.

23   D. E. Paterson and C. K. Job, 'Bone changes and absorption in leprosy; a radiological, pathological, and clinical study' in R. G. Cochrane and T. F. Davey (eds.), *Leprosy in theory and practice*, 2nd ed., pp. 425–46, Bristol: J. Wright, 1964.

24   C. J. Hackett, 'The human treponematoses' in D. Brothwell and A. T. Sandison (eds.), *Diseases in antiquity*, pp. 152–69, Springfield, Ill.: C. C Thomas, 1967.

25   E. H. Hudson, 'Christopher Columbus and the history of syphilis', *Acta trop.*, Basel 1968, **25**, 1–16.

26   G. S. Rost, 'Roentgen manifestations of bejel ("endemic syphilis") as observed in the Euphrates river valley', *Radiology* 1942, **38**, 320–5.

27   C. J. Hackett, *Bone lesions of yaws in Uganda*, Oxford: Blackwell, 1951.

28   H. U. Williams, 'The origin and antiquity of syphilis: the evidence from diseased bones. A review, with some new material from America', *Arch. Path.* 1932, **13**, 779–814, 931–83.

29   J. N. Hyde, 'A contribution to the study of pre-Columbian syphilis in America', *Am. J. med. Sci.* 1891, **102**, 117–31, see pp. 124–8.

30   M. Weber, 'Schliffe von mazerierten Röhrenknochen und ihre Bedeutung für die Unterscheidung der Syphilis und Osteomyelitis von der Osteodystrophia fibrosa sowie für die Untersuchung fraglich syphilitischer, prähistorischer Knochen', *Beitr. path. Anat.* 1927, **78**, 441–511. There is a typescript of an English translation in the Library of the Royal Society of Medicine, London.

31   L. Michaelis, 'Vergleichende mikroskopische Untersuchungen an rezenten, historischen und fossilen menschlichen Knochen. Zugleich ein Beitrag zur Geschichte der Syphilis' in L. Aschoff, M. Borst, M. B. Schmidt, L. Pick and W. Koch (eds.), *Veröffentlichungen aus der Kriegs- und Konstitutionspathologie* (Jena: G. Fischer) 1930, **6**, Heft 1. There is a typescript of an English translation in the Library of the Royal Society of Medicine (La 8°. Tr. 4808).

32   S. F. Wilhelm, 'Osteitis fibrosa and the hyperostotic form of bone syphilis; a comparative anatomical and roentgenological study', *Surg. Gynec. Obstet.* 1925, **41**, 624–39.

33   C. Wedl, 'Über einen im Zahnbein und Knochen keimenden Pilz', *S. Akad. Wiss. Wien* (Math.-naturwiss. Classe) 1865, **50**, Abt. I, 171–93.

34 W. Roux, 'Über eine im Knochen lebende Gruppe von Fadenpilzen (Mycelites ossifragus)', *Z. Wiss. Zool.* 1887, 45, 227–54.

35 C. A. Baud and P. W. Morgenthaler, 'Recherches sur l'ultrastructure de l'os humain fossile', *Archs. suisses Anthrop. gén.* 1952, 17, 52–65.

36 R. J. Werelds, 'Observations macroscopiques et microscopiques sur certaines alterations post mortem des dents', *Bulletin du Groupement international pour Recherche scientifique Stomatologie* 1961, 4, 7–60.

37 R. J. Werelds, 'Nouvelles observations sur les dégradations post mortem de la dentine et du cément des dents inhumées. (Etude des dents recueillies dans les ruines de l'ancienne Abbaye de Vivegnis [1235–1790] près de Liège', ibid. 1962, 5, 554–91.

38 C. Wells, 'Pseudopathology' in D. Brothwell and A. T. Sandison (eds.), *Diseases in antiquity*, pp. 5–19, Springfield, Ill.: C. C Thomas, 1967.

39 E. Lancereaux, *A treatise on syphilis. Historical and practical*, transl. G. Whitley, 2 vols., vol. 1, pp. 235–44, London: New Sydenham Society, 1868.

7 Disease, Micro-Evolution and Earlier Populations: an Important Bridge between Medical History and Human Biology

DON BROTHWELL

It is a part of the progressive winds of change in medical biology that scientists from other disciplines are being increasingly drawn into some research fields. It is good to see this also happening in medical history where, although literary ties have always been strong, biological links have been all too infrequent. In my own experience, there has even been resistance to this interdisciplinary cooperation. My contribution to this volume will I hope help to show that medical history and human biology now share common ground, important to both. Pre-war physical anthropology has given rise to a discipline far more aware of disease as a selective pressure in human communities; and it is now the turn of medical history to realize that the spectrum of disease—if placed in correct perspective —needs to be considered against the background of human biological and cultural change.

From the recent evidence of potassium-argon dates, it seems probable that the earliest hominids have evolved over some two million years, and there is no doubt that the mosaic of disease he set out with is very different from that known today. There is also no doubt that the conquest of disease during human evolution has influenced and been influenced by human variation, adaptability, and increasingly complex cultural levels. A further important factor has no doubt been bacteriological micro-evolution, at times perhaps associated with major biocultural advances in man. In view of the taxonomic chaos extant in the study of this group of organisms,[1] I do not intend to comment further on this subject. Eventually, however, the whole question of the potential rate of change in pathogenic organisms over the past few million years will have to be seriously considered, for surely it is really a little absurd to con-

tinue to write on the history and epidemiological progress of 'syphilis', or 'leprosy', or 'tuberculosis' in earlier man as though the
micro-organisms were unchanging. In actual fact, some of the
palaeopathological lesions already known may really be 'pre-' or
'proto-' 'syphilis' and so on, if taxonomic distances could be determined rather than just considering similarity of bone lesions.

But to return to the main subject of this paper. I want to outline
some of the common ground between medical history and human
biology, and in so doing to show a field of medical history which is
so far poorly explored. We are concerned with disease in earlier
communities, and in the two-way relationship between disease,
population variability, and cultural change.

II

DISEASE AND HUMAN VARIATION, A BRIEF HISTORY OF AN ASSOCIATION

It would be wrong to assume, because the past few decades have
seen such progress in human biology, that resistance and adaptation
to disease in man are subjects of only recent interest. The beginnings
are well founded in nineteenth-century writings, in works on
anthropology no less than in studies on the geography of earlier
diseases. Admittedly, comparative observations were scanty, and
Prichard, in his detailed *Researches into the physical history of mankind*,[2] cited C. W. Hufeland who urged that '...the comparative
pathology of living tribes and species must be more attentively
studied and more fully elucidated than it has yet been, before we
can render complete our acquaintance with their physical history.
The diseases and predispositions to disease peculiar to certain races,
constitute as much a part of the physical description and enter as
fully into the aggregate of distinctive characters belonging to these
races, as any feature in their anatomical structure' (p. 150).

Earlier works than this of course consider diseases in different
human populations, and, for example, '...the hereditary transmission from parents to children of a constitutional liability to pulmonary disease, and especially to consumption'[3] was also being
discussed. Prichard[2] elaborates on this, concluding that '...a tribe of
people, by long residence in a given district, are capable of acquiring a
peculiar hereditary and national variety of constitution, predisposing

them to a particular disease from which other tribes of the same original stock are altogether or very nearly free' (p. 155).

Nott and Gliddon[4] allocate a whole chapter to the influence of climate and diseases on human populations. In particular, yellow fever is discussed in detail, and a case is presented for a varying susceptibility to this disease in different peoples. Pouchet[5] also considers yellow fever, and 'marsh-fever', from the point of view of differential susceptibility and the possible heritability of acquired resistance to disease. Hirsch,[6] who contributed much in his *Handbook of geographical and historical pathology*, seemed doubtful of the 'congenital' basis of immunity, at least to malaria. In this he was challenged by Reid[7] who argued for some heritable 'resisting power' (p. 278) over half a century before certain haemoglobin variants were found to afford some protection against malaria! These earlier writers, both medical and biological, showed varying degrees of clarity and confusion regarding the question of inherited resistance to disease versus acquired immunity. Nevertheless, one can see in their work the first attempts to think dynamically about the possible changing status of a disease in relation to varying human populations, and to suspect that heritable factors were involved in the resistance to some diseases.

By the early years of this century, the possible genetic basis of certain of the less common anomalies was being studied, in particular by the Galton-Pearson School in London. Present interest, however, might be seen to stem principally from the writings of J. B. S. Haldane,[8] who stressed the possible importance of disease resistance as a factor in natural selection. Not until the 1950's was it realized to what extent variation in certain human biochemical polymorphisms might somehow be related to some disease frequencies.

III

GENES, DISEASE AND MICRO-EVOLUTION,
THE EXTENT OF THE PROBLEM

In a recent symposium of the International Biological Programme on 'Natural selection and transmissible disease', Professor L. S. Penrose emphasized the difficulty in analysing the contribution of genes to disease resistance in man.[9] Inborn and acquired immunity are not easy to distinguish, and direct transmission of a pathogen from mother to child has been confused with the transmission of genes. Nevertheless, some studies (both on families and twins) give support to the view that genetical factors are involved in resistance— in some diseases at least. So far, associations with disease have mainly been tentatively suggested for certain blood group charac- ters (the antigens, similar to ones in the parasites, perhaps impeding immunological response), and for haemoglobin traits. This work is generally well reviewed,[10,11,12,13] so that only brief remarks need be made here.

Of the blood group systems and disease, the majority of work has so far centred around the ABO system. Although beginnings were made in the 1920's, the first large-scale survey was being published as recently as 1953, and was concerned with cancer of the stomach and its significant correlation with group A.[14] Further claims for associations between disease and blood groups are listed for brevity in Table 1, sample sizes varying from over 3500 cases to about 150.

TABLE 1. Some claimed (but by no means proven) associations between blood group phenotypes and disease

Disease	Associated ABO or secretor phenotype
Bubonic plague	0
Smallpox	0, N
Syphilis	B and AB
Infantile diarrhoea	A
Influenza virus A_2	0
Bronchopneumonia	A or AB
Diabetes mellitus	A
Paralytic poliomyelitis	B (and excess of non-secretors)
Rheumatic fever	A, B (and non-secretors)
Pernicious anaemia	A
Duodenal ulcer	0
Cancer of stomach	A
Gastric ulcer	0
Salivary gland tumours	A
Tumours of the ovary	A
Cancer of the cervix	A
Pituitary adenoma	0
Cancer of the prostate	A
Cancer of the pancreas	A

It will be seen that both bacterial and viral diseases have been considered, as well as non-infective disorders, in particular peptic ulcer and a variety of malignancies. Although such associations can only be regarded as very tentative, the growing evidence is as a whole quite impressive. But, even when far more is known, anyone wishing then to try to make sense of the patterns of human disease and genetic variation—especially with a hope of projecting such relationships back into historic or prehistoric time—still has many troubles ahead. To begin with, as F. Vogel[9] has pointed out, the picture may be obscured to some extent by the fact that one disease might be pushing the frequency of a gene in one direction, but another disease might be exerting pressure in the opposite direction. Population movement, at times over great distances, and varying degrees of intermixing of peoples, are other factors which blur the true nature of micro-evolutionary patterns. But the fact remains that this is an exciting field worthy of more exploration, and the eventual findings will have significance for medical history as well as human biology. It is certainly rich in possibilities, and even in a recent severe critique of claimed associations between disease, diet and blood groups, Charlotte Otten[15] could not resist the temptation of a little more speculation:

No one has yet ventured to suggest an association between blood group frequency and diet by way of the gut, but several factors indicate that a look in this direction may not be completely unwarranted. *Escherichia coli* and the Proteus ('putrefying') group, both largely associated with a carnivorous diet, are reported to carry B antigenic activity, at least in some strains...Do, then, blood type B individuals make better carnivores than blood type A folk? Do intestinal environments differ immunologically with regard to their receptivity to one organism or another? Will one species of microbe, more easily established for immunological reasons, increase the growth and vitality of its particular host, while another species proves deleterious? (p. 215)

The classic example of a simple genetic situation influencing the pattern of an infective disease is, of course, that of haemoglobin S (sickle cell trait) and malaria. Despite the fact that both heterozygotes and homozygotes for this haemoglobinopathy have varying degrees of anaemia, the allele has been maintained in some populations at relatively high frequencies. Malaria is thought to be responsible for this haemoglobin polymorphism, the heterozygotes being considered more resistant to *Plasmodium falciparum* malaria. Thalass-aemia has similarly been thought to be associated with malaria. In both anaemias marked skeletal changes may result,[16] which gives us an opportunity perhaps to study the spread of these inherited traits through time. Angel[17,18] is one of the few to consider this question so far, with regard to bone changes in early skeletons, and more work is needed, especially on early African series. As regards Angel's findings so far, he concludes:[18]

If the thalassemias, sicklemia and other abnormal hemoglobins and also favism (G6Pd deficiency) all depend on a new and almost lethal *falciparum* parasite then these protective mutations could have occurred and started to increase in anopheline foci around the Eastern Mediterranean by Upper Palaeolithic times: the area of greatest mutational variety is a logical place to look for the origin of these polymorphisms and their first balance against falciparum malaria. The tendency of the first farmers to settle in marshy areas (soft soil) like the Konya and Macedonian plains would explain the extremely high development of porotic hyperostosis (thalass-emia and sicklemia presumably) in skeletons at Catal Hüyük and Nea Nikomedeia as contrasted with those at Khirokitia (dry valley), Kephala on Kea (rocky headland), Karatas-Semayük (Lycian mountain valley). (p. 387)

Other polymorphic characters which are being investigated for possible associations with disease, include ear-wax types, where wet cerumen may more often occur with arteriosclerosis in the absence of hypertension, but not when it is present.[19] In addition, the ability to taste phenylthiocarbamide (PTC)[20] is being studied in relation to thyroid disease, glaucoma, and even oral disease. Although PTC is itself an artificial product, the broader question of taste polymorphism, primitive communities and food tolerance in the past, is an interesting one.

IV

So far, I have been concerned with human variation/disease relation-ships in which the genetics was not complex, but many such problems revolve around multifactorial characters; for a good general review, see Sorsby.[21] Conditions as divergent as tubercu-losis[22] and osteoarthritis[23] have been considered for possible herit-able factors. Information on twins continues to appear. In the study of 2537 twin pairs by Marshall, Hutchinson and Honisett,[24] they concluded that in 12 of 24 common diseases investigated in this twin series, there was evidence of an hereditary factor. Although these possible genetic factors seem likely to be multifactorial and complex, it would be wrong to ignore them in any consideration of the adaptability of man, during his evolution, to diseases.

One instance of polygenic variation in human populations, which seems to confer some degree of protection against climatic severity, is skin pigmentation. With the reduction of body hair in man, some time during the Pleistocene Period, there was an increase of excessive exposure of the skin to ultra-violet radiation. It is now well established that such radiation induces skin cancers, and that the more light-skinned individuals are far more likely to develop these cancers in regions of strong sunlight; see Blum[25] for a review of the subject. In some regions, therefore, there is probably a considerable selective advantage in possessing moderate or considerable amounts of epidermal melanin. This is perhaps simplifying the position rather, and it would be more exact to conclude that human pigmentary variation is '...a compromise between the conflicting demands of protection from skin cancer and sunburn, thermo-regulation and synthesis of Vitamin D'.[26] Incidentally, in the case of eye pigmentation which is also very variable in man, disease may have exerted a selective influence in other ways; for instance, iris pigmentation appears to be correlated in some areas with the degree of ocular onchocerciasis.[27]

Primates and protohominids

Before further discussion of recent human populations, it is pertinent to this review to consider disease at the non-human primate level. Although only a crude indicator, it is nevertheless a worthwhile method of showing the types of infection which could well have been 'carried through' into the hominid evolutionary line. Some aspects of this question have already been touched on by a variety of authors,[28,29,30,31,32] and the patchy nature of the data does not permit more than a tentative survey. Richard Fiennes, in particular, has recently considered in breadth the zoonoses of primates,[31] and I have used this work as a primary reference source. In Table 2, selected parasites and diseases are given with a view to emphasizing the wide range of zoonoses in non-human wild primates which are

TABLE 2. Some zoonoses of wild Old World primates, early hominids or recent man. Arrows tentatively indicate possible continuity of infection from an ancestral primate stock through to man (allowing for species change in the parasites). Primate data adapted from Fiennes.[31] The symbol 'U' is to suggest that the zoonosis may have been very restricted or uncommon in extent.

Zoonosis	Old World primate	Proto-hominid	Man
(a) *Ectoparasites*			
Fleas, lice, mites	?U ————	?U ———	U
(b) *Arthropod vectors*			
Ticks	U ————	?U ———	U
(c) *Endoparasites*			
Trematodes			→
Cestodes			→
Nematodes			→
Filarioidea			→
(d) *Protozoa*			
Entamoeba histolytica			→
Trypanosoma rhodesiense		?U ———	→
Leishmania		?U ———	→
Plasmodium			→
(e) *Fungi*			
Dermatophytoses			→
Aspergillosis			→
(f) *Bacteria*			
Spirochaetosis	?U ————	?U ———	→
Leptospirosis	?U ————	?U ———	→
Treponematoses	?————		→
Cocci infections			→
Enteric infections			→
Tuberculosis	U ————	?U ———	→
Q fever	?U ————	?U ———	→
(g) *Viruses*			
Yellow fever			→
Mumps, measles	?	? ———	→
Influenza		? ———	→
Poliomyelitis	?	? ———	→
Rabies	?U ————	?U ———	U
Herpes-virus simiae	————→	?	
Herpes-virus simplex	- - -	? - -	→
Infectious hepatitis	?U ————	?U ———	→

also found, or have their related counterparts, in man. In order to suggest the sort of continuum which occurred from non-human primates to recent man, the first column (wild Old World primates) is followed by tentative indications as to whether early hominids might be expected to have 'inherited' from primate ancestors the particular zoonosis; and finally there is the present situation in *Homo sapiens*. The limitations to this sort of scheme are as follows:

(a) The recent non-human primates may have only been infected with some of these diseases within thousands, or even hundreds, of years, rather than millions of years ago.

(b) The severity of a particular disease in early hominid individuals and the amount of mortality cannot be reconstructed from epidemiological information on recent primates, including man.

(c) Frequency of occurrence in recent primates is no certain indicator of the extent of susceptibility to the particular disease in emerging hominid populations.

Accuracy of assessments in Table 2 will inevitably vary, some errors being likely to contract when more data become available on living primates. In the case of external parasites such as fleas, ticks and so on, it seems most unlikely that they have ever been totally absent from the hominid line; but what we cannot hope to establish is to what extent 'grooming' habits a million or more years ago restricted their frequency, or to what extent they were then a health threat in terms of the spread of spirochaetal diseases. In the case of tapeworm infestation, the important human genus *Taenia* might not have been present to any extent in early Pleistocene man, and its present life-cycle is far more likely to have been successful following the domestication of pigs and ruminants during Neolithic times.

Leishmaniasis seems unlikely, on present evidence, to be frequent in wild primates, but with the evolution of an erect posture for ground living and with the probable reliance of the early hominids on a hunting-collecting-scavenging existence, transmission of *Leishmania* by sandflies may have become a threat for the first time. The question of the antiquity of malaria has been discussed at some length by Bruce-Chwatt,[30] Fiennes[31] and others. Without going further into the confusing state of affairs regarding the classification of primate malarias. it seems likely that malaria was established by the emergence of the hominoid super family. Perhaps with the special adaptive changes of the early hominids, and their radiation into different regions of Africa and Asia, further species changes also took place in *Plasmodium*. However, it was following the vast cultural, and in part environmental, changes which resulted from the Neolithic Revolution that malaria probably became a serious health threat to human populations.

As a final example of palaeo-epidemiological reconstruction back to non-human primates, we might consider trypanosomiasis. After a careful consideration of the whole question, Lambrecht[29] concludes that the progress of this disease in primates probably became critical during early Pleistocene times. His views on the differentiation of *T. gambiense* and *T. rhodesiense* are shown in Table 3 (p. 122). He sums up the position by saying:

Trypanosomes, two species of which cause African sleeping sickness today, are blood parasites of great antiquity. Their presence in Africa at the time of the first stages of human evolution may have been of great consequence, at first acting as a discriminating agent between resistant and non-resistant types of hominids, and later also in shaping migration routes and settlement patterns. As a possible clue as to why man arose in Africa, the author postulates that trypanosomes may have precluded the development of certain ground-dwelling faunas, allowing certain more resistant primates to fill the empty ecological niches. Some of these primates, thus becoming ground-dwellers, became the precursors of the hominid branch. (p. 22)

Much of our knowledge of the sequence of disease from non-human primates to early hominids, or of special disease adaptations following this evolutionary phase, is likely to remain highly speculative. Nevertheless it is worthy of consideration, and is essential to a proper perspective of disease in man.

V

TIME, CULTURE, PLACE, AND DISEASE

The emergence of the genus *Homo* probably dates to more than a million years ago, and for much of this time man has been passing through one or other of the Palaeolithic culture phases. Although a lot is known about changing forms of stone artifact, one of the few lasting parts of any prehistoric culture, only very tentative guesses can be made as to how much more economically successful the late

Palaeolithic peoples were compared with earlier Pleistocene groups. In terms of food, all were dependent upon hunting and collecting. It is possible, however, that hunting efficiency may have increased as better tools were devised, and this could have resulted in a slowly increasing human population.[33] By, perhaps, twenty or thirty thousand years ago, numbers were sufficiently large—and dispersal in the Old World sufficiently great—for movement into the New World to commence. This probably occurred only by means of the Bering Straits land bridge until late prehistoric times, that is, when there may have been trans-Pacific movements, followed eventually by European contacts.

TABLE 3. Schematic representation of the evolution of human trypanosomiasis. Adapted from Lambrecht (p. 13)[29]

Forest	Period	Savannah
Primates in trees have no contact with Glossina	Pliocene	Evolution of trypanosomes in savannah animals carried by savannah tsetse flies
	Lower Pleistocene (development of hominid species)	Contact between hominids and trypanosome-carrying tsetse flies
Contact between forest tsetse flies and trypanosome-carrying hominids	Middle Pleistocene (partial invasion of forest by hominids)	Trypanosomes of the *rhodesiense* type evolve in hominids
Establishment of man-adapted *T. gambiense* in forest tsetse flies	Upper Pleistocene (occupation by man of both biotopes)	*T. rhodesiense* maintained in animals by game flies. Occasional return in man

Survival of these Palaeolithic groups depended upon the nomadic 'harvesting' of wild plant and animal foodstuffs, the bands remaining small (see Kerley, pp. 148–9). The size of the breeding population was probably also small—on recent ethnographic evidence—perhaps with an average of about four hundred individuals. The progress of a disease was likely to have been somewhat delimited by the size of these fairly isolated units, and as Hare[34,35] has already pointed out, new intrusive infections, especially highly virulent ones, may be conceived as burning themselves out without affecting more than a few hundred people. By Upper Palaeolithic times, one might therefore visualize a thinly spread world population, varyingly restricted in group numbers and fertility by food availability and climate, in which a few diseases—such as *Salmonella* and *Clostridia* infections, certain of the cocci, and dysentery—could have been widespread and recurring. Superimposed on this primary disease stratum would be other diseases acquired by contacts with other populations, and also by contact with the animals hunted. It might be mentioned here that health studies of the few surviving primitive groups today, for instance the Bushmen of Southern Africa,[36] are unlikely to give reliable information as to the health status of earlier Stone Age peoples. As Cook[37] has pointed out, these recent groups have been pushed into inferior or restricted territories and suffer, often in the extreme, from diseases transmitted from contacts with advanced cultures.

It was towards the close of the Mesolithic period in Europe and south-west Asia that profound cultural changes began to occur, and from this experimental phase there emerged the Neolithic Revolution. Of special significance was the domestication of animals and plants, beginning perhaps as early as 10 000 B.C. and continuing as regards one species or another through to the present day. This vast change in economic organization encouraged population expansion far beyond that permitted by the simpler hunting and collecting economies. In turn, the expanding groups moved in search of more cultivatable or productive land and began to influence as never before the fauna and flora around them. Settled communities—villages, towns and eventually cities—were now possible, and with them came new health threats and diseases. Garn[38] sums up the human biological significance of these changes when he says:

We may view much of recent human evolution as a series of local adaptations (primarily in food-producing peoples) to disease situations arising out of food producing. In some cases man has made room for his diseases simply by favoring the insect or rodent vectors of the disease. In other cases man has moved to potential disease areas in actual pursuit of some particularly food-producing economy. In general he has favored disease by increasing his numbers and by increasing the number of contacts with other populations. And he has favored disease-selection by developing dietaries that are themselves growth limiting, and inimical to the maintenance of an optimum immunochemical (defense) system. (p. 235)

From the point of view of nutrition, the Neolithic period might be regarded perhaps as the beginning of the misuse of food. For the first time, populations could rely on food combinations, especially high carbohydrate diets, which prevented starvation but were nutritionally inadequate. It is therefore only in the last few thousand years that rickets, scurvy, kwashiorkor, and the vitamin A and B complex deficiencies are likely to have occurred in any frequency. I have discussed this question in some detail elsewhere,[39,40] and need not elaborate further here. The other health/genetic repercussions which have followed in the wake of the agricultural developments and population increase of the past few thousand years might be listed under four distinct categories.

1. *Non-nutritional disease implications of the Neolithic Revolution*

Closer contacts between man and animals occurred in two ways; as a result of breeding and herding domestic varieties, and by the scavenging activities of wild animals at habitation sites. Bovine tuberculosis may have become a serious health threat in this respect, and it may be significant that a number of Predynastic or early Dynastic cases of possible spinal tuberculosis in man are known from Egypt,[41] one of the regions of early civilization.

There is some evidence that brucellosis and anthrax were further hazards of farming. Rodent infestation of towns and villages could have been established early, with the result that plague and spirochaetal jaundice might for the first time have reached epidemic proportions. As Polunin[42] has suggested in his studies of Malayan aborigines, forest clearances and shifting cultivation provide a suitable environment for *Anopheles maculatus*, which is reflected in an increased frequency of malaria among these people. In a similar way, the spread of mite-borne scrub typhus may have been encouraged.

2. *Changing survival differentials*

The profound cultural changes of the past 10 000 years have in some ways been a conquest against the way of life in existence for much of human evolution. Changes in fertility, community size, habitation, clothing and the advent of pottery and cooking are some of the means by which adaptive pressures have been modified. As Penrose[43] says, 'The process of civilization undoubtedly alters the fitness conferred by different genes. A peculiar individual may be unfit to survive if he has to fend entirely for himself, but may contribute to the survival of a group to which he belongs; for example, a person with severe myopia might be incapacitated for actual hunting but might be able to make very sharp arrows or knives for others' (p. 131).

3. Relaxed selection

In a series of recent studies,[44,45,46] R. H. Post has emphasized the need to consider relaxed selection as a possible reason for some of the variation we see in man today. In his words, '...it is suggested that the rigor of natural selection in eliminating hereditary and deleterious abnormalities has relaxed in populations with longer histories of civilization as contrasted with "primitives" who are still living in hunting or food collecting culture-habitats'[46] (p. 101).

In one series of anomalies studied, deformed nasal septa,[46] it was possible to work with skulls, and there is thus a hope of substantiating these first results with further studies of earlier populations. Certainly, Post's results so far suggest that 'civilized' communities are more likely to show higher frequencies of deformed septa. Similarly, in a further study of this evolutionary question, he concludes: 'The fact that high rates of breast cancer, high frequencies of hypolactators, and very ancient histories of domestic animal milk are found in Caucasian populations and in no other suggests that problems of etiology and epidemiology may well be investigated under the hypothesis of relaxed selection'[45] (p. 27).

In the case of colour blindness, Post[44] and others have suggested that here also, the frequency pattern supports this hypothesis. However, Penrose[43] has suggested that this condition might, in some situations, be advantageous even in primitive hunting communities. Clearly there is plenty of room for differences of opinion, in view of the paucity of data, but the question is one which can no longer be ignored in any consideration of abnormality through time.

4. Social stratification

With the increasing expansion of post-Neolithic societies, divisions of labour and authority occurred. Simpler social structures gave rise to complex ones in which trades, castes, religions and political hierarchies were some of the phenomena which split communities. In some cases these must have acted as barriers to, or routes for, the initiation or transfer of disease. Leprosy, the antiquity of which in China[47] seems established earlier than in the West, could well have been brought back and 'injected' into Europe and North Africa by Roman traders and explorers. Although large numbers of ancient skeletons have been searched for evidence of this disease, there are no bone changes from Europe or Africa which might indicate this disease to be older than the sixth century A.D.

In the case of socioeconomic stratification and disease frequency differences, there is to my knowledge no good data yet from early historic or prehistoric times which might be used to exemplify this relationship. Such stratification may nevertheless have assisted in the differential survival of some levels of earlier societies and the greater mortality of other strata. Where gene frequency differences had already occurred in such strata, then further micro-evolutionary change would take place—relative to the population as a whole—with the disproportionate survival of certain social levels. Changes in cranial morphology in England, following the high mortality, perhaps, of the poorer segments of society during the Great Plague of London (1665), has been suggested as an example of differential survival, but this needs cautious testing.

With regard to socioeconomic aspects of early disease frequency variation, survival differentials would not be acting in the same way for all disease conditions. This might be illustrated by reference to cancer incidences in a recent population[48] (Table 4).

TABLE 4. Incidence* of cancer in Puerto Rico (1953–54), by two socioeconomic classes (from Marcial, 1960)[48]

		Age group (years)			
		20–24	25–34	34–44	45–54
Cervix	Indigent	1.1	16.2	44.3	59.9
uteri	Nonindigent	1.0	11.7	42.4	40.8
Breast	Indigent	1.5	2.2	8.9	15.1
	Nonindigent	1.0	2.3	15.7	20.4

* Per 100 000.

In the case of cancer of the cervix, the indigent sample shows higher values, and this may be related to the larger families and much poorer hygiene. On the other hand, breast cancer shows significantly higher values in the older age group, in the nonindigent series, and this may be associated with generally smaller families and a tendency to refrain from breast feeding.

VI

PALAEODEMOGRAPHIC PROBLEMS

Palaeodemography may be defined as the study of the demography of earlier peoples, especially of prehistoric and protohistoric cultures. I have discussed elsewhere[49] the breadth of topics embraced by palaeodemography, of the problems inherent in the analysis of such data, and of the differences between the procedures of this discipline and the demographic methodology of recent populations. The important point is that we are usually only dealing with skeletal series, which impose various limitations on conclusions to be drawn from their vital statistics. But all is not lost, and what I wish briefly to consider here is some of the information which has been assembled and which is pertinent to studies on the health of earlier man.

1. *Mortality and age group*

In any surveys of age frequencies one must first be aware of the potentially biasing effects of bad soil conditions operating against the preservation of infants' skeletons, and of social factors which might distort age-group data. Sample size is also all too often smaller than desirable. Differences between early groups nevertheless occur, and although mortality within any age group is the sum of multiple disease factors, these 'death patterns' are a useful adjunct to other assessments of community disease loads. Age data can be presented in various ways; for instance, in age groups, with the sexes separated, as child/adult ratios, or in terms of the mean life expectancy of adults, children, or both. A few studies have been made through time and in one region. At present, the most important need is to assemble larger samples of burials (cemetery groups) belonging to different regions and cultures. Also to apply the most recent age-estimation procedures to these series.

2. *Mortality and sex-ratio*

The sexing of immature skeletons is still a matter of controversy, and the whole question is urgently in need of attention, preferably with computer assistance. However, a consideration of adults is at least possible, and differences in the sex-ratio of various age-group samples for a cemetery series can be demonstrated. Moreover, even in the presented limited data, one can see possible inter-group differences. For instance, Chiarelli and his colleagues[50] find in early Egyptian material a female mortality peak in the 20- to 30-year-old period, which they relate to increased hazards of childbearing in females of that age. In marked contrast, the prehistoric series from Indian Knoll, Kentucky,[51] actually shows a decline in female deaths during this age period. To what extent such findings truly represent the people of that area and culture can only really be decided by further studies on other relevant series.

3. *Detecting inbreeding isolates*

Although for the most part questions of migration and isolation, in relation to population health and vital statistics, are beyond the bounds of the palaeodemographer, I think there is one aspect which might yield some meaningful information. Isolation tends to lead to diversification in relatively small groups, and through inbreeding, mutation and genetic drift, even abnormal characters may be markedly increased in frequency. In the highly inbred population of Tristan da Cunha,[52] congenital abnormalities including retinitis pigmentosa and the syndrome of deafness, high palate and pinna deformity syndrome are unusually common. Some of the other defects involve parts of the skeleton: hypertelorism, short terminal phalanges, pronounced micrognathia. In an isolate living in Maryland, U.S.A., the defects included the severe dental anomaly of dentinogenesis imperfecta.[53] Yet a further example, also one where the skeleton is affected, is the increased frequency of familial spastic paralysis on the Adriatic island of Krk.[54]

The point I wish to make is that such isolation, inbreeding, and increase in congenital defects are not just a phenomenon of civilized communities. The dramatic occurrence of Kuru[55] in the Fore tribe of New Guinea is a clear demonstration of this, if any is needed. This degenerative disorder of the central nervous system is restricted to the one tribe, and incidentally results in a 2 : 1 sex-ratio in favour of males. It seems to me only a matter of time before evidence appears in early skeletal material suggesting inbreeding. Indeed we might already have some evidence of this, although as yet slender. For example, in a series of Nubian skeletons belonging to the Christian colony which settled around the temple of Philae, five cases of similar hip-joint deformity were noted by Elliot Smith and Wood Jones,[56] while in nearly six thousand bodies from other Nubian cemeteries, only two further cases were noted. In view of this frequency difference, and the fact that dysplastic hip incidences can increase in isolates,[57] we should clearly consider these early Nubian cases as possibly indicative of group inbreeding.

4. *Disease movement, time and space*

It is all too easy when approaching the question of infective disease in the past, to present suitable hypotheses which seem to 'fit' the cultural and environmental facts. Where the parasite leaves no trace, our conclusion may perhaps always be extremely tentative, but where evidence of certain ancient disease may be found in human remains, then there is hope of substantiating an hypothesis. This might be illustrated, as yet very patchily, by reference to tuberculosis. Morse[58] and others seem satisfied that Pott's deformity of the spine may be tentatively identified in early vertebrae, and thus by careful surveys of large numbers of spinal columns from different regions and periods, we might hope to see a changing frequency pattern for this disease. One would expect the earliest evidence to occur in regions of early cattle breeding and milk use, that is, the eastern Mediterranean area. In fact we have very early evidence from Egypt and Nubia.[41] Although there is one questionable case from Germany,[59] it is, in fact, not until Saxon times in central and northern Europe that we begin to get a significant number of possible cases of bony tuberculosis. This change is unlikely to be solely due to differences in sample sizes, though this may be a factor, and it could well be that we have here concrete evidence of the gradual and late spread of tuberculosis into northern Europe—at least to the extent when it was a more common health threat.

VII

I have endeavoured to show in this discussion that there is common territory between medical history and human biology, and that it is a largely unexplored field for both sides. Changing patterns of disease have been important influences in human evolution and adaptability, and thus on the genetic composition of populations. On the other hand, human bio-cultural changes have considerably influenced some diseases, and in particular the Neolithic Revolution marked the beginning of great changes in man and his parasites.

Other subjects which deserved consideration, had sufficient pertinent data been forthcoming, include aspects of the evolution of the human brain and the emergence of crowd psychopathology. Although our brains have doubled in capacity since the differentiation of the early hominids, few have considered the critical subject of brain expansion relative to pelvic form,[60] though obstetrical difficulties must have acted as selective factors. Ethnopsychiatric studies on primitive peoples, such as the Australian aborigines,[61,62] are still only in their early stages, but may eventually help to define abnormal traits with a long human history, from the traits of 'civilization' and crowds such as war, crowd panic, religious mania, and so on; ancient texts can also be revealing in this respect.[63,64] Human behaviour may seem a long way from the subject of disease and microevolution, but it must be remembered that mental as well as somatic variation occurs in man, and that the processes of change, adaptability, and abnormality apply to both.

REFERENCES

1 P. H. A. Sneath, 'New approaches to bacterial taxonomy: use of computers', *Ann. Rev. Microbiol.* 1964, 18, 335–46.
2 J. C. Prichard, *Researches into the physical history of mankind*, 3rd ed., 3 vols., vol. 1, 'Section VI. Third head of the analogical investigation of species. Pathological considerations', pp. 150–60, London: Sherwood, Gilbert and Piper, 1836–41.
3 A. Combe, *The principles of physiology applied to the preservation of health, and to the improvement of physical and mental education*, 4th ed., p. 218, Edinburgh: Maclachlan and Stewart, 1836.

4   J. C. Nott, 'Acclimation; or, the comparative influence of climate, endemic and epidemic diseases, on the races of man' in J. C. Nott and G. R. Gliddon, *Indigenous races of the earth, or, new chapters of ethnological inquiry*, etc., pp. 353–401, London: Trübner, 1857.

5   G. Pouchet, *The plurality of the human race*, transl. and ed. (from 2nd ed.) H. J. C. Beavau, 'Chapter IV. Anatomical, physiological, and pathological varieties', pp. 43–61, London: Longman, Green, Longman, and Roberts, 1864.

6   A. Hirsch, *Handbook of geographical and historical pathology*, transl. (from 2nd German ed.) C. Creighton, 3 vols., London: New Sydenham Society, 1883–86.

7   G. A. Reid, *The present evolution of man*, pp. 273–80, London: Chapman and Hall, 1896.

8   J. B. S. Haldane, 'Disease and evolution', Supplement of *La Ricerca Scientifica* 1949, 19, 68–76.

9   N. A. Barnicot, 'Natural selection and transmissible disease', *Nature, Lond.* 1965, 208, 535–6. Also, unpublished comments on the International Biological Programme meeting on 'Natural selection and transmissible disease' held in June 1965 (circulated by the convener of the Human Adaptability Project).

10 C. A. Clarke, 'Blood groups and disease' in A. G. Steinberg (ed.), *Progress in medical genetics*, vol. 1, pp. 81–119, New York and London: Grune and Stratton, 1961.

11 F. B. Livingstone, 'Natural selection, disease, and ongoing human evolution, as illustrated by the ABO blood groups', *Hum. Biol.* 1960, 32, 17–27.

12 A. G. Motulsky, 'Metabolic polymorphisms and the role of infectious diseases in human evolution', *Hum. Biol.* 1960, 32, 28–62.

13 A. C. Allison, 'Abnormal haemoglobin and erythrocyte enzyme-deficiency traits' in G. A. Harrison (ed.), *Genetical variation in human populations* (Symposia of the Society for the Study of Human Biology, vol. IV), pp. 16–40, Oxford: Pergamon, 1961.

14 I. Aird, H. H. Bentall and J. A. F. Roberts, 'A relationship between cancer of the stomach and the ABO blood groups', *Br. med. J.* 1953, i, 799–801.

15 C. M. Otten, 'On pestilence, deit [*sic*], natural selection, and the distribution of microbial and human blood group antigens and antibodies', *Current Anthropology* 1967, 8, 209–26.

16 J. Caffey, 'The skeletal changes in the chronic hemolytic anemias (erythroblastic anemia, sickle cell anemia and chronic hemolytic icterus)', *Am. J. Roentg.* 1939, 37, 293–324.

17 J. L. Angel, 'Osteoporosis: thalassemia?', *Am. J. phys. Anthrop.* 1964, 22, 369–73.

18 J. L. Angel, 'Porotic hyperostosis or osteoporosis symmetrica' in D. Brothwell and A. T. Sandison (eds.), *Diseases in antiquity. A survey of the diseases, injuries and surgery of early populations*, pp. 378–89, Springfield, Ill.: C. C Thomas, 1967.

19 M. Miyahara and E. Matsunaga, 'Association of ear-wax types with

susceptibility to arteriosclerosis—a preliminary report', *Ann. Rep. Natn. Inst. Genet. Tokyo* 1966, 17, 127–9.

20 H. Kalamus, 'Genetical variation and sense perception' in G. E. W. Wolstenholme and C. M. O'Connor (eds.), *Biochemistry of human genetics*, pp. 60–75, see pp. 67–71 (Ciba Foundation. Symposium jointly with the International Union of Biological Sciences), London: Churchill, 1959.

21 A. Sorsby (ed.), *Clinical genetics*, London: Butterworth, 1953, pp. [603].

22 R. Turpin, 'De l'influence de l'hérédité sur la sensibilité de l'homme à la tuberculose', *III Congresso Internazionale de Medicina neo-ippocratica* 1956, pp. 209–31.

23 R. M. Stecher, 'Heredity of osteoarthritis', *Arch. phys. Med.* 1965, 46, 178–86.

24 A. G. Marshall, E. O. Hutchinson and J. Honisett, 'Heredity in common diseases; a retrospective survey of twins in a hospital population, *Br. med. J.* 1962, 1, 1–6.

25 H. F. Blum, *Carcinogenesis by ultraviolet light*, Princeton, N.J.; Princeton University Press, 1959, pp. 340.

26 G. A. Harrison, 'Pigmentation' in Harrison, 1961, op. cit. (above, note 13), pp. 99–115, see p. 110.

27 D. P. Choyce, 'Ocular onchocerciasis in Central America, Africa and British Isles', *Trans. R. Soc. trop. Med. Hyg.* 1964, 58, 11–47.

28 A. Cockburn, *The evolution and eradication of infectious diseases*, pp. 68–105, Baltimore: Johns Hopkins Press, 1963.

29 F. L. Lambrecht, 'Aspects of evolution and ecology of tsetse flies and trypanosomiasis in prehistoric African environment', *J. Afr. Hist.* 1964, 5, 1–24.

30 L. J. Bruce-Chwatt, 'Paleogenesis and paleo-epidemiology of primate malaria', *Bull. World Hlth. Org.* 1925, 32, 363–87.

31 R. Fiennes, *Zoonoses of primates. The epidemiology and ecology of Simian diseases in relation to man*, London: Weidenfeld and Nicolson, 1967, pp. 190.

32 A. H. Schultz, 'The occurrence and frequency of pathological and teratological conditions and of twinning among hon-human primates' in H. Hofer, A. H. Schultz, D. Starck (eds.), *Primatologia, Handbuch der Primatenkunde*, vol. 1, pp. 965–1014, Basel: S. Karger, 1956.

33 C. S. Coon, 'Race and ecology in man', *Cold Spring Harb. Symp. quant. Biol.* 1959, 24, 153–9.

34 R. Hare, *Pomp and pestilence. Infectious disease, its origins and conquest*, London: Gollancz, 1954, pp. 224.

35 R. Hare, 'The antiquity of diseases caused by bacteria and viruses, a review of the problem from a bacteriologist's point of view' in Brothwell and Sandison, 1967, op. cit. (above, note 18), pp. 115–31.

36 B. Bronte-Stewart, O. E. Budtz-Olsen, J. M. Hickley and J. F. Brock, 'The health and nutritional status of the Kung Bushmen of South West Africa', *S. Afr. J. Lab. Clin. Med.* 1960, 6, 187–216.

37 S. F. Cook, 'Survivorship in aboriginal populations', *Hum. Biol.* 1947, 19, 83–9.

38 S. M. Garn, 'Culture and the direction of human evolution', *Hum. Biol.* 1963, **35**, 221–36.

39 D. Brothwell and P. Brothwell, *Food in antiquity*, London: Thames and Hudson, 1969, pp. 248.

40 D. R. Brothwell, 'Dietary variation and the biology of earlier human populations' in P. Ucko and G. Dimbleby (eds.), *The domestication and exploitation of plants and animals*, London: Weidenfeld and Nicolson, 1969.

41 D. Morse, D. R. Brothwell and P. J. Ucko, 'Tuberculosis in ancient Egypt', *Am. Rev. resp. Dis.* 1964, 90, 524–41.

42 I. Polunin, 'The effects of shifting agriculture on human health and disease', *Symposium on the impact of man on humid tropics vegetation*, pp. 388–93, Goroka, Territory of Papua and New Guinea, September 1960, UNESCO Science Co-operation Office for South East Asia, n.d.

43 L. S. Penrose, 'Changes in the quality of human populations' in J. B. Cragg and N. W. Pirie (eds.), *The numbers of man and animals*, pp. 131–7, Edinburgh: Oliver and Boyd, 1955.

44 R. H. Post, 'Notes on relaxed selection in man', *Anthrop. Anz.* 1965, **29**, 186–95.

45 R. H. Post, 'Breast cancer, lactation, and genetics', *Eugen. Q.* 1966, **13**, 1–29.

46 R. H. Post, 'Deformed nasal septa and relaxed selection', *Eugen. Q.* 1966, **13**, 101–12.

47 Lu Gwei-Djen and J. Needham, 'Records of diseases in ancient China' in Brothwell and Sandison, 1967, op. cit. (above, note 18), pp. 222–37.

48 V. A. Marcial, 'Socioeconomic aspects of the incidence of cancer in Puerto Rico', *Ann. N.Y. Acad. Sci.* 1960, 84, 981–8, see Table 2.

49 D. R. Brothwell, 'Palaeodemography' in W. Brass (ed.), *Biological aspects of demography*, Oxford: Pergamon, 1970, in press.

50 B. Chiarelli, M. Masali and D. Davide, 'Richerche sulle collezioni antropologiche egiziane dell'Istituto de Antropologia di Torino, II. Dati demografici sugli adulti', *Riv. Antrop.* 1966, **53**, 67–76.

51 F. E. Johnston and C. E. Snow, 'The reassessment of the age and sex of the Indian Knoll skeletal population: demographic and methodological aspects', *Am. J. phys. Anthrop.* 1961, 19, 237–44.

52 J. A. Black, H. E. Lewis, C. K. M. Thacker and A. K. Thould, 'Tristan da Cunha: general medical investigations', *Brit. med. J.* 1963, ii, 1018–24.

53 R. J. Hursey, Jr., J. Witkop, Jr., D. Miklashek and L. M. Sackett, 'Dentinogenesis imperfecta in a racial isolate with multiple hereditary defects', *Oral Surg.* 1956, 9, 641–58.

54 Z. Dolinar, 'Prispevek k dednosti spastične familiarne paralize na otoku Krku' ['A contribution to the problem of inheritance of spastic familial paralysis on the island of Krk'], *Biološki Vestnik (Ljubljana)*, 1963, **11**, 115–21.

55 D. C. Gajdusek, 'Kuru', *Trans. R. Soc. trop. Med. Hyg.* 1963, **57**, 151–69; R. L. Kirk, 'Population genetic studies in Australia and New Guinea' in

P. T. Baker and J. S. Weiner (eds.), *The biology of human adaptability*, pp. 395–430, see pp. 418–20, 'C. Specific disease syndromes', Oxford: Clarendon Press, 1966.

56 G. E. Smith and F. W. Jones, *Report on the human remains*, vol. II of *The Archaeological Survey of Nubia, Report for 1907–1908*, Cairo: National Printing Dept, 1910, pp. 378.

57 C. Corrigan and S. Segal, 'The incidence of congenital dislocation of the hip at Island Lake, Manitoba', *Canad. med. Ass. J.* 1950, 62, 535–40.

58 D. Morse, 'Tuberculosis' in Brothwell and Sandison, 1967, op. cit. (above, note 18), pp. 249–71.

59 P. Bartels, 'Tuberkulose (Wirbelkaries) in der jüngeren Steinheit', *Arch. Anthrop.* 1907, 6, 245–55.

60 F. A. Mettler, *Culture and the structural evolution of the neural system*, New York: The American Museum of Natural History, 1956.

61 J. E. Cawte, 'Australian ethnopsychiatry in the field: a sampling in north Kimberley', *Med. J. Aust.* 1964, 1, 467–72.

62 J. E. Cawte, 'Tjimi and Tjagolo. Ethnopsychiatry in the Kalumburu people of north-western Australia', *Oceania* 1963–4, 34, 170–90.

63 G. C. Moss, 'Mental disorder in Antiquity' in Brothwell and Sandison, 1967, op. cit. (above, note 18), pp. 709–22.

64 J. V. Kinnier Wilson, 'Mental diseases of ancient Mesopotamia' in Brothwell and Sandison, 1967, op. cit. (above, note 18), pp. 723–33.

8 Recent Advances in Palaeopathology

ELLIS R. KERLEY

Most human diseases, malformations and reparative processes are much older than recorded history. There is adequate evidence of prehistoric pathology to substantiate this statement and a few examples will be given before reviewing recent trends and new techniques in palaeopathology.

Some of the earliest human fossils prove that disease and injury occurred several hundreds of thousands of years ago. The baboon remains at Sterkfontein and Makapansgat, generally dated as late Villafranchian (Lower Pleistocene) between 600 000 and 1 000 000 years old, as well as some of the skulls of the Australopithecines, have depressed fractures which appear to be ante-mortem. A blow to a living bone results in a fracture directly below the point of impact and the fragments, although forced into the cranial cavity, are held in place by the periosteal membranes and so are wedged together in the shape of the striking implement. Dry bone of the skull, however, shatters into irregularly shaped fragments. Thus by contrasting fractures in the living with those produced in the laboratory, it may be possible to reconstruct the events responsible for the death of individuals nearly a million years ago.

In one of the earliest fossils that is undoubtedly human, *Pithecanthropus erectus* (the Java femora and skulls, not the whole species of *Homo erectus*) dating from the Middle Pleistocene, about 500 000 years old, there is an exostosis on the femur identical with that seen in present-day myositis ossificans; it must, therefore, indicate an old muscle injury.[1] A slightly younger *Homo erectus* representative (Early Pleistocene) from Kanam, Africa, has a lesion of the mental symphysis at first thought to be a chin eminence. Brothwell[2] and others on the basis of the macroscopic appearances of the

135

bone, have suggested, however, that it is an osteosarcoma, although it is also possible that it could be a benign tumour of the dental series. Later in the Pleistocene, Neanderthal material has several instances of pathology and injury. The skeleton from La Chapelle-aux-Saints is from the Würm glacial period, or about 50 000 years old. First described by Marcelin Boule, it became the type specimen for Neanderthal. More recent examination, however, by Straus and Cave suggests that it is not 'typical' and that it is pathological in several respects: ante-mortem loss of molar teeth with mandibular bone resorption, and also osteo-arthritis.[3] At Skhul Cave near Mount Carmel, in a 'progressive' Neanderthal group, an old healed injury, either crushing or penetrating, of the foot with a pseud-arthrosis has been discovered. Again, in the skeleton of one of the Neanderthal people of Shanidar, Iraq, there is evidence of either surgical or traumatic amputation of the arm.[4] Whichever it was, the individual lived for several years thereafter, suggesting that a handicapped person could survive in this particular community, estimated to have existed 45 000 years ago. The Broken Hill speci-men of Rhodesia also possesses abnormalities: extensive caries and two cranial holes due perhaps to the canine teeth of a large car-nivore, to a weapon, or to independent events such as the bony destruction of otitis media together with a fatal blow on the head.[5] In more recent prehistoric times examples of pathology have been encountered in all parts of the world, but especially in Egypt,[6] Greece,[7] and in many archaic and more recent American Indian sites.[8,9,10] In most of these locations old fractures, osteomyelitis, loss of teeth, and caries are common. There is thus a wealth of palaeopathological material, much of which awaits adequate inter-pretation.

II

THE DEVELOPMENT OF PALAEOPATHOLOGY AS AN AREA OF INVESTIGATION

Although the first mention of disease in prehistoric animal skeletal remains ante-dates the earliest discovery of human fossil specimens, palaeopathology did not become an area of investigation until the end of the nineteenth century.[11] Rudolf Virchow was one of the first palaeopathologists and most of his work in the field was published in the last decade or two of the century. The outstanding feature of these early days of the study of prehistoric disease was the recognitive abilities of a few experienced physicians with access to known bony pathology. Since the autopsy table serves for documentation and collection, the pathologist was, therefore, on the whole, the best prepared to evaluate skeletal lesions. But with the increasing use of X-rays at the turn of the century, the radiologist was soon in a better position to compare those of prehistoric specimens with his increasing collection of verified bone diseases, than was the pathologist who compared gross specimens with the few diagnosed lesions in his museum or memory.

The early part of the twentieth century saw an increase in the number of prehistoric excavation sites with the more frequent use of more precise and well-documented methods. Consequently, there were many new communities with numerous instances of pathology to be investigated. G. Elliot Smith,[12] Warren Dawson[13] and Marc Ruffer[6] were among those who studied large numbers of Egyptian mummies and skeletal remains. In the extensive collection of Egyptian material, not only were bones and desiccated soft tissues available, but there were also descriptions of a few diseases and treatments to be found in the surviving papyri.[14] The use of X-rays was particularly helpful in diagnosing skeletal lesions in both exposed bones and wrapped mummies.

Aleš Hrdlička, a physician and physical anthropologist who for many years was Curator of Physical Anthropology at the U.S. Museum of Natural History in Washington, D.C., participated very actively in the pathology of the American Indian, both living[15] and prehistoric.[16] These research interests and his medical training placed him in a unique position during the early part of the present century to compare prehistoric pathology with modern diseases, and with cultural practices in the living descendants of those who showed evidence of disease or trauma. Another investigator whose research and writings had a widespread effect on the study of palaeopathology during the first quarter of the twentieth century was Roy Moodie. The publication of his comprehensive survey of the entire field in 1923[17] has remained a major contribution to the understanding of the subject and the most important early twentieth-century summary of palaeopathology. His interest was not limited to any one human group or to any one species, or to any particular disease and so he was able to deal effectively and in depth with a wide range of disorders and cultural groups, and was particularly suited to write his classic.

Several students of palaeopathology from the early 1930's to the present, have described the pathological conditions of the skeletal remains of certain prehistoric populations.[11] These may have included the Egyptians,[6,12,13,18] Nubians,[19] Ancient Greeks,[20,21] Pre-Incas,[16,18] and various Indian communities of both North and South America. Some authors have dealt with specific methods of treatment in various prehistoric populations,[22,23,24,25] and these papers have dealt fairly extensively with surgery and with the handling of injuries. Other investigators have pursued the origins and distributions in prehistoric times of specific diseases;[26,27,28] the pre-Columbian distribution of syphilis and yaws, and the early distribution of tuberculosis and leprosy have been of particular interest to them.

The comparison of healed but untreated prehistoric diseases with their treated modern counterparts has been extremely useful in diagnosing unknown conditions, but there are obvious limitations to this technique imposed by the influence of therapy. In order to understand untreated disorders and their causes in prehistoric communities, it has been necessary to examine the pathology of modern primitive people and Adolph Schultz[29,30] and others have extended this to the study of free-ranging non-human primates. These observations, combined with recent experimental studies of the nutritional, developmental, and pathological variation in various non-human primates are providing a better understanding of the general primate biological and social background from which man and his diseases have originated (see Brothwell, pp. 114–21).

III

A GENERAL TREND IN THE STUDY OF PALAEOPATHOLOGY

One of the most notable recent trends in the development of palaeopathology has been to turn from the description of individual specimens to a consideration of entire populations.[31] Included here are not only those specimens discovered in geographical areas or in specific archaeological sites, but also those found at different levels of the same site. Thus at any given time, the number of individuals

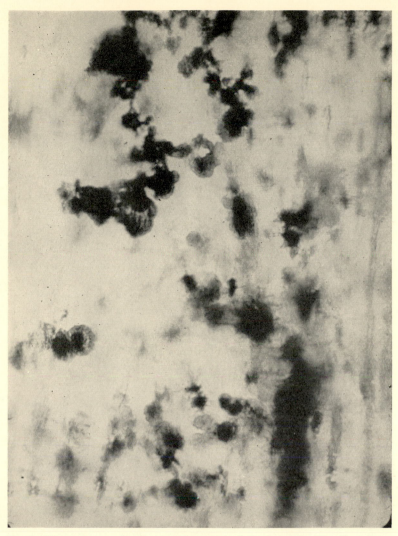

FIG. 1 Photomicrograph of a ground section of rib from Shanidar Cave, Iraq, about 45 000 years old. Osteocytic lacunae have been enlarged by the leaching activity of acid-rich ground water or by bacterial action in peripheral areas of the bone. (Polarized light.)

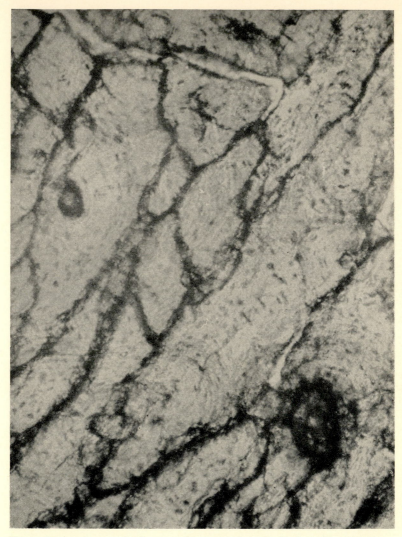

FIG. 2 Photomicrograph of a ground cross-section of a rib from Shanidar Cave, Iraq, about 45 000 years old, showing multiple micro-fractures. (Specimen through the courtesy of T. Dale Stewart, U.S. National Museum of Natural History.)

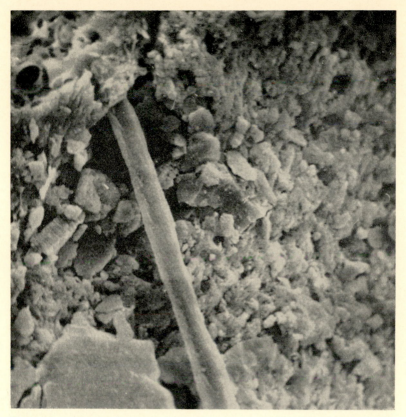

FIG. 3 A stereoscan electron micrograph of an area of massive swelling in the
tibia of an American Indian showing the presence of an unidentified spicule
(x3200). (Courtesy of Don Brothwell, British Museum (Natural History),
London.)

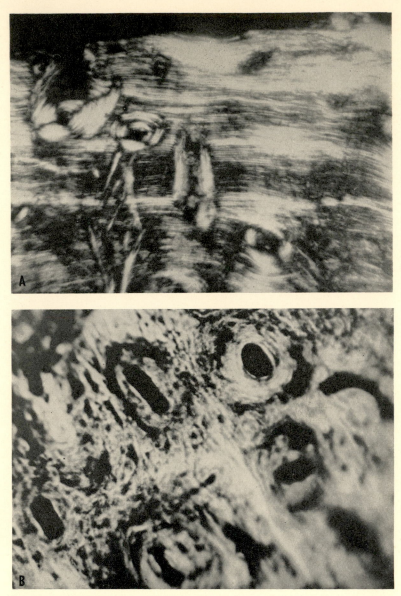

FIG. 4 A ground section of fresh bone (A) showing normal biologic distribution of bone minerals, as seen by polarized light. (B) A microradiograph of archaeological bone from Indian Knoll, Kentucky, about 5 000 years old. Non-biologically deposited post mortem calcium can be seen as light areas. Leached out areas of low calcium concentration appear dark.

who died and are representative of a community then living must be considered, rather than trying to deal with the entire site as a neatly packaged entity. In the case of hereditary diseases, of course, one would expect to find them distributed from the top to the bottom of a burial area since the genes would be passed from one generation to the next. In examining the site, evidence of conditions that have occurred over a long period of time, say several hundreds or thousands of years, would have to be interpreted as possibly hereditary, in particular developmental disorders. There are many present-day hereditary diseases of bone which can be readily identified from other bony lesions and in an archaeological site the same types can be seen at its different ages. On the other hand, where a disease or group of lesions is discovered only in one level, but in several remains at that level, famine or infection resulting from migration and contact with other peoples must be considered a possible, if not probable, explanation.

We look at a demographic analysis of an archaeological population for some indication of the latter's size at any given time, its geographical spread, its density and its social structure. To some extent this information can be inferred from the skeletal remains, particularly if there are instances of pathology of an hereditary or epidemic nature. The size of a community is of some importance since in the large, crowded and very compact city-state type, infectious diseases would be expected to be more rampant, and plague, for example, more common than in those that were smaller and more widely spread. On the other hand in smaller groups of twenty or thirty individuals who were essentially hunters and food-gatherers, the sudden appearance and subsequent disappearance of evidence of infection in the skeletal remains at a given time might suggest migration and contact with neighbouring peoples. In larger societies, stability might be inferred from the presence of hereditary diseases at a fairly fixed rate over a long period of time in any given site. Thus, the occurrence of a condition such as the viable, hereditary form of achondroplasia might occur at about the same rate from early to late dates in a city site or cemetery. The rate of occurrence for achondroplasia of this type is surprisingly similar in many large populations. There is also the problem of congenital anomalies of bone, reviewed by Brothwell and Powers.[32]

IV

TECHNIQUES OF EXAMINATION

In recent years emphasis has been placed on the use in palaeo-pathology of new techniques of examination borrowed from medicine and biology and this has brought about an important advance in the subject. As refinements in the equipment and methods for examining pathological specimens have occurred, so they have been applied to prehistoric specimens as often as the available material has permitted. Improved techniques of prepara-tion and preservation have, for example, converted skeletal frag-ments, previously impossible to investigate, into informative samples amenable to histology and microradiography.

1. *Gross examination*

Of all the methods of investigating palaeopathological material, however, macroscopical inspection is still the most important and informative. A particular disease may leave only representative stigmata on the skeleton but the involvement may have extended far beyond these and the extent can best be evaluated by gross examina-tion of the bone, especially of its surface. Thus the nature of new bone formation can often be determined; whether smoothly rounded and reactive and formed in a mass of necrotic material, whether finely spiculated early callus as in the early stages of repair, or whether composed of highly disorganized, hastily-formed, irregular spicules such as in an osteosarcoma.

One of the best methods of carrying this out is to compare ancient lesions with verified disease processes from a modern pathological collection, such as the one at the Armed Forces Institute of Pathology in Washington, D.C., comprising three thousand specimens of diagnosed osseous disorders. For the inter-pretation of the range of appearances of skeletal lesions, the experi-ence of the examiner derived from the study of well-substantiated examples of each bone disease is of prime importance in determining his ability to diagnose pathological changes in ancient bones (with regard to syphilis, see Hackett, pp. 105–8).

The use of X-rays is also essential for the adequate interpretation of the nature, extent and course of skeletal pathology, whether modern or prehistoric.[33] There is available an enormous store of radiological data on all bone disorders, whereas the collections of gross specimens are limited in most medical schools. It is, therefore, much easier to compare the X-ray appearances of prehistoric lesions and those of diagnosed patients than it is to compare macroscopical manifestations. The growth-arrest lines of Harris will be discussed below (p. 106).

2. *Microscopical examination*

A. *Light microscopy*. One of the earliest applications of microscopy to palaeopathology was reported by Ruffer in 1911,[34] and this investigation of the microscopical changes in arteries was an early diagnostic innovation. He reported again in his monumental study of pathology in Ancient Egyptians which was limited to mummified remains.[6] Until recently, however, this technique has been used relatively infrequently for the examination of prehistoric pathological material because in general the results have proved to be disappointing (Hackett, pp. 106–7). Obviously in most palaeopathological specimens the cells have long since disappeared and the histologist is left, for example, with only dry bone which frequently may be uninformative because it fragments and is lost during preparation. Moreover microscopical changes include local destruction of bone around osteocytic lacunae (Fig. 1),* possibly due to bacterial action or to concentrations of acid in small, local areas of the soil in contact with parts of the bone. Some fossil specimens which appear to be intact although friable, may be found to have numerous micro-fractures (Fig. 2), due possibly to repeated moistening and drying out, or, in northern regions, to temperature variations in near-surface bone.

More recently, microscopy has been employed not so much to interpret cellular changes but rather to equate the appearances of structures examined at low power with their macroscopical and radiological manifestations. When utilized in this fashion the technique has proved rewarding.[35] Even more important, microscopical, in conjunction with the gross and radiological, measurements of a lesion and the comparative dimensions of pathological and normal bone can provide a great deal of additional information concerning the age of a particular disease process. Measurements can readily

* Figs. 1–4 will be found between pages 138 and 139.

be made with a micrometer stage on the microscope or with an ocular reticule or micrometer.

Light microscopy depends largely upon methods of preparation standard in most pathology laboratories, but they are not suitable for many specimens of prehistoric bone, which require instead decalcification and subsequent staining of small samples from a lesion. In many instances, specimens are heavily infiltrated with groundwater calcium or on the other hand much of the calcium may have been leached out and replaced by other minerals. They are often, therefore, friable and difficult to prepare by normal histological techniques. In such cases, a ground bone section may be more informative, particularly where none of the soft tissue and cellular components remains. This procedure has resulted from the development of plastics; pieces of bone can be embedded and sections then cut with precision machines without fear of destruction. One of the best methods of examining ground bone sections is by polarized light because the birefringence of calcified bone makes the osteons and each individual collagen lamella readily discernible. Consequently, the examination of prehistoric specimens is greatly enhanced by the use of a microscope with a low-power scanning lens and polarizing equipment. Other special lighting effects may be equally useful. Thus if post-mortem calcification is not too extensive, dark field examination may give additional information concerning the rates of bone formation or destruction. A special light source high in infra-red, together with an infra-red analyser or a camera loaded with infra-red film, provides yet another means of assessing the effects of disease on the microscopical structure of bone.

The standard binocular laboratory microscope is very useful for examining ground sections of decalcified bone, but the stereoscopic dissecting instrument can be even more helpful in understanding the three-dimensional features of lesions beyond the macroscopical and radiological level. The high-power lenses and the flat field of the standard microscope are efficient for the enlargement of cell detail, but when the cells have disappeared the structural relationships can be seen best in depth at ten to thirty magnifications.

B. *Electron microscopy.* Recently, more and more applications of the electron microscope have been made to palaeopathological material. Although the preparation of prehistoric bone for electron microscopy is often difficult, methods nevertheless have been worked out for procedures such as decalcification. Brothwell, amongst others, has used them.[36]

The electron microscope can also be employed for the examination of recently mummified skin, hair, and remnants of other tissues,[37] as well as occasionally for the identification of organisms dating from long before the earliest appearance of prehistoric man.[38] It is also useful for the study of collagen; Ascenzi[39] and others have examined this in bone, shell and in amorphous material from ancient sites. It is relevant here that one use of the electron microscope not yet fully exploited could be the analysis of coprolites (fossilized faecal remains) in order to determine the balance of dietary animal and vegetable substances, as well as the quality of the protein in collagen (see p. 145).

Foreign elements other than bacteria have also been discovered by electron microscopy, as Brothwell has demonstrated.[36] Using the new scanning instrument (the *Stereoscan*) with a fine probe to examine bulky, solid bone samples, he has observed previously unsuspected spicular structures (Fig. 3). Their significance is not at present clear but until they are demonstrated in the bones of patients with known diseases, it must be assumed that they are post-mortem alterations rather than pathological changes.[40] The scanning electron microscope is a potentially valuable tool for the assessment of palaeopathological materials and it will be applied to them with increasing frequency in the future.

The electron micro-probe is a new addition to the instruments which reveal ultra-microscopical structure and one that may prove unusually informative in analysing fossilized bone. Like X-ray diffraction, it can identify individual elements, but, in addition, it measures the relative amounts of the various elements it detects and it deals with sub-microscopical samples. It consists of a stream of electrons in a very narrow, focusable beam able to scan very small areas of a field. The beam excites photons in the specimen and their wave-length is specific for the element. The number of photons of any given wave-length can be counted automatically and the quantity of the substance in an area thus determined. Don Ortner of the Smithsonian Institute in Washington, D.C., has applied the technique to fresh bone. He has also examined pathological material and has found interesting differences between the mineralization of normal bone and that affected by fluorine poisoning.[41] The microprobe has not yet been used on archaeological bone to any extent. However, it offers considerable potential in the estimation of the time since death. The calcium/phosphorus ratio should indicate relative age in specimens from the same site and also provide a basis for absolute dating in specific geological areas.

3. *Microradiographical examination*

In the past few years techniques for taking X-rays of microscopical sections, particularly of bone, have been developed. These provide detailed information on the mineral content of various parts of an osseous lesion.[35] In some conditions, such as osteogenesis imperfecta, rickets and osteomalacia, the demineralization is due to deficiencies in the formation of the osteoid matrix and it is therefore conceivable that microradiographs will show similar abnormalities in archaeological specimens, even though they may have been buried for a long time in soil relatively rich in calcium.

In specimens from the same site where the ground-water conditions are fairly constant, it is often possible to estimate the relative age of bone fragments by the microscopical and microradiographical examination of their mineral content. Microradiographs, for example, show clearly the amount and distribution of calcium. In fossilized, or partly fossilized, bone the distribution of ground-water calcium carbonate (calcite) is in a non-biological pattern, instead of being dispersed concentrically within osteons and cementum lines (Fig. 4). There may, however, be variations in ground-water distribution in an archaeological site, which can result in excessive fossilization of one skeleton but leaching out of the normal calcium phosphate in another of the same era. Both fossilization and leaching are readily identifiable and quantifiable by the use of microradiographical techniques but considerable caution in interpreting variations is essential.

An area of increasing interest in recent years has been the microscopical and microradiographical analysis of these post-mortem bony changes;[35] that is, the increase in calcium carbonate in non-biological distributions and the leaching out of calcium phosphate by the repeated action of ground water. Under certain circumstances other minerals may also be discovered in prehistoric bone. Thus in parts of Florida at the same archaeological site, bones rich in iron and magnesium may be encountered below the level of ground-water and calcium-depleted, leached-out specimens. Microradio-graphical analysis can determine areas of post-mortem deposits of calcium or other minerals and it readily reveals their non-biological distributions. If enough is known about the ground-water content of a site over a long period of time, it is possible to make very rough estimates of the time since death by means of microradiographs and polarized-light microscopy.[35]

4. *Immunological studies*

Candela[42] and other investigators[43] have been able to determine the blood groups of the ABO system in prehistoric bone and muscle. In the case of the former, the method is essentially the absorption of known Type A or B blood antibodies by a titred solution of pulverized cancellous bone taken from a haemopoetic area. It has been applied successfully to mummified bone several thousands of years old from Egypt, Peru, Alaska and from other parts of the world. In more recent samples, however, the technique may be affected by post-mortem conditions, particularly by the presence of certain bacteria, and may therefore be unreliable.[44] As new and improved laboratory methods become available, it is likely that the determination of blood types other than the ABO system will be feasible. In fact it is not beyond the realms of possibility that we may one day be able to diagnose specific types of anaemia from the marrow infarcts of cancellous bone. Certainly from the gross and radiological examination of this sort of material it is often possible to detect individuals who suffered during life from sickle cell or Cooley's anaemia,[45] although these cannot be differentiated by means of the bone alone. While for the present immunological studies of prehistoric bone have been somewhat unrewarding, there is every reason to hope that in the future they may be applied to bone, just as they have been recently applied to *in vivo* proteins by Morris Goodman[46] in the examination of the phylogenetic relation-ships among primates.

5. *Electrophoresis of proteins and dating techniques*

The electrophoresis of serum and tissue proteins in the living has yielded considerable data on the genetic associations of populations and on the individual haemoglobin phenotype of patients with here-ditary anaemias.[47] It may be some time before it is possible to examine prehistoric haemoglobins or haptoglobins in the way that blood can be typed but it is reasonable to expect that changes in the electrophoretic patterns of proteins from decalcified ancient bone or mummified muscle will provide a means of estimating the time since death. Other modern ways of dating material include techniques employing the radioactive half-life of carbon-14[48] including its use to date collagen residues in bone,[49] potassium/argon analysis,[50] and the chemical estimation of the amount of fluorine in bone.[51] Combinations of these methods have proved most useful when dealing with prehistoric groups or with individual specimens.[52]

6. *Entomology and parasitology*

This is a field that now offers an additional source of knowledge concerning prehistoric disease. The study of insects and parasites found in grave sites, burial pits, village sites, kitchen middens and so forth can give a great deal of information concerning the nature of infestations in prehistoric communities.[53] Gilbert[54] has shown that the presence in burials of the exuvia of certain fly pupae denotes the time of year during which the remains were interred. Some species of flies today, for instance, do not appear before the first of June in certain geographical areas and may not be present after the first frost. Consequently, any burial containing their exuvia must have occurred during the summer months. On the other hand, of course, their absence does not necessarily indicate a winter funeral. The same inferences can be made concerning prehistoric interments, unless evidence of drastic climatic change in the area can be shown to have occurred. The investigation of the remains of lice found in habitation sites, in old buffalo robes of recent prehistoric Indians, or in the dirt surrounding burials, may indicate the infestation of a population with specific types of lice, some of which have been known in historic times to carry diseases. Man has had the companionship of lice and other parasites for most of his existence and it is probable that in Neolithic cities the closely packed inhabitants were particularly susceptible to lice- and rat-borne diseases.

In the case of other parasites, their presence in coprolites affords important studies. The remains of intestinal varieties in their ova have been demonstrated and as more advanced methods of investigation become available, it will be possible to identify individual types with increasing accuracy.[55] Some parasites, like the trichina nematode, are sufficiently widespread in muscle and organs to be found in the mummies of individuals infested by them. The encysted parasites are distinctive and should be readily identified by the microscopical examination of reconstituted muscle.

V

OTHER ADVANCES IN PALAEOPATHOLOGY

1. *Geographical factors*

Quite often, when pathologists are called upon to examine prehistoric remains for the interpretation of possible abnormalities, they are not able to assess the effects of cultural practices unfamiliar to Western European society, much less the effects of geographical variation. Thus in many widespread prehistoric American Indian populations deformation of the skull can be seen at all ages. Because of its occasional asymmetry and the severe degree found in some groups, one may be tempted to interpret it as a pathological and even hereditary condition, when, in effect, it is the result of binding the infant's head to the flat back of the cradle board during the period of rapid skull growth. Again, in certain parts of the world, trephination of the skull has been practised extensively by various races,[56] and in some primitive African societies today it is still carried out.[57] In cases where the holes are old and their edges healed, they are often misinterpreted as old wounds or occasionally as defects. X-rays of old healed trephinations in both modern and primitive societies often show the outlines of the original hole and microscopic sections may indicate the confines of the original defect by changes in the lamellar structure and in the orientation of osteons in the bone that fills in or surrounds the edge of the drilled or incised area.[24]

Geographical influences on disease can be seen in modern as well as in prehistoric communities.[58] Thus it has been well documented recently that the presence of calcium fluoride in drinking water affects not only the incidence of dental caries but also the occurrence of skeletal pathology in general, particularly of osteoporosis.[59] In primitive peoples living at moderately high altitudes there is a tendency towards peripheral vascular disease and anaemias are more severe.[60] In the case of hereditary anaemias such as Cooley's and the sickle cell variety, it has been demonstrated that there is a high correlation between their geographical distribution and the occurrence of *falciparum* malaria (see Brothwell, pp. 116–17). Furthermore, glucose-6-phosphate dehydrogenase distribution has been associated with favism, a hereditary susceptibility to poisoning by the fava bean.[61] That these conditions occurred in prehistoric times and have persisted into the present is most probable. Areas with low concentrations of ground-water iodine have long been endemic for goitre and presumably were so in prehistoric times also; thus, in the iodine-poor Ohio River Valley drainage area, there is an Adena figurine that suggests thyroid deficiency. Recently, the importance of trace elements such as zinc, copper, and so forth has been amply demonstrated because of their role in promoting growth. In areas where these are deficient, marked growth retardation can be seen, and it is unlikely that they were appreciably more abundant in prehistoric times.

2. *Dietetic factors*

In addition to specific geographical conditions such as altitude, parasitism, and ground-water mineral distribution, there is the problem of diet which depends upon a combination of soil richness, rainfall, and climate in general, and upon other ecological factors, but also upon the technological status of the society in question.[62] In prehistoric times, many communities consisted of hunters and gatherers who were totally dependent upon the natural fauna and flora of their ecological zone. However, they were forced to migrate in response to the movements of game and to alter their diet to accommodate seasonal changes and the effects of animals upon naturally occurring fruits and vegetables. In the more advanced Neolithic cultures most of the major groups were essentially agrarian and the diet was very susceptible to change during periods of famine when crops failed sometimes for several successive years. In the later Neolithic populations, methods for storing grain and other vegetable products against times of want tended to eliminate or minimize starvation or semi-starvation in the winter months or when the crops failed.

Most of man's prehistoric existence, however, was spent on a 'feast-or-famine' existence, when small bands of hunters and gatherers ate richly when the game was plentiful and eked out a bare existence when it was not and also during the winter season when naturally occurring vegetable staples could not be obtained. Since most primitive societies have inefficient methods for the storage of meat products, they generally fluctuated between a purely marginal existence in winter and early spring, and a time of abundance during the summer and early autumn. It is not uncommon in such populations to find a high proportion of the growth-arrest lines of Harris in X-rays of the long bones. It is less well known that they can also be detected in microscopic section, occurring not only around the periphery of growing, long bones where sub-periosteal bone deposition is halted temporarily, but even in the structure of the osteons themselves. Moreover they may be demonstrated in some specimens by microradiography, as well as by polarized light. Until the full significance of these lines has been determined with certainty, however, they must be interpreted with caution. Their variability, which Marshall has recently demonstrated,[63] is in particular a cause for circumspection. Nevertheless it is known that they can be produced by the ingestion of heavy metals, especially lead and phosphorus, by excessive radiation, by severe illness of some duration, and by certain dietary deficiencies.[64] Concerning the last of these aetiological agents, Harris's lines in intermittently malnourished early communities have yet to be evaluated.

The examination of coprolites should afford valuable information regarding diet. While many are isolated discoveries, in quite a few archaeological sites they represent the accumulated excrement of the entire community. Detailed microscopical analysis of their components at several prehistoric sites has provided considerable data concerning dietary patterns,[65] and this may help to confirm or to explain the nature of malnutrition when malformations or deformities of the skeletal remains have given evidence of its presence.

3. Art forms

Palaeopathologists have long sought information concerning disease in the paintings, figurines, statuaries and other art forms of prehistoric people. Many show obvious evidence of disease or injury which can be readily diagnosed but there are others which are less easy to interpret. This is the case, for example, with the clay figurines from prehistoric Mexico[66] which reveal a variety of human disorders, both pathological and traumatic in origin, but in some a precise diagnosis cannot be made. Some of the earlier wall paintings in European caves show wounds inflicted by spear and by bow and arrow, and in certain early Greek statues pathological conditions are also clearly depicted, as are disorders such as achondroplasia in the hieroglyphics and tomb-wall paintings of Ancient Egypt; diseases of the endocrinological and reproductive systems are, for obvious reasons, more common.[67]

The interpretation of ancient art forms can thus be informative if sufficient detail and specificity are present to enable the palaeopathologist to identify abnormalities with confidence. Where this is not so, the possibility of misconstruing an artistic convention or a symbolic representation is a very real danger. This hazard is well illustrated by the differences of opinion, recently recorded,[68] concerning the significance of a symbolic Eskimo mask showing marked facial asymmetry. One observer maintains that this depicts 'a classic lower motor neurone facial palsy' (Bell), whereas the other states that it represents the 'half-man, half-animal' spiritual being common in western Alaska! Clearly, a more critical approach, notably absent at the moment, is needed for the interpretation of art forms in relationship to palaeopathology.

VI

Palaeopathology has been an area of concentrated interest for a number of years and it has intrigued, and incorporated the interests of, many investigators from various disciplines.[1] Most of the recent trends in this discipline have been the result of making new instruments and new techniques of examination available, or of applying older instruments, such as the microscope, to new specimens or structures. The electron microscope and related instruments are creating new horizons, and recent knowledge of the role of heredity has provided a basis for understanding the distribution of diseases in communities and between them over long periods of time (see Brothwell, pp. 114–21). Future developments in the subject will probably include demographic research, the more precise identification of specific diseases, particularly infectious ones, in prehistoric communities, and the study of the prehistoric distribution of these diseases in time and space. As new instruments and techniques are developed they will be applied to the elucidation of these problems relating to prehistoric skeletal material but for the time being, and in the foreseeable future, the most important method of examining and interpreting prehistoric lesions remains a knowledgeable comparison of them with the gross, the radiographic, and the microscopical appearances of verified, present-day pathological entities.

The academic status of palaeopathology and its formal relationships with the various disciplines it impinges upon, have yet to be determined, but all would agree with Temkin that '...medical historians should be greatly interested in a vigorous growth of palaeopathology in close contact with historical pathology, in particular, and with the history of medicine, in general'.[69] Finally, there is Stewart's challenging call-to-arms, 'The field is wide open. I repeat this to everyone. Anyone who goes into this field can make a great contribution to knowledge.'[70]

REFERENCES

1 E. R. Kerley and W. M. Bass, 'Paleopathology: meeting ground for many disciplines', *Science* 1967, **157**, 638–44.
2 D. Brothwell, 'The evidence for neoplasms' in D. Brothwell and A. T. Sandison (eds.), *Diseases in antiquity. A survey of the diseases, injuries and surgery of early populations*, pp. 320–45, Springfield, Ill.: C. C Thomas, 1967.
3 W. L. Straus and A. J. Cave, 'Pathology and posture of Neanderthal man', *Q. Rev. Biol.* 1957, **32**, 348–63.
4 T. D. Stewart, 'Restoration and study of the Shanidar I Neanderthal skeleton in Bagdad, Iraq', *The American Philosophical Society Year Book*, 1958 [published 1959], pp. 274–8.
5 C. B. Courville, 'Cranial injuries in prehistoric man' in Brothwell and Sandison, 1967, op. cit. (above, note 2), pp. 606–22.
6 M. A. Ruffer, *Studies in the paleopathology of Egypt*, Chicago: University of Chicago Press, 1921. See also A. T. Sandison, 'Sir Marc Armand Ruffer (1859–1917) pioneer of palaeopathology', *Med. Hist.* 1967, **11**, 150–6.
7 J. L. Angel, 'Population, size and microevolution in Greece', *Cold Spring Harb. Symp. quant. Biol.* 1950, **15**, 343–51.
8 E. A. Hooton, *The Indians of Pecos Pueblo. A study of their skeletal remains*, New Haven: Yale University Press, 1930, pp. 391.
9 J. S. Miles, 'Diseases encountered at Mesa Verde, Colorado. II. Evidences of disease' in S. Jarcho (ed.), *Human palaeopathology. Proceedings of a*

Symposium...held in Washington, D.C., January 14, 1965..., pp. 91–7, New Haven and London: Yale University Press, 1966.

10   C. E. Snow, 'Indian Knoll skeletons of site OH2, Ohio County, Kentucky', *University of Kentucky Reports in Anthropology* 1948, 4, 371–554.

11   H. E. Sigerist gives an excellent survey of the early phase of palaeopathology in *A history of medicine*, vol. 1, *Primitive and archaic medicine*, pp. 38–66, New York: Oxford University Press, 1951. For British contributions to palaeopathology, see D. Brothwell, 'The palaeopathology of early British man: an essay on the problems of diagnosis and analysis', *Jl. R. anthrop. Inst.* 1961, 91, 318–44. For a survey of the outstanding American work, see S. Jarcho, 'The development and present condition of human palaeopathology in the United States' in Jarcho, 1966, op. cit. (above, note 9), pp. 3–42, which includes the discussion. An excellent French review is that of L. Pales, *Paléopathologie et pathologie comparative*, Paris: Masson, 1930; it has the best bibliography for it contains 660 titles.

12   G. E. Smith, *The royal mummies*, Catalogue général des antiquitiés égyptiennes du Musée du Caire, Nos. 61051–61100, Le Caire: L'Institut Français d'Archéologie Orientale, 1912, pp. 118.

13   G. E. Smith and W. R. Dawson, *Egyptian Mummies*, London: Allen & Unwin, 1924, pp. 190.

14   W. R. Dawson, 'The Egyptian medical papyri' in Brothwell and Sandison, 1967, op. cit. (above, note 2), pp. 98–111; C. D. Leake, *The Old Egyptian medical papyri*, Lawrence, Kansas: University of Kansas Press, 1952.

15   A. Hrdlička, *Physiological and medical observations among the Indians of Southwestern United States and Northern Mexico*, Washington, D.C.: Smithsonian Institution, 1908, Bureau of American Ethnology, Bulletin 34, pp. 460.

16   A. Hrdlička, *Anthropological work in Peru in 1913, with notes on the pathology of the Ancient Peruvians*, Washington, D.C.: Smithsonian Miscellaneous Collection, vol. 16, No. 18, 1914, pp. 69.

17   R. L. Moodie, *Paleopathology*, Urbana, Ill.: University of Illinois Press, 1923, pp. 567.

18   R. L. Moodie, *Roentgenologic studies of Egyptian and Peruvian mummies*, Chicago: Field Museum of Natural History, Anthropology, Memoirs, 1931, vol. III, pp. 66.

19   F. W. Jones, 'Chapter VII. General pathology (including diseases of teeth)', pp. 263–91, 'Chapter VIII. Fractured bones and dislocations', pp. 293–342, in G. E. Smith and F. W. Jones, *Report on the human remains*, vol. II of *The archaeological survey of Nubia. Report for 1907–1908*, Cairo: National Printing Dept., 1910.

20   J. L. Angel, 'Osteoporosis: thalassemia?', *Am. J. phys. Anthrop.* 1964, 22 (N.S.), 369–72.

21   J. L. Angel, 'Porotic hyperostosis or osteoporosis symmetrica' in Brothwell and Sandison, 1967, op. cit. (above, note 2), pp. 378–89; see also J. B. Moseley, 'The paleopathological riddle of "symmetrical osteoporosis"', *Am. J. Roentg.* 1965, 95, 135–42.

22 E. H. Ackerknecht, 'Primitive surgery', *Am. Anthrop.* 1947, 49 (N.S.), 25–45.

23 E. A. Hooton, 'Oral surgery in Egypt during the Old Empire', *Harv. Afr. Stud.*, Varia Africana I, 1917, 1, 29–32; see also F. F. Leek, 'Reputed early Egyptian dental operations, an appraisal' in Brothwell and Sandison, 1967, op. cit. (above, note 2), pp. 102–5, who is critical of Hooton's article and of other evidence concerning the treatment of apical abscess by the Ancient Egyptians.

24 S. L. Rogers, 'The healing of trephine wounds in skulls from pre-Columbian Peru', *Am. J. phys. Anthrop.* 1938, 23, 321–40.

25 T. D. Stewart, 'Stone Age skull surgery: a general review, with emphasis on the New World', *Annual Report of...the Smithsonian Institution*, pp. 469–91, Washington, D.C., 1957 [published 1958: publication number, 4333].

26 C. J. Hackett, 'The human treponematoses' in Brothwell and Sandison, 1967, op. cit. (above, note 2), pp. 152–69.

27 V. Møller-Christensen, 'Evidence of leprosy in earlier peoples' in Brothwell and Sandison, 1967, op. cit. (above, note 2), pp. 295–306.

28 H. U. Williams, 'The origin and antiquity of syphilis: the evidence from diseased bone. A review, with some new material from America', *Archs. Path.* 1932, 13, 779–814, 931–83.

29 A. H. Schultz, 'Notes on diseases and healed fractures of wild apes and their bearing on the antiquity of pathological conditions in man', *Bull. Hist. Med.* 1939, 7, 571–82; reprinted in Brothwell and Sandison, 1967, op. cit. (above, note 2), pp. 47–55.

30 A. H. Schultz, 'The occurrence and frequency of pathological and teratological conditions and of twinning among non-human primates' in H. Hofer, A. H. Schultz, D. Starck (eds.), *Primatologia. Handbuch der Primatenkunde*, vol. 1, pp. 965–1014, Basel: S. Karger, 1956.

31 See, for example, J. G. Roney, Jr., 'Palaeoepidemiology: an example from California' in Jarcho, 1966, op. cit. (above, note 9), pp. 99–120 which includes the discussion, and also 'Palaeopathology of a California archaeological site', *Bull. Hist. Med.* 1959, 33, 97–109.

32 D. R. Brothwell and R. Powers, 'Congenital malformations of the skeleton in earlier man' in D. Brothwell (ed.), *The skeletal biology of earlier human populations* (Symposia of the Society for the Study of Human Biology, volume VIII), pp. 173–203, Oxford: Pergamon Press, 1968; see also J. E. Anderson, 'Skeletal "anomalies" as genetic indicators', ibid., pp. 135–47.

33 C. Wells, 'The radiological examination of human remains' in D. Brothwell and E. Higgs (eds.), *Science in archaeology. A comprehensive survey of progress and research*, pp. 401–12, London: Thames & Hudson, 1963; D. R. Brothwell, T. Molleson and C. Metreweli, 'Radiological aspects of normal variation in earlier skeletons: an exploratory study' in Brothwell, 1968, op. cit. (above, note 32), pp. 149–72.

34 M. A. Ruffer, 'On arterial lesions found in Egyptian mummies (1580 B.C.–525 A.D.)', *J. Path. Bact.* 1911, 15, 453–62.

35 J. Blumberg and E. Kerley, 'A critical consideration of roentgenology and microscopy in palaeopathology' in Jarcho, 1966, op. cit. (above, note 9), pp. 150–70. See this survey for further literature.

36 D. Brothwell, 'The study of archaeological materials by means of the scanning electron microscope; an important new field', in D. Brothwell and E. Higgs (eds.), *Science in archaeology. A survey of progress and research*, pp. 564–6, 2nd ed., London: Thames & Hudson, 1969; R. F. Macadam and A. T. Sandison, 'The electron microscope in palaeopathology', *Med. Hist.* 1969, **13**, 81–5.

37 T. S. Leeson, 'Electron microscopy of mummified material', *J. Stain. Techn.* 1959, **34**, 317–20; P. K. Lewin, 'Palaeo-electron microscopy of mummified tissue', *Nature, Lond.* 1967, **213**, 416–17.

38 R. Hare, 'The antiquity of diseases caused by bacteria and viruses, a review of the problem from a bacteriologist's point of view' in Brothwell and Sandison (1967), op. cit. (above, note 2), pp. 115–31; L. W. Schopj, E. S. Borghoorn, M. D. Maser and R. O. Gordon, 'Electron microscopy of fossil bacteria two million years old', *Science* 1965, **149**, 1365–7.

39 A. Ascenzi, 'Some histochemical properties of the organic substance in Neandertalian bone', *Am. J. phys. Anthrop.* 1955, **13** (N.S.), 557–66; see also this author's 'Microscopy and prehistoric bone' in Brothwell and Higgs, 1969, op. cit. (above, note 36), pp. 526–38.

40 For the general problem of difficulties in the interpretation of palaeopathological material, see C. Wells, 'Pseudopathology' in Brothwell and Sandison, 1967, op. cit. (above, note 2), pp. 5–19, and his book on *Bones, bodies and disease: evidence of disease and abnormality in early man*, London: Thames and Hudson, 1964; A. T. Sandison, 'Pathological changes in the skeletons of earlier populations due to acquired disease, and difficulties in their interpretation' in Brothwell, 1968, op. cit. (above, note 32), pp. 205–43.

41 D. Ortner, personal communication, 1969.

42 P. B. Candela, 'Blood group tests on stains, mummified tissues, and cancellous bone', *Am. J. phys. Anthrop.* 1939, **25**, 187–214.

43 L. G. and W. C. Boyd, 'Blood group reactions of preserved bone and muscle', ibid. 1939, **25**, 421–34; M. S. Glemser, 'Palaeoserology' in Brothwell and Higgs, 1963, op. cit. (above, note 33), pp. 437–46; J. P. Garlick, 'Blood groups and prehistory', ibid., pp. 447–64.

44 F. P. Thieme and C. M. Otten, 'The unreliability of blood typing aged bone', *Am. J. phys. Anthrop.* 1957, **15** (N.S.), 387–97.

45 J. E. Moseley, 'Radiographic studies in hematologic bone disease: implications for palaeopathology' in Jarcho, 1966, op. cit. (above, note 9), pp. 121–30.

46 M. Goodman, 'Deciphering primate phylogeny from macromolecular specificities', *Am. J. phys. Anthrop.* 1967, **26** (N.S.), 255–75.

47 F. B. Livingstone, 'Anthropological implications of sickle-cell gene distribution in West Africa', *Am. Anthrop.* 1958, **60** (N.S.), 533–62; idem., 'Aspects of the population dynamics of the abnormal hemoglobin and

glucose-6-dehydrogenase deficiency genes', *Am. J. hum. Genet.* 1964, **16**, 435–50.

48 E. H. Willis, 'Radiocarbon dating' in Brothwell and Higgs, 1969, op. cit. (above, note 36), pp. 46–7; but see also M. A. Tamers and F. J. Pearson, Jr, 'Validity of radiocarbon dates on bone', *Nature, Lond.* 1965, **208**, 1053–5.

49 H. Sellstedt, L. Engstrand and N.-G. Gejvall, 'New applications of radiocarbon dating to collagen residue in bones', *Nature, Lond.* 1966, **212**, 572–4.

50 W. Gentner and H. J. Lippolt, 'The potassium-argon dating of Upper Tertiary and Pleistocene deposits' in Brothwell and Higgs, 1969, op. cit. (above, note 36), pp. 88–100.

51 See, for example, K. P. Oakley, 'Fluorine, uranium, and nitrogen dating of bone' in E. Pyddoke (ed.), *The scientist and archaeology*, pp. 111–19, London: Phoenix House, 1963; idem, 'Analytical methods of dating bones' in Brothwell and Higgs, 1969, op. cit. (above, note 36), pp. 35–45.

52 R. J. Braidwood, *Prehistoric man*, 7th ed., New York: W. Morrow, 1968.

53 A. W. Pike, 'The recovery of parasite eggs from ancient cesspit and latrine deposits: an approach to the study of early parasite infections' in Brothwell and Sandison, 1967, op. cit. (above, note 2), pp. 184–8.

54 R. M. Gilbert, 'Seasonal dating of burials at the Leavenworth Site (39CO9), with the use of fly pupae', *Plains Anthrop.* 1966, **11**, 172.

55 A. W. Pike, 'Recovery of helminth eggs from archaeological excavations', *Nature, Lond.* 1968, **219**, 303–4; J. G. Moore, G. F. Fry and E. Englert, 'Thorny-headed worm infection in North American prehistoric man', *Science* 1969, **163**, 1324–5.

56 There is a large literature, but see Stewart (1958), op. cit. (above, note 25); F. P. Lisowski, 'Prehistoric and early historic trepanation' in Brothwell and Sandison, 1967, op. cit. (above, note 2), pp. 651–72.

57 E. L. Margetts, 'Trepanation of the skull by the medicine-men of primitive cultures, with particular reference to present-day native East African practice' in Brothwell and Sandison, 1967, op. cit. (above, note 2), pp. 673–701, with extensive bibliography; see also I. G. Russu and V. Bologa, 'Trepanationen im Gebiet des heutigen Rumanien', *Sudhoffs Arch.* 1961, **45**, 34–66.

58 See, for example, M. T. Newman, 'Adaptation of man to cold climates', *Yearb. phys. Anthrop.* 1953–61, **9**, 214–19; Sigerist has summarized the earlier work on the geography of disease in op. cit. (above, note 11), pp. 77–85, and Sir Dudley Stamp, *Some aspects of medical geography*, London: Oxford University Press, and E. H. Ackerknecht, *History and geography of the most important diseases*, New York: Hafner, 1965, deal with some of the more recent.

59 Wells, 1964, op. cit. (above, note 40), p. 112.

60 C. S. Coon and E. E. Hunt, *The living races of man*, pp. 273–6, London: Cape, 1966; R. Kampier, 'Splenic infarction due to sicklemia and air travel', *Sth. med. J.* Nashville 1957, **50**, 277–8.

61 H. Lehmann and R. G. Huntsman, 'Chapter 16. Glucose-6-phosphate dehydrogenase (G-6-PD)' in *Man's haemoglobins including haemoglobinopathies and their investigation*, pp. 182–90, see pp. 184, 186–7, Amsterdam: North-Holland Publishing Co., 1966.

62 For antiquity, see D. Brothwell and P. Brothwell, *Food in antiquity*, London: Thames and Hudson, 1969.

63 W. A. Marshall, 'Problems in relating the presence of transverse lines in the radius to the occurrence of disease' in Brothwell, 1968, op. cit. (above, note 32), pp. 245–61.

64 E. A. Park and C. P. Richter, 'Transverse lines in bone: mechanism of their development', *Johns Hopkins Hosp. Bull.* 1953, 93, 234–48; H. McHenry, 'Transverse lines in long bones of prehistoric California Indians', *Am. J. phys. Anthrop.* 1968, 29 (N.S.), 1–18.

65 E. O. Callen, 'Diet as revealed by coprolites' in Brothwell and Higgs, 1969, op. cit. (above, note 36), pp. 233–43; R. F. Heizer, 'The anthropology of prehistoric Great Basin human coprolites', ibid., pp. 244–50.
R. F. Heizer and L. K. Napton, 'Biological and cultural evidence from prehistoric human coprolites. The diet of prehistoric Great Basin Indians can be reconstructed from desiccated fecal material', *Science* 1969, 165, 563–8.

66 A. I. Weisman, 'Pre-Columbian artifacts portraying illness', *Bull. Menninger Clin.* 1966, 30, 39–44. Physicians are often willing to make bold diagnoses when they discover bodily abnormalities in art forms but often they cannot be substantiated. A restrained and reasonable handling of ancient artistic material is that of J. Gourevich, 'Recorded in clay', *Abbottempo* (Weert) 1965, 3, 16–21. See also D. Duran Martinez, 'Surgery of the Mayas', ibid. 1963, 1, 14–20.

67 A. T. Sandison and C. Wells, 'Endocrine diseases' in Brothwell and Sandison, 1967, op. cit. (above, note 2), pp. 521–31; idem., 'Diseases of the reproductive system', ibid., pp. 498–520.

68 E. Holtzman and D. J. Ray, Letters in *Science* 1968, 160, 252.

69 O. Temkin, 'Palaeopathology and the history of medicine', in Jarcho, 1966, op. cit. (above, note 9), pp. 30–5, see p. 35.

70 T. D. Stewart, 'Some problems in human palaeopathology' in ibid., pp. 43–55, see p. 55.

9 History of Science and History of Medicine

MARIE BOAS HALL

To the historian of science, history of medicine is a bewildering mixture of the familiar and the bizarre, of assimilable and alien facts, of the knowable and the unknowable. Inherently, history of medicine is perhaps no more complex than history of science; but tradition, the almost mystic aura surrounding an art ultimately or directly connected with healing the sick, and centuries of compilation of histories of medicine by diverse hands have rendered the subject difficult to grasp by outsiders. There is besides the old and (in many cases) well-founded belief that only trained physicians should attempt the history of their subject, a belief which has often made those not medically qualified reluctant to attempt a discipline for which they may be found inadequately prepared.

However, none of these attitudes and complexities need hinder the historian of science from acting as critic of a completed performance, nor from trying to indicate to his fellow historian what problems and approaches can be of use to his own discipline. Although true history of medicine can probably claim to be older than history of science—certainly it was better established in the late nineteenth and early twentieth centuries—yet the latter appears to have established its place in intellectual and academic life in the past quarter of a century much more securely and lastingly. And it also appears to have acquired the necessary self-confidence to permit its practitioners to proceed without overmuch doubt or self-analysis, a confidence which history of medicine at the moment patently lacks.

This is a paradoxical situation, for it is only a little over thirty years ago that the position seemed markedly different. At that time, history of medicine seemed the more secure, and George Sarton could write in a mixture of envy and indignation that it was unfairly well treated, being in the possession of the 'institutes' which history of science lacked, and could also complain of a complacent tendency which he observed in historians of medicine to claim that their subject was 'the best part' of history of science.[1] And although Henry Sigerist wrote apologizing for the production of a good deal of bad history of medicine, and for possible arrogance on the part of some of its practitioners, he too saw good grounds for complacency about the state of his discipline.[2] Yet so much had the situation changed even in the few years that followed, that in 1950 Sigerist could look back at his earlier article as a defence of his subject, characterizing it as an attempt 'to show that the history of medicine is not a mere chapter in the history of science but has intrinsic problems of its own'.[3] That he felt the need to defend history of medicine as an independent discipline should today surprise historians of science and historians of medicine alike, but it perhaps indicates certain complexities in the subject to which the outsider may be more sensitive than is the practitioner.

II

By and large the historian of science probably finds it easier to see where the two disciplines coincide than does the historian of medicine, for he sees (or should see) that many aspects of history of medicine consort well with his conception of his own subject, while, equally, many other aspects lie outside it. Roughly, the 'medical sciences', however defined, belong to both forms of history, while such topics as the art of medical practice, hygiene, therapeutics, the social aspects of the medical profession, diagnosis, medical education, all belong exclusively to the history of medicine.[4] The line of demarcation is not and cannot be sharp and fixed, for the historical development of all aspects of medicine has caused the interrelation to fluctuate with historical periods. When medicine was one of the few 'scientific' professions, and a medical education the only education pretending to instruct a man in scientific subjects outside mathematics, then a large number of scientists were either practising physicians or medically qualified. In such periods, the content of medical education is of equal relevance to the histories of science and medicine. Similarly, in the sixteenth and seventeenth centuries, the incorporation into the pharmacopoeia of metallic and mineral drugs renders materia medica a subject of direct interest to the historian of chemistry. Sometimes the beginnings of a medical subject seem more directly related to history of science than its later and more advanced development: so anatomy of the sixteenth and early seventeenth centuries is generally discussed by historians of science, though that of the eighteenth or later centuries is not; they will mention Bichat's work on tissues, but not that of later histologists like His; they will discuss the case histories of Hippocrates, but not those of modern physicians. Often the choice must seem arbitrary, perhaps dictated in part by the limited medical knowledge of the historian, but there is a certain validity in the concept which dictates that the first great leap forward is of more general relevance than orderly progression along a well-defined path.

It is evident that the development of the medical sciences must and does have its place in history of science; here indeed both forms of history share equally. Physiology is the most obvious example: it is no accident that the historian of science finds the *Natural faculties* the Galenic text most relevant to his interests, that he expects his students to read Harvey's *De motu cordis* more thoroughly than any other medical text, nor that he is more at home with the work of Claude Bernard than with that of his pupils. An interest in the development of physiology is no more strange to him than an interest in the development of botany or zoology; that *human* physiology is in question is less relevant than that it is an aspect of *animal* physiology. Conversely, there are subjects which belong more to him than to the historian of medicine, yet are truly important for both fields; microscopy, for example, or physiological optics, or the study of the role of air in respiration, or even the investigation of spontaneous generation—a topic of purely scientific interest until its solution, when it was perceived to have dramatic medical applications. In all these cases both subjects are involved and neither can or should wish to claim a monopoly. Finally there are purely scientific subjects which the historian of medicine must nevertheless consider: botany (for materia medica); chemistry (for materia medica and physiology); physics (mechanics as applied to physiology, optics, thermometry) and so on; Hippocrates showed that even meteorology had some bearing upon medical practice. In all these cases the line of demarcation between the disciplines is shifting and uncertain, and neither can fairly claim the advantage.

159

Equally clearly there are other areas which belong entirely, or almost so, to the historian of medicine. Pathology is an obvious example: it is both the case that its development can be little understood by most historians of science and that it has little direct interest for the development of non-medical science. Pathology was indeed for long one of those strangely isolated aspects of medicine; until well on in the eighteenth century it was not often correlated with clinical observation and consequently had no very beneficent effect upon the development of medical practice.[5] This is not to say that its findings were ignored, but rather that they were applied to the elaboration of medical theory rather than connected with any aspect of disease. Since the lesions of organs could only be observed *ex post facto*, their detection in a cadaver offered no guidance to practitioner or patient, and rather fostered than diminished that excessive tendency towards systematization of disease theory so characteristic of late eighteenth- and early nineteenth-century medicine. Not that there was any question of a clear-cut, *a priori*-empiricist dichotomy; empiricism was usually carried to equal excess and equally extreme over-simplification.

Another obvious area reserved for the medical historian is diagnostics. Here the situation is complex; for the historian needs both an understanding of diagnostic complexities and a sharp critical faculty, a combination unfortunately rare. The historian of science cannot but notice, and if he be at all curious, deplore, the tendency of medical history towards hagiolatry in this field. The great clinicians of the past—were they truly gifted with a perception greatly in advance of their time, so that they were able to perceive a totality of symptoms in a way denied to most men for generations thereafter, or is it rather the case that they were quick, keen and careful observers who noted symptoms in such detail that the modern historian can perceive the relevant symptoms, consciously or unconsciously discarding the irrelevant ones? The truly conscientious historian must not only be aware of which view he is taking, but must make his action clear to his audience. For otherwise he is not writing history as most historians understand it, but is rather praising famous men, viewing the past in the light of the present. This can be exciting and provides an agreeable exercise in the admiration of our ancestors which may suitably provoke awe, admiration and the desire for emulation on the part of medical

students. But it is not history, and the historian of science is bound
to reject it as such.

An even more striking example is to be found in the area of
therapeutics. It has long been a tradition in the history of medicine
(as often in the history of science as well) that to be a 'modernist'
and an iconoclast is necessarily to be 'modern' and therefore praiseworthy. Aside from the fact that it is more than time that we discarded the Victorian naïveté which insists upon awarding marks to
those great men who appear likely to be successes in our own day,
this can readily lead to sheer obscurantism and even unconscious
suppression of the truth. Was it desirable that herbal remedies
should be replaced by chemical ones? Were antimony or calomel
really in some way superior (they were certainly potentially more
powerful) than black hellebore or senna or rhubarb? Was tartar
emetic the great saviour of the sick that it was thought to be through
the nineteenth century? I do not know; but I should like to know,
and have often appealed in vain to histories of medicine to tell me.
Surely historians of medicine when they are qualified medical men
should know the answers and, more important, be prepared to
examine critically what they learn and teach about the administration of drugs. Even in the simplest cases it is often impossible to
establish whether accepted treatment had any basis in fact. To take
a well-known and (as far as I have ever been able to discover) un-
resolved example: was there any way of curing, or even alleviating,
the symptoms of syphilis before the discovery of salvarsan? Nineteenth-century medical writers who still prescribed mercurials
naturally thought that the sixteenth-century treatment was un-
exceptionable, except when it turned to guaiacum. Does mercury
cure syphilis? And if so, is the administration of large doses of
calomel effective, as nineteenth-century popular medicine clearly
believed?[6] Indeed, the layman historian would like to know not
only the answers to such questions as these, but also, where possible,
how the administration of mercury might be expected to affect the
patient's symptoms. There has been over the past hundred years a
very thorough study of the chemical pharmacopoeia and textbook
from the chemical point of view, so that it is relatively easy to find
the *chemical* nature of specific drugs, and the value of the chemical
procedures adopted in their preparation. But there has been little or
no medical analysis of such preparations. As a slightly absurd

example, consider Jean Beguin's 'burning spirit of Saturn', first described in his *Tyrocinium chymicum* of 1610. Chemically, it has been known since about 1660 to contain no lead; for over a century it has been known to be acetone, and is so denominated in histories of chemistry. I am aware of no similar *medical* consideration—perhaps unnecessary in this case, where even a layman can safely assume that it does not, as Beguin stated, render a man impotent, and that, as he also stated, a few drops are unlikely to prove effective in desperate cases.

A layman would rejoice to find a competent and thorough analysis of the medical aspects of seventeenth-century—and later—pharmacopoeias. This perhaps will call for the development of a specialized branch of the history of medicine, for one cannot easily find sources to provide the answer, unlike anatomy, where correctness of earlier judgement can be determined by consultation of a modern work of reference. Human anatomy has not changed over the centuries, but pharmacopoeias and methods of medical treatment have, wiping out the past in their progress. Hence the history of therapeutics is an intrinsically more difficult subject than the history of anatomy, calling for special skills which must be developed by trial and error methods. It is a subject also which calls for the exercise of great care and judgement, since it can be reconstructed only theoretically and imaginatively—it cannot be undertaken practically to any great extent, unlike microscopic biology which, as Edwin Clarke has recently shown,[7] can with great perseverance be reconstructed historically by laborious and ingenious trials with old instruments. Yet it is a subject which has much to offer both the history of science and the history of medicine; and the former will be much in the debt of anyone who tries to investigate this almost wholly neglected field.

III

Both history of science and history of medicine suffer from a peculiarity in the nature of their basic literature: for many years it has been an important, fashionable and increasingly expensive component of the rare-book world. Successful scientists, engineers and physicians have found that the collection of first editions of the classics of their fields provided a satisfying and absorbing avocation and pleasure. To the extent that such collections have been presented to public bodies, the historian has gained; otherwise he finds himself precluded by financial restrictions from buying for himself, and for libraries to which he has convenient access, essential tools of his trade. In return, the wealthy collector has often, like Fulton or Klebs,[8] turned bibliographer and provided his poor colleague with useful, detailed bibliographies of books he may never handle. Medical or scientific bibliography can prove useful; it can also prove something of a snare for the historian, whose values must differ from those of the bibliographer. The latter, especially if he be a collector, values a book either for its actual rarity, or because it contains a new fact or discovery (whether immediately recognized or not). The historian is, on the one hand, more critical, judging a book by the importance of any fact, discovery or theory contained in it; on the other hand he is often more interested in a book with many, readily available editions than a book with one scarce one, for multiplicity of editions shows that the book was widely read and hence influential, while many (though obviously not all) scarce books are so because little cherished. The historian must always remember that for him rarity implies possible neglect, and that a discovery known to no one except the author tells us nothing about the historical development of a subject, only about the personal development of the author. So a study of Leonardo da Vinci's wonderful anatomical drawings tells us much about the refinement of Leonardo's technique and interest with the years, but very little about the history of anatomy. (We can to some extent gauge thereby the amount of anatomical knowledge commonly available to artists in Leonardo's day and the inherent anatomical potentialities of the period, but as his drawings were virtually unknown to contemporaries, and totally unknown to anatomists in the generations after his death, what he did could not bear fruit.)

Rarity, indeed, can only have a negative value in suggesting what was unlikely to be known, which in itself may, indeed, be of some interest. Though historians of medicine and science have often been reluctant to accept this sort of evidence there is good reason, for example, to believe that a medieval manuscript known in only one or two copies was not influential, whereas one known in many copies was. And here, too, one must differentiate between text and author.

163

Certainly Galen would not have become the historian of medicine's 'anti-hero' (as Aristotle did for the historians of science of two or three generations ago) if more discrimination had been exercised in this respect. We have no excuse since Charles Singer's careful studies[9] for lumping Galen's texts together and saying that 'all' Galen was studied in the medieval university medical schools. We know, or should know (though even Singer never quite realized the significance of his own later work), that neither *The use of the parts* nor the *Anatomical procedures* nor the *Natural faculties* was available to thirteenth-century medical students; that *The use of the parts* became known in good time to be read by Leonardo; and that the *Anatomical procedures* and the *Natural faculties* were virtually new books in the early sixteenth century. This puts an entirely different complexion upon the development of sixteenth-century anatomy from the conventional account, and upon the Galenolatry of Linacre and Caius. Related to this approach is the confusion arising from the temptation to ascribe originality to someone who in fact 'modernized' the ancients: a good case in point is Sherrington's famous and fascinating study of Jean Fernel.[10] This is a valuable study of sixteenth-century medicine with one major defect: Sherrington had obviously never read Galen's *Natural faculties* with the same lack of prejudice he employed when reading Fernel, and so did not perceive how much Fernel drew from Galen, nor of how little value were the anti-Galenical protests of sixteenth-century writers like Fernel, or even Vesalius. Clearly the history of sixteenth-century medicine in its widest sense needed rewriting in terms of such scholarly discoveries, and is indeed slowly being so rewritten.

Similarly one cannot but feel that medieval medicine needs to be submitted to the kind of meticulous scholarship recently devoted to the history of medieval physical science. As long as studies are either concerned with collecting (illustrations, manuscripts, titles, translations and so on), so long will the history of medieval medicine remain in a primitive state. We need the printing and translation of texts, informed and critical commentary on those texts, and the relation of illustration to text. Only thus will it be possible to understand such problems as the relation of post-mortems to anatomical dissections, to name but one example among many. Above all, medieval medical texts need to be approached in a true historical manner, and neither treated as quaint examples of a past age nor taken for direct precursors of the modern world, but regarded as what they truly are, the product of a particular historical age with its own culture, values and modes of procedure. How this method can be profitably and excitingly combined has been amply demonstrated by Owsei Temkin in his splendid series of articles on the influence of philosophical concepts upon nineteenth-century medical ideas.[11] Here an historian of medicine has taught grateful historians of science, who have only recently begun to consider the influence of *Naturphilosophie* for example upon both nineteenth-century physics and nineteenth-century biology.[12] And there have been many other studies of this kind, most recently of Harvey.[13] This is a most admirable example of 'history of ideas', of too general an interest to be exclusively classified as either history of medicine or history of science.

History of medicine has often suffered from the disability that for long plagued history of science: both have too often been merely the relaxation of the elderly, successful practitioner regarding history as intrinsically simple, something to be 'picked up' by any intelligent educated man. Though this has provided many useful books and articles, it has also produced much positivistic, Whig history, and many ahistorical judgements. Historians of medicine, like historians of science, need to have their subject recognized as independent, and would-be historians of any branch of intellectual history must have a firm grasp of historical methods and historical feeling. The history of science has achieved this at a more rapid rate than the history of medicine, and may serve both as a warning and as an encouraging example.

Both history of science and history of medicine, as historical subjects, require a thorough knowledge of the general aspects of life and thought of the period in which the particular ideas, events or books under consideration existed. They cannot be written about or studied in isolation; without a real feeling for general history on the part of a writer any subject becomes mere chronicling at best, and inaccurate popularization at worst. Only such an historical sense on the part of their exponents can make these subjects genuinely professional or 'scientific' in the Continental sense; mere qualification in the subject-matter (medicine, zoology, physiology, or whatever) is not and cannot be enough, though it is a very necessary preliminary. Would-be historians of medicine, like

would-be historians of science, must therefore always be doubly
sensitive to the exigencies of their subject-matter. Of course this
sensitivity can be, and often has been, acquired by those writing
only as an avocation, and has, regrettably, sometimes escaped otherwise admirably prepared 'professional' historians; but it is a thing
that must always divide the layman and the true professional in
the history of a subject, as it does in the subject itself.

IV

The discussion above has concerned itself mainly with the bookish
aspects of the history of medicine: with medical sciences, therapeutics, anatomy, theory of disease, physiology—all subjects
enshrined in books. But there are of course many other aspects often
difficult to assess precisely because they are not specifically literary.
These are the more nearly social aspects, those which have led one
historian of medicine to declare,[14]

It so happens that medicine, in the ordinary sense, represents a group
of the biological sciences, but that medicine as an art is closely related to
the social sciences.

And another to insist,[15]

Medicine is not a *branch of science* and never will be. If medicine is a
science then it is a social science.

The concept of medicine as an 'art' (in the craft sense) is, of
course, as old as Hippocrates, and not presumably new in his day.
The critical success of 'scientific medicine' in the second half of the
nineteenth century, a period when the positivistic concept of science
was at its height, has tended to obscure this aspect for all but a
handful of historians of medicine, and from this has stemmed
a number of possible errors and distortions. If medicine is purely a
science, then successful and famous physicians must have been so
because they effected cures; consequently their theories and
methods of treatment must have been 'correct', or at least more so
than those of their contemporaries; and hence the biographer or
historian must justify such theories and methods. But is it necessarily so? Did every physician of the past always literally follow the
theory of treatment he wrote about and lectured upon? Did patients

recover because of his treatment or in spite of it? What makes a successful practitioner—science at all times, or sometimes psychology? In the days before proper nursing, the doctor must have served in a double capacity, both prescribing and inspiring confidence and the will to overcome disease.

In these respects, as in some others, history of medicine is closer to history of technology than to history of science. Like history of technology it has scientific aspects, it has craft techniques, and it has social and economic influences and aspects. The history of technology is in many ways a newer subject than history of medicine, but it is a very self-conscious one which is currently endeavouring to develop sound methods of approach. The two subjects could readily learn from one another. The historian of technology, particularly of the period before the eighteenth century, has the same difficulty as the historian of medicine in evaluating brilliant practitioners whose success (or apparent success) need not have had a sound basis in theory—though history of medicine does not have to allow for the strongly imaginative element present in, for example, many technological inventions of the Renaissance.

Once again, critical examination and interpretation of actual medical practice must to a large extent rely upon sound medical knowledge; but not exclusively so, nor does medical knowledge suffice. It is one thing to note what a physician claimed as his method of treatment and evaluate that; it is another to compare this with his actual practice, for which no medical competence is necessarily required. Certainly it is possible to admire and approve of Sydenham's expressed preference for milder methods of treatment than those advocated by many of his more heroic contemporaries; but do his case histories show that he practised in as mild a fashion as historians sometimes claim to be the case? It does not seem to me that he was in fact so whole-hearted in dispensing with blood-letting as some of his biographers appear to think he was. Case histories need studying, evaluating, in many cases editing and publishing, either for the first time or for the first time *in toto*. Publication by itself provides useful (and, preferably, inexpensive) raw material for the student; but critical, scholarly and thorough editing is necessary to make such case histories useful in a larger sense. Only so will it be possible to build up a comprehensive history of *actual* medical treatment over the centuries, to supplement the

167

history of the *theory* of medical treatment which already, at least in part, exists today.

The situation is similar for surgery, though here, for the pre-nineteenth century at least, theory was so primitive that theory and practice more often than not went hand in hand. The greatest gap is probably in the analysis of the therapeutic aspects of surgery. What plasters, unguents, caustics and so on were actually applied, and what effect might these be expected to have upon the wounds for which they were prescribed? A surgeon like the sixteenth-century William Clowes can provide a rich source of material for such an examination, but though his case histories exist in sixteenth-century editions, and useful modern extracts have been reprinted, no thorough study of his complete work has, I believe, ever been attempted.[16] Clowes is also interesting as an example of how a wealthy patient might monopolize a surgeon's time—a fact casting an important light upon the state of his practice and the varying medical attention awarded to different social classes.

There was, indeed, a very sharp division in this respect between social classes. We presumably know most about the treatment of the rich in large cities (it is difficult to remember, for example, how much the College of Physicians was a group of *London* physicians), and next most about the treatment of the very poor in large cities, for they of necessity came for succour to the great hospitals which served as a source for instruction and research. We know less, until the last hundred years, about medical treatment of the city middle classes and superior artisans, who presumably relied largely upon apothecaries and empirics. (From literary sources we know that in the early nineteenth century the wealthy in England summoned physicians for themselves, apothecaries for dependants and servants.) Here sources are difficult to interpret, for many are diatribes against unlicensed practitioners by the properly qualified, and vice versa; what elements of truth these diatribes contain can only be determined by very careful analysis. For the eighteenth and nineteenth centuries there are useful literary sources, especially novels; diaries where they exist are useful for all ages. We know little, normally, about country practitioners and least of all about what is loosely called 'folk medicine'. This latter (which of course still exists today) should more properly be called non-professional medicine, consisting as it does of medical advice offered freely by friends of the patient, in country villages often by reputed wise men or women, in all places and times by those with a reputation for special interest or knowledge. In the seventeenth century so much treatment was of this kind, even in the wealthy classes, that a great deal of information can be obtained from letters and diaries; the same probably applied in later periods as well. This is not really very different from the advice sought from the 'wise woman' in a village: the language is different and the approach more sophisticated, but allowing for the difference in class and education both sorts of advice are aspects of the same popular medical tradition.

Related to both the social aspects of medicine and the history of technology is the history of the progress of instrumentation in medical practice. This is relatively neglected; we know the way in which instruments were developed, but less about the way in which they were applied in day-to-day medical practice. It is easy to discover the stages in the invention of particular instruments—the first account of the pulsilogia, the standardization of the thermometer, the invention of the stethoscope—but how much and when these and other instruments were commonly utilized in medical practice and what effects their use had is more difficult to ascertain. Here once again the sources are fragmentary, but by no means impossibly difficult to analyse profitably, and they would well repay study in the wake of the historians who have dealt with the development of the instruments themselves.

Another social aspect of history of medicine that will repay further study is the relation of the physician to the public, both the public relations of medical men and the view held by society of the potentialities and possibilities of medicine. A fair amount has already been written about this subject for the modern period. It is the theme of Richard Shryock's *The development of modern medicine* that there was a crisis in public confidence in the first half of the nineteenth century; he saw medicine as progressing 'scientifically' in the seventeenth century until, as he put it,[17]

All that seemed necessary, in order to realize the hopes of philosophers, was for medical science to continue steadily along the way of the physical disciplines, and for medical practice to follow closely after...a strange and tragic thing happened...Medicine at first faltered, and then fell behind; physic failed to keep up with physics.

And, as he admirably showed, so far was this the case that by 1800 the public as well as the philosophers were losing faith in orthodox medicine (especially in the United States where medical theory drew upon traditional European concepts and carried them to dogmatic extremes) and sought relief elsewhere, to be saved only by the application of the discoveries of medical science after about 1850. Although Shryock's work touches on problems from 1600 onwards, his main interest was in the period after 1750 and the chapters on the earlier periods chiefly provide the scientific background. Similar analyses for earlier periods would be equally rewarding: there is much need for what Henry Sigerist planned to do in his projected eight-volume *History of medicine*, as shown by his remarkable first volume, the only one he lived to complete.

V

It should be obvious, but I believe it is not entirely so, that history of medicine, like history of science, requires specialization. No one since George Sarton has even thought of trying to write a large, thorough history of science; probably no one since Sigerist has thought of trying to do the same for the history of medicine. Each aspect requires so much special knowledge and preparation that, if either subject is to progress, it must have the benefit of the development of experts. And if experts are to appeal to more than a narrow panel of other experts they must learn, in Collingwood's phrase, to ask the right questions.[18] As he rightly said, interesting and stimulating historical answers—whether in history of science, history of medicine, naval history, or the history of Roman settlement in Britain—can only be given in response to interesting and stimulating questions. In the absence of these, history is merely past fact or fiction, rather than the recreation of a past that has made the present, as all historians must hope to make it.

REFERENCES AND NOTES

1   G. Sarton, 'Second preface to volume XXIII: the history of science versus the history of medicine', *Isis* 1935, 23, 313–20. I cannot trace the source of the remarks which irritated Sarton. Arturo Castiglioni certainly spoke

of the history of medicine and the history of science indifferently, though he was much concerned with preserving the history of what he called the 'art' of medicine. See *A history of medicine*, 2nd ed., p. v ('Author's Preface', 1940), New York: A. A. Knopf, 1947.

2   Henry E. Sigerist, 'The history of medicine *and* the history of science: an open letter to George Sarton, Editor of *Isis*', *Bull. Hist. Med.* 1936, 4, 1–13.

3   Henry E. Sigerist, *A history of medicine*, 1, 34 n. 9, New York: Oxford University Press, 1951.

4   As Sigerist (1936) wrote, 'Science is one aspect of medicine and there are a great many other aspects', op. cit. (above, note 2), p. 5. Later (1951) he went further, writing, 'medicine is not a natural science, either pure or applied', op. cit. (above, note 3), p. 14.

5   Cf. R. Shryock, *The development of modern medicine: an interpretation of the social and scientific factors involved*, p. 65, New York: A. A. Knopf, 1947.

6   Cf. Richard Henry Dana, *Two years before the mast*, New York: Harper, 1840, where he speaks of calomel as the only thing which in his belief can possibly save the life of his gravely ill Sandwich Island friend on the beach near San Diego, California.

7   E. Clarke and J. G. Bearn, 'A seventeenth century microscope', *Med. biol. Illust.* 1967, 17, 74–80.

8   J. F. Fulton's bibliography of Robert Boyle (1932, 1961) is his best-known work of this genre, but he composed many others, including those on Lower and Mayow. A. C. Klebs, 'Incunabula scientifica et medica: short title list', *Osiris* 1937, 4, 1–359.

9   See especially Charles Singer and C. Rabin, *A prelude to modern science*, Cambridge: The University Press for the Wellcome Historical Medical Museum, 1946, and *Galen on anatomical procedures*, transl. Charles Singer, London: Oxford University Press for the Wellcome Historical Medical Museum, 1956.

10 Sir Charles Sherrington, *The endeavour of Jean Fernel*, Cambridge: The University Press, 1946.

11 O. Temkin, 'On the interrelationship of the history and philosophy of medicine', *Bull. Hist. Med.* 1956, 30, 241–51; 'Materialism in French and German physiology of the early nineteenth century', ibid., 1946, 20, 322–7; 'The philosophical background of Magendie's physiology', ibid., pp. 10–35.

12 Cf. L. Pearce Williams, 'The physical sciences in the first half of the nineteenth century: problems and sources', *History of Science* 1962, 1, 1–15, and Everett Mendelsohn, 'Physical models and physiological concepts: explanation in nineteenth-century biology', *Br. J. Hist. Sci.* 1965, 2, 201–19.

13 Walter Pagel, *William Harvey's biological ideas: selected aspects and historical background*, New York: Hafner, 1967.

14 Shryock, op. cit. (above, note 5), p. 38.

15 Sigerist, op. cit. (above, note 2), pp. 4–5.

16 William Clowes, *Profitable and necessarie booke of observations* [facsimile],
    ed. DeWitt T. Starnes and Chauncey D. Leake, New York: Scholars'
    Facsimiles & Reprints, 1945; and *Selected writings of William Clowes
    1544–1604*, ed. F. N. L. Poynter, London: Harvey & Blythe, 1948.
17 Shryock, op. cit. (above, note 5), p. 17.
18 See especially R. G. Collingwood, *An autobiography*, pp. 36–9, 127–46,
    Oxford: The University Press, 1939, 1951.

10 Medical Lives and Medical Letters: a Chapter in the History of Scientific Biography

J. Z. FULLMER

To compress between the covers of a book the bitter-sweetness and complexity of the life of one man is impossible. The great biographers have all realized the hopelessness of their assignment, yet biographies continue to appear because it is in the biographer's nature to try, at least, to give some idea of what it must have been like to be a certain person, living in a certain time, and doing certain things. Not only do biographies continue, but a survey of a large number of them shows that they are as varied in aim, structure, content, style and tone as the subjects with which they deal. Virginia Woolf said that 'We have lives that are all ceremony and work, and lives that are all chatter and scandal.'[1] Had she examined the large number of lives devoted specifically to men of medicine and science, she could well have expanded the list to include lives that are all romance, all pious adulation, all hortatory didacticism, as well as lives that are tissues of half-truths, and lives that reveal more of biographer than of biographee. The complexity of life itself is mirrored in the myriad ways in which it has been dealt with by the practising biographer.

It is interesting to inquire why the biographical craft—or art—has varied so widely. Surely it might be argued that lives of great figures share so many features that any literary diversity would eventually disappear. During certain periods some biographical models have dominated the *genre*, and reading a large batch of them written under the influence of a particular model can generate a superficial impression of uniformity. Yet, by and large, biographies do differ markedly from one another, and in ways which are not all ascribable to their individual subjects. Part of the diversity arises because biographers, like all writers, bend both consciously and unconsciously to the trends of taste pursued by their contemporaries. In addition, the biographer of a scientist is buffeted by changes in scientific fashions. He can reflect by his emphases and by his silences what he and his contemporaries think are important topics in science and medicine. What may be regarded as scientifically apropos or chic by one generation may appear to the next as esoteric or dull. It is this pervasive influence of intellectual *milieux* which makes the writing of scientific biography[2] so varied and so difficult. A biographer perforce writes of events in the past, but he cannot escape his own present, no matter how strong his will to do so.

As a result, reading a series of biographies devoted to a single subject is doubly beguiling. If the biographers were conscientious men, it is fascinating to see how increasing scholarship brings increasing knowledge of a subject. It is equally fascinating to see how different social and intellectual climates mark biographers. Recognizable period fashions in scientific biography emerge. This essay has as its purpose a description of some of those changing fashions. Examples will be drawn chiefly from works about William Harvey and about John Hunter. The lives of both were such, and their achievements of such an order of magnitude, that biographers are repeatedly drawn to them.[3] Placing their biographies in chronological order, much as paintings or sculptures are sometimes displayed, illuminates, in part, how scientific biographical practice has varied.[4] To be sure, such an array of biographical effort, like the array in an art gallery, may occasionally disconcert the man of taste—there are efforts which it may be kinder to ignore, since they are truly unworthy of being included within any artistic canon. Nonetheless, in order that the total record may be understood, honesty demands the exhibition of all specimens, however short some of them may fall from a preconceived aesthetic standard. Further, such an array makes it possible for us to profit as craftsmen from past achievements, for a chronological appraisal, with its attendant judgements, speaks to the point of what we now ask of scientific biographers.

Casual survey shows us that biographies have not been produced at a constant rate with respect to time. Periods of great biographical activity are interspersed with decades and even generations when such activity is very slight. Intermittent production is, first, a clue to the wellspring of biography, and, second, a hint about the way biographers react to their own times. The two factors are inextricably intertwined. The purpose of the biographer is close to that of the man of medicine; both aim to cheat or delay death.[5] Moreover, something akin to the classical law of supply and demand operates in the making of books, as well as in the production of more utilitarian goods. As in all human endeavours, several agencies surely are at work to condition the demand. Nicholson[6] discussing a long period of biographical silence has argued that in times of great religious faith, when the promise of an after-life was very real, biographies disappeared and hagiographies replaced them. The hagiographer hoped to encourage his readers to earthly lives of such piety and manifest good works that the blessings of the promised after-life would be assured. In periods of scepticism, however, Nicholson said the enduring hope for a life after death found expression in reading and writing biographical portraits. Even then a taste for moral didacticism may linger and so great a biographer as Dr Johnson saw as part of his task providing his readers with virtuous exemplars.

From time to time not only has general biographical activity ebbed, but interest in a particular figure or group of figures may also fall off. Selective declines can take place in a period when a large number of biographies are being produced. Sometimes a 'definitive' biography was published, temporarily discouraging further efforts; or it may be, too, that the man or his work temporarily lost intellectual favour. An additional factor may operate. As the appendix shows (p. 189) there were no nineteenth-century book-length biographies of William Harvey[7] before the 1870's. Harvey was not out of fashion at the time, nor had a definitive biography of him appeared; rather, the materials available to putative biographers could not be forced to fit the going biographical model. The 'lives-and-letters' format to which the nineteenth century clung could not easily be applied to Harvey.

Given a suitable biographical subject, biographers react in disparate ways to the demands of their times. A biographer may avoid or minimize certain aspects of his subject's work and life, for example, and since no one ever wants to write a dull book, silence may be accorded those things the biographer and his contemporaries regard as commonplace. Philosophical, intellectual or social taboos, as well, may operate as hidden censors. Of William Harvey's two

175

great works, *De motu cordis*[8] and *De generatione animalium*,[9] nearly all biographers used to discuss only the first. Those biographers who conceived Harvey as important only because of his announcement of the circulation of the blood found little in his other work to please them. What led Harvey to his great discovery, his frankly Aristotelian approach to the living system and his overt emphasis on the role of the circle, was glossed over or ignored, especially at times when the Aristotelian tradition was deplored or discounted. The dimmer status awarded *De generatione* or its omission from the Harvey canon occurred when practical results were in demand, since that work could be taken as markedly deficient in any 'correct' applications or conclusions. It was, further, a lack easily ascribable to Harvey's Aristotelian bias. However unjustly, the work was either mentioned and excused as the meandering lucubrations of a very old man,[10] or given a cursory appraisal that ignored the central position of the ideas Harvey there expressed, ideas which he held for much of his productive life.

For John Hunter other kinds of censorship were applied. Whatever else might be said of him, he was singularly lacking in the scholarly background thought by some to be a necessary prelude to a life of great accomplishment. One necrologist, pressed by the demands of his contemporaries and chafed by Hunter's lack of classical panache, invented it, and awarded it to him posthumously:

As a man of letters, independent of his profound scientific studies, he had traced the practice of surgery to the earliest ages. He was well acquainted with every practitioner mentioned by Pliny; with all the Greek and Roman authors who had written on the subject...

As a man well versed in antient history, the Egyptian chronology was familiar to him, as far as it related to the antiquity of anatomy. As a scholar distinguishably classic, he knew that Homer was an anatomist (at least that he had ideas of anatomy) as well as an Epic poet; nor less did he know that this noble science was entirely overwhelmed with barbarism by the Goths and Vandals, and most happily restored in the fourteenth century.[11]

Hunter, who found the classics pale stuff, indeed, might have been outrageously profane had he been able to read of his alleged classical distinction. His biographers, too, virtually ignored Hunter's syphilis, while exhaustively discussing other of his ailments, although Hunter's writings show that he deliberately infected himself with the disease to study it. That syphilis had consequences for him there can be little doubt, yet even those nineteenth-century biographers who mentioned his infection did not note it had changed the man's life in any way.

Early biographies and obituaries often do much to set a tone and establish a reputation on which subsequent treatments depend.[12] In this respect William Harvey was exceedingly fortunate, for his first biographer was John Aubrey, that sprightly commentator and acute observer who established English biography as one of the lively, minor arts.[13] Aubrey had been commissioned by Anthony Wood[14] to compile data for Wood's *Athenae Oxonienses*, a complex tapestry of a work demonstrating the wit and wisdom of post-Reformation Oxonians. Aubrey's magpie mind led him to assemble every telling scrap he could about his subjects. He made a great effort to verify what he had been told, and, even though at times he was too credulous, his naïveties cannot efface his genuine achievements. In the case of Harvey the results were especially happy, for not only had Aubrey known him for many years, but the two men were good friends. Aubrey produced a portrait of Harvey as economical as some Japanese brush paintings, and as incisive; he shows us William Harvey, a real man, in a real world. His biographical technique repays study, even today.[15]

While Harvey was fortunate in his first biographer, John Hunter encountered total disaster. Jessé Foot was a London surgeon associated for a time with the Middlesex Hospital, and then in private practice in Salisbury Street, Strand, and in Dean Street in Soho. Convinced of his own merits, he sought to rival the fame of John Hunter. Perhaps he was thwarted by his own limitations, for he certainly was never recognized to anything like the degree that Hunter had been. In frustrated revenge he attempted to undercut Hunter's reputation. His biography, an unremitting scurrilous scream, claimed Hunter's works to be useless plagiarisms, pinched, in part, from Tobias Smollett. Dipping his pen in vitriol Foot etched a picture of an embittered Hunter, belligerent and stupid.[16] Foot's canards were repudiated by subsequent biographers, but his performance did guarantee him the notoriety for which he so obviously hungered while alive. Posterity remembers four kinds of biographers: those who write a first, or an 'official' biography; those who produce a work which time reveals to have been patently false;

those who debunk a reputation; and, finally, those who produce a work of such captivating innovation that their efforts become models for succeeding generations of biographers. Foot was of the first three kinds, and every subsequent biographer of Hunter (despite the fact that copies of the work are now extraordinarily hard to come by) feels compelled to refute at least some of Foot's coarser allegations. Jessé Foot, if he is remembered at all, is infamous for his bile. It is the hard-working biographer's consolation that the name of John Aubrey has lasted, too, and with more gracious and endearing associations.

Even if subsequent biographers had no difficulty showing that Hunter was not as Foot has painted him, Hunter's personal habits still gave them pause. Early and mid-nineteenth-century biographers laboured like Hercules with the problem of Hunter's speech, for by the turn of the century, a great biographical reformation was in full swing. In 1791 James Boswell's incomparable life of Dr Samuel Johnson appeared. Johnson had been famous long before he died; his biography would have been widely read by his contemporaries even if it had been a poor performance. Boswell was, however, the consummate biographical artist and the work has become the most influential English biography ever written. Largely through judicious quotation and anecdotes Boswell presented Johnson as he saw him, scrofulous, untidy, portly, witty, literate, humane and lovable. So warm was the light in which Johnson was bathed that some have claimed him to be Boswell's creation. Moreover, so compelling is the biographical technique and the reader so caught in the portrait-narrative that it is easy to forget that the work treats Johnson in penetrating detail for only about a third of his life, and that in that period Boswell was with him for only a little more than two hundred days. This biography is a classical example of a correct union between method and subject, for the exhaustive reporting Boswell exploited and developed was essentially a literary device, uniquely suited to a literary man. The fun, the grandeur and the warmth of Johnson's reproduced speech comes, in part, from the sparkling array of rhetorical devices, the apt similes and metaphors, and the stunning sentence constructions which spellbound his hearers and charmed Boswell's readers. The quality of Johnson's thought, often arresting for its own sake, was enhanced by the frame in which Boswell exhibited it. Response to Boswell's achievement

178

was both immediate and continuing; the lesson derived from its success was that maximum portraiture resulted if the subject could be quoted directly. For a subject whose achievements were other than literary, however, or for a biographer who had not taken the precaution of assiduously capturing verbatim quotations from his subject's own lips, direct reporting presented obstacles. To fill the imagined void biographers resorted to concocted pastiches of excerpts from printed works, letters and diaries; the resulting in-artistic *découpages* were fobbed off on a public hungry for 'true-to-life' accounts.

Hunter's unrelieved profanity complicated any attempt to treat him according to the Boswellian pattern. Nineteenth-century bio-graphers who had known him, or who could interview those who had, limited by a canon of taste related to that which ruled the earlier, classical-minded necrologist, could not quote Hunter ver-batim. Attempts to report edited conversations were saltless, and, as a result, lives of Hunter often risked being as soggy and pallid as milk toast. For William Harvey the Boswellian method could not even be attempted. Beyond what Aubrey left there were no reported conversations of any length, and Harvey's scientific writings were mostly in Latin.

From our point of view, even when biographers resorted to quoting chunky excerpts from papers, lectures and letters, the effort misfired. The mid-nineteenth century had many scruples (or so it appears today) but they did not include accurate and verbatim quotation. Sections of letters and diaries thought too personal, or unflattering, or judged slanderous to those still alive, were deleted or altered, often without any indication that changes had been made. Our scholarly standards require painstaking attention to matters such as these; a subsequent biographer must regard Victorian quotations warily, until he has been able to check the originals for himself.

John Hunter was less unfortunate in his 'official' biography than the foregoing might imply. Drewry Ottley's *Life of John Hunter* published in 1835[17] is linearly organized, opening with Hunter's birth and closing with his death. It is to Ottley's credit that although the holocaust of Hunter's papers had already occurred, and Clift's accusations against Sir Everard Home as plagiarist were already widely circulated,[18] Ottley did not permit the story to destroy the general proportions of his life of Hunter. Nonetheless, a sense of proportion aside, the work is stolid and almost unrelieved. It sputters to life momentarily when Ottley quotes Hunter's letters to his friend and former student, Edward Jenner, for those letters show us to some extent what manner of man Hunter was. He emerges lively, ungrammatical, dogged in the pursuit of an experimental plan, and alive with a quizzical curiosity for all of the odd creatures of God's universe. That the misapplication of Boswell's method led to much biographical abuse there can be no doubt, but, in the case of Ottley's *Hunter*, the Boswell model served a good end.

Of course there were biographies written during the nineteenth century which ignored the Boswellian format. In fact, for medical biography, exceptions to the format were more numerous than they were, for example, in literary or political biography. Since many of the biographers were themselves medical men they must often have been unaware of prevailing literary fashions. Joseph Adams's *Memoirs of the life and doctrines of the late John Hunter, Esq.*[19] is a good case in point. That this work went through at least two editions testifies to popular interest in John Hunter, since even in 1818 some readers must have been aware of the drawbacks of the book. Although Adams stood outside the biographical mainstream, he did foreshadow one of its major preoccupations. The book is more than two hundred pages long; approximately one-third of them are comprised in the section 'Mr. Hunter's complaints and death' (pp. 139–201). Hunter's death was not without drama, and it certainly was of great interest to the medical fraternity, for he died of a heart attack while defending a policy position at a hospital board meeting. Adams's morbid interest was explainable, since Adams was himself a doctor. We write best what best we know, and doctors as biographers are no exception to the rule. Why does a biographer choose one subject and not another? What does a biography celebrate? Surely the answers are partly based on the accomplishments of the subject during his lifetime. It is a hard lesson for a biographer to remember, even though it has all the appearances of a dreary commonplace. Extended post-mortems are not necessarily biographically instructive. Nowadays dissection of life style and of the mind's adventure is considered far more illuminating.

Adams also provides convenient examples of how standards of the biographer's own times may affect his judgements and emphases.

In trying to account for Hunter's marriage to Ann Home, his chief concern (in a paragraph) was to explain why Hunter had been drawn to this gay, bright and charming young woman, although he did say, in one sentence, why she had married him:

...the gratification was reciprocal, as far as Mr. Hunter's studies were consistent with female delicacy: for, however dull many of the details of comparative anatomy might be, yet the habits of various tribes of animals never fail to interest every feeling mind. (pp. 65–6)

All evidence points to the marriage as a happy one; life with Hunter did indeed mean living under the same roof with a zoo and a museum, so one must conclude that if Ann Hunter had a burning interest in 'the habits of various tribes of animals' it must have helped. Are the details of comparative anatomy, or, for that matter, of any branch of learning, ever dull? Ann Hunter, intelligent mother of five, could not have found them so. But if this were the only basis for a sound marriage it must be unique in the long history of marriages. Regency-conditioned Adams granted women a minor role, their intelligence and interest hemmed in by their 'female delicacy', whatever that might be. Adams preferred the world of men and manly feeling, for he spent two pages discussing the long estrangement between John Hunter and his older brother, Dr William Hunter. He overbalanced that portion of his text, however, by the six pages he needed to delineate John's grief when his brother died. The catalogue might be continued. Adams succeeds in showing more of the concerns of 1818 than what it must have been like to have been John Hunter. We can only lay the book aside in frustration and disappointment, the promise of the title, *Memoirs of the life and doctrines*, betrayed by Adams's performance.

Whether nineteenth-century biographers wrote within or outside the Boswellian tradition, they had much in common, over and above their general preoccupation with last words and death-bed agonies. To explain certain characteristic traits of their subjects many of them relied on genealogical histories which descended in stately progression through their opening chapter or chapters. The youthful hero was shown as the culminating star in a crown handed down through a long line of worthies; the childlike versions of the traits that were to bring him adult fame were the result of the happy and almost purposive combination of those same traits by his forebears. Ancestral proclivities might be made to account, for example, for a hero's great interest in natural history, but it was more usual to emphasize inheritance of traits like courage, perseverance and devotion to duty, since it was these which were thought decisive in bringing a hero to greatness. Moreover, most biographers were concerned only with the external, the 'public' man. What went on in the recesses of the subject's mind was his own affair (excluding, nonetheless, certain manly emotions) into which the public should not pry. Intellectual and aesthetic motivations, or experimental aims, were usually ignored. It was this point of view as much as any other which fostered the nineteenth-century myth under which we labour still, that of the lonely, creative rebel, buttressed by his individuality against the common horde. The innovator appeared to rise unbidden (except for his judiciously selected ancestors), worked according to secret or hidden lights, usually counter to or ahead of his time, and then died. This point of view guided the biographer in the construction of the centre portion of the life. Here his dependence on the Boswellian method might become extreme, for the biographer became, not an interpreter, but a compiler of excerpts; if the subject were a scientist, biographers were usually content to report selected published, experimental conclusions. Had the hero suggested anything since shown to be scientifically 'wrong', chances were good that his biographer might omit it. In mid-century the biographers often failed to understand that to reject was to impoverish, although the whole direction of their biographical thrust was to burnish the image of their hero.

The two final chapters were reserved to make up for any deficiencies such delicate embargoes might have produced. Dying was what went on in the penultimate chapter; over-all character analysis was the topic for the last. After the biographer swept together a grab-bag of remarks about his subject's physical appearance and extra-scientific achievements in sports or cultural pursuits, the life was crowned with wreaths of testimonial letters. If the biography were especially well-made, the author reverted to providing additional proof for the moral traits that genealogical earnestness had catalogued in the opening. Supporting letters were usually supplied by the great and near-great who had known the deceased. The tone of these volumes is nearly as predictable as their format. Almost defiantly eulogistic, they marched steadily through the years, filling shelves with weighty panegyric. To be sure, these two- and three-volume compilations guaranteed a memorial to their subject almost as elaborate as that which Queen Victoria dedicated to her Consort, but it has also been claimed that the possibility of their creation must have added an extra dimension of horror to a potential subject's anticipation of death.

So unsatisfactory a pattern could not long endure. As the nineteenth century drew to a close concern for the life of the inner man began to show itself in small ways in the writing of biographies. The model persisted, to be sure, but the prohibitions of mid-century were slowly discarded, and the oppressive 'lives-and-letters' format was gradually replaced by a more fluid organization. If death still had its sting—and who would deny it?—the reader was subtly reminded that the adventure of the scientific mind is exciting, fascinating and complex. Moralistic grandeur and purposive forebears gave way to a consideration of more viable influences. Stephen Paget's *John Hunter, man of science*,[20] Robert Willis's *William Harvey*,[21] and the Harvey biography by D'Arcy Power,[22] as well, serve as good examples. From the many biographies produced towards the close of the century it almost appears that there was a general realization of how much the achievement of Boswell's *Johnson* depended on Boswell. There was far more to life than chunky quotations could reveal. For scientific biographers there was, however, a marked handicap, a handicap which persists. Loss of Boswell as model left the scientific biographer modelless; what was required was an innovator, a biographical artist, who could create a work uniquely designed to show the life of a man of science.

Perhaps the closest there came to such an innovator was Edmund Gosse, who in 1907 published his *Father and Son*.[23] The work intermingles autobiography with biography, but, in spite of the personal element, it is objective in tone and apparently without sentimentalization. Although only twenty-one years of the joint lives are covered, the reader is convinced that he knows what agonies 'The Father' suffered, and what were the conflicting elements that shaped 'The Son's' rebellion. The firm background of an extreme Calvinist faith heightened this 'record of a struggle between two temperaments, two consciences and almost two epochs'. In spite of the sharpness of the confrontation, the writing is illuminated, as is life itself, with incidents of genuine humour, merriment, and flashes of zest and desire for life. The work is a *tableau vivant* of, among other things, the impact of Darwinism on a traditional and devout, Fundamentalist biologist. It is biography of the highest sort.

Great as Gosse's work was, it could not become a model for scientific biography. For one thing, not every scientist labours in an era of tremendous theoretical upheaval—although it is surprising to realize how many have. Moreover, it is vouchsafed to few biographers to be privileged and intimate witnesses to and partners in so shattering a polarization. Gosse's biography-cum-autobiography remains a solitary eminence, without imitators, although study of it by a potential biographer is very rewarding.

What influence Gosse might have had was overshadowed by two other influences on the biographical mainstream. The first was the introduction of novelistic, or fiction-techniques (a usage which Gosse certainly prefigured) and the second was the appearance of what has since been termed 'Stracheyism'. In what follows each of these will be dealt with in turn. Both of the trends made discontent with the Victorian format greater, and that discontent increased the work a biographer had to do. Readers demanded that the biographer interpret, rather than eulogize. Interpretation could produce breaks from the linear construction on which biography had previously depended, since the structure of the biography could be used to heighten an interpretive pattern.

Moreover, novelistic or fictional techniques existed to hand, ready for borrowing by the biographers. Why they were available is not hard to discover. Concern with the inner, mental life and the subsequent widespread fascination with Freudian concepts led many novelists to exploit, or, at least, to give the appearance of exploiting autobiographical incidents. Literary critics developed the apparatus for dealing with these ostensibly biographical episodes within their fictional setting. Further, for a novelist to create a character it was no longer necessary to delineate him from birth to death. In the hands of a gifted writer selected portions of a fictional life were enough to create, for the reader, a man or woman in the round. The character talked, moved, and, above all, thought, in the world in which the novelist had placed him. It is not surprising that biographers, too, would turn similar techniques to account. If hypothetical characters could be endowed with verisimilitude, real lives should become graphic through the same kinds of treatment.

In the twentieth century biographers dealt with their subjects in these kinds of ways, but another biographical influence, that modelled on Lytton Strachey's creative performance in *Eminent Victorians* and later works also became important. Strachey had attached to his first biographical book an essay that served almost as a manifesto for subsequent biographers. In practice he sought to bring down certain heroes and heroines from their Victorian Olympus. What before might be regarded as biographical 'loosening' became, under the impact of Strachey, a mighty expansion; taboos which heretofore had been fastidiously skirted were now defiantly tossed aside. Psychological insights and 'honesty' were the writer's first obligation. Widespread as these ideals became, as well as the 'debunking' to which they led when grossly applied, they were initially of little use to scientific biographers. Strachey himself had failed twice in the application of his own tenets; once, when he wrote about Elizabeth and Essex, far remoter in time than Florence Nightingale or Dr Thomas Arnold; and, secondly, when he had planned his *Eminent Victorians* to include twelve subjects, half of whom were to be scientists. For them he intended a laudatory tone. His talents, perhaps, did not lend themselves to praise nearly as well as they did to the puncturing of over-inflated reputations, and he abandoned his original scheme. Strachey must also be regarded in this instance a victim of his own environment, for he lived in a period which openly admired science and scientists. Strachey was not alone in being unable to treat scientific figures in a mocking way. In spite of the subsequent rash of 'debunking' biographies, few of them dealt with scientists. Both Harvey and Hunter, for example, escaped that pillory, although biographical interest in them endured. Science and scientists, medicine and medical men continue to be well-regarded; we reserve our most trenchant criticism for the military, for the organization man, for the Snopeses, for the Widmerpools, or for pompous bureaucrats. Surely some of the tremendous acclaim given Strachey came about because he crystallized critical opinions almost before we realized that they were, indeed, our opinions. Nonetheless, as has been said, so critical an attitude could not conveniently be deployed upon scientists—they were, it was thought, humble or even crude persons, sprung from humble folk, working on humble problems. There is little to debunk in a man who spends most of his time in a littered or dirty laboratory. No one

185

would deny the scientist his own vision of the sublime, but it is a vision forever tied to earthly things for which even now some experience repugnance or aversions. Debunking medical men is often an impossibility, partly for psychological reasons. In the final analysis every biographer, like every other man, understands that some day he will be at the mercy of the arts and skill of a man of medicine; psychologically he cannot afford to debunk a prototype of those very practitioners on whom he may have to depend for physical comfort, or for a few extra months or years of life. While the reputation of the medical fraternity has indeed suffered eclipses in public esteem, in the past seventy years its sun has been in general ascent. Biographers cannot free themselves from that rising respect to become debunkers any more than they can purge themselves of their own ultimate dependence on medical practitioners.

Debunking aside, Strachey's influence permeated medical and scientific biography almost as much as Boswell's had. Intellectual biography is not only acceptable, but demanded by the twentieth-century reading public. It may well be that the revelation of what goes on in a man's mind accounts for our present-day fascination with biography. Where does the biographer get that kind of information? Fortunately for him, decades of scholarship have released vast hoards of material with which he can work. He can usually find —with assiduous searching in some cases—letters, diaries, and note-books by his subject, and he can supplement his discussion of this material with impressions and comments left by his subject's contemporaries. The biographer's task is now one of sensitive selection and arrangement, and, above all, of interpretation. If the success of the former requires the biographer as craftsman, the success of the latter depends upon the biographer as artist. The written record is essentially a neutral one. As the biographer contemplates a mass of neutral papers he realizes how dependent we are on the small gestures, on intonation, for our knowledge of the living person and for forming our judgements. Only acute insights will allow him to judge, for example, if a note has been made in haste, or with deliberation; in sorrow, or with bounding jubilation; in a casual moment, or with studied intent. Perhaps the rise of oral histories will help future biographers in their interpretive role, but past experience teaches us, too, that they may lead the biographer to new problems of complex and subtle kinds.

186

Further, it is not now unusual for a biography to 'read like a story', any more than it is unusual for a story to 'read like a biography'. Use of novelistic techniques is not without its dangers, for, in the hands of a less than inspired writer, the reader may lose both worlds. Louis Chauvois in a short life of Harvey published in 1957[24] opened his work with a chapter to describe a day in the life of Harvey. Borrowing heavily from D'Arcy Power's earlier work, and from his readings about the social conditions in Harvey's time, he sought to supply his readers with a glimpse of how Harvey might have lived. The method failed. If an opening chapter is to set the tone for what follows, one is here prepared for a domestic life, a *mise en scène* against which scientific matters will play, which is certainly not the case. After the supposed trivia of Harvey's day have been revealed (and some of Chauvois's account has since been shown to be factually wrong) the linear arrangement appears. Chauvois read Aubrey and used what he read, but much of Aubrey's original sprightliness has been lost. The effect of the first section is so deadening that only writing of the liveliest sort could have overcome his initial and self-imposed handicap.

John Kobler's *Reluctant surgeon: the life of John Hunter*[25] also used novelistic techniques. The work opens with a short section designed to portray imaginatively the young John Hunter, and to hint at some of the intellectual problems that he was to face as an adult. The introductory passage is not long, and the book moves quickly into the more usual biographical mode. The extent of Kobler's departure from the novelist's format (which the introduction promises) can be seen in the expositional passages designed to show the reader what medical practice was like before and during the days of the Hunters. True novelistic technique would doubtless have revealed much of the same material less directly than the straight exposition Kobler employed. It is to Kobler's credit that he avoided making up conversations to support his biographical interpretation. In general, whenever such supposed conversations are contrived in a biography they convey an interpretation about the subject that is either too simplistic or completely wrong. Having finished the book Kobler's readers certainly know more of what it must have been like to have been John Hunter, and have some insight, too, into how Hunter worked, both as a medical man and as a comparative anatomist. Is the work the definitive biography of

187

Hunter for our time? The answer is clearly 'No'. It is the play of the biographer's imagination which kindles and enlivens a subject; but for scientific biographies his imagination must forever be bound by the stern discipline of verifiability. Novelistic techniques do, indeed, have a role in the writing of biographies, but, if used less than prudently, the biographer runs the risk of finding his work neglected by the very audience he hoped to address.

Not all contemporary biographers have adopted novelistic techniques. Sir Geoffrey Keynes's *Life of William Harvey*[26] patiently corrects the older biographical records and presents much newly discovered material with painstaking scholarship. Future biographers of Harvey—and that there will be future biographers cannot be doubted—will have to begin with Keynes. Walter Pagel's *William Harvey's biological ideas*[27] published a year after Keynes's work exhibits our predilection for intellectual history. The mind's adventure for Harvey presents a fascinating panorama into which every reader enters with profit.

Modern biographers, as Pagel demonstrates, realize that the mind, however detached or ahead of its time, does not work in a vacuum. If scientific biographies have been popular in the past, and some of them have been very popular, it is partly because we realize that the biographical mode can most usefully explore all the factors which impinge upon intellectual achievement. The model biography of this sort has still to be written, and it may well be that it never will, but that cannot discourage us. Scientific biographies are needed; for many major figures we presently can rely only on older works, not a few of which suffer from some of the same drawbacks we have encountered in works devoted to Harvey and Hunter. The minds of scientific men are both complex and various, and herein lies the secret of our endless fascination with biography. Art galleries, in addition to what they display, hold forth always the bright promise of future works. Portraits, still-lifes or sculptures—we know that we have not yet exhausted them all, and that our own intellectual adventure will be enriched by those scientific biographies yet to come.

APPENDIX

Biographies, in chronological order, of William Harvey (1578–1657) and John Hunter (1728–93) on which this study is based.

I. WILLIAM HARVEY

John Aubrey, *Brief Lives*, see Keynes (1966, op. cit., below, note 17, pp. 431–7) for the complete transcription of the text.

James Paget, *Records of Harvey: in extracts from the journals of the Royal Hospital of St. Bartholomew*, London: J. Churchill, 1846, pp. 43.

J. H. Aveling (coll. and ed.), *Memorials of Harvey: including a letter and autographs in facsimile*, London: J. and A. Churchill, 1875, pp. 27.

Joh. Hermann Baas, *William Harvey, der Entdecker des Blutkreislaufs und dessen anatomisch-experimentelle Studie über die Herz- und Blutbewegung bei den Thieren*, Stuttgart: F. Enke, 1878, pp. 116.

R. Willis, *William Harvey: a history of the discovery of the circulation of the blood*, London: Kegan Paul, 1878, pp. 350.

D'Arcy Power, *William Harvey*, London: T. Fisher Unwin, 1897, pp. 283 (Master of Medicine Series).

S. Weir Mitchell, *Some memoranda in regard to William Harvey, M.D.*, New York [privately printed], 1907, pp. 45.

S. Weir Mitchell, *Some recently discovered letters of William Harvey with other miscellanea. With a bibliography of Harvey's works by Charles Perry Fisher*, Philadelphia [privately printed], 1912, pp. 59.

R. B. Hervey Wyatt, *William Harvey (1578-1657)*, London: L. Parsons, 1924, pp. 214 (The Roadmaker Series).

Archibald Malloch, *William Harvey*, New York: P. B. Hoeber, 1929, pp. 103.

Wilmot Parker Herringham, *The life and times of Dr. William Harvey*, New York: P. B. Hoeber, [1933], pp. 83 [reprinted from *Annals of Medical History*].

H. P. Bayon, *William Harvey, physician and biologist: his precursors, opponents and successors*, Parts i–v, London: Taylor and Francis, 1938–39, pp. 185 [reprinted from *Annals of Science*].

Geoffrey Keynes, *The personality of William Harvey*, Cambridge: The University Press, 1949, pp. 48.

Louis Chauvois, *William Harvey: his life and times: his discoveries: his methods*, London: Hutchinson, 1957, pp. 271.

Kenneth J. Franklin, *William Harvey, Englishman 1578-1657*, London: MacGibbon and Kee, 1961, pp. 151.

Kenneth D. Keele, *William Harvey: the man, the physician, and the scientist*, London: T. Nelson, 1965, pp. 244.

Geoffrey Keynes, *The life of William Harvey*, Oxford: Clarendon Press, 1966, pp. 483.

Walter Pagel, *William Harvey's biological ideas: selected aspects of historical background*, New York: Hafner, 1967, pp. 394.

189

II. JOHN HUNTER

Jessé Foot, *The life of John Hunter*, London: T. Becket, 1794, pp. 287.

Everard Home, 'A short account of the author's life, by his brother-in-law' in John Hunter, *A treatise on the blood, inflammation, and gunshot wounds*, pp. xii–lxvii, London: G. Nicol, 1794.

Joseph Adams, *Memoirs of the life and doctrines of the late John Hunter, Esq.*, 2nd ed., London: J. Callow and J. Hunter, 1818, pp. 262.

Drewry Ottley, 'The life of John Hunter, F.R.S.' in James F. Palmer (ed.), *The works of John Hunter F.R.S. with notes*, vol. 1, London: Longman, Rees, Orme, Brown, Green & Longman, 1835, pp. xv–xxiv, 1–198. There is also a separate publication, *The life of John Hunter, F.R.S.*, Philadelphia: Haswell, Barrington & Haswell, 1839, pp. 139.

George R. Mather, *Two great Scotsmen: the brothers William and John Hunter*, Glasgow: J. Maclehose, 1893, pp. 251.

Stephen Paget, *John Hunter: man of science and surgeon (1728–1793)*, London: T. Fisher Unwin, 1897, pp. 272 (Masters of Medicine Series).

George C. Peachey, *A memoir of William and John Hunter*, Plymouth: W. Brendon, 1924, pp. 313.

Jane M. Oppenheimer, *New aspects of John and William Hunter. I. Everard Home and the destruction of the John Hunter manuscripts. II. William Hunter and his contemporaries*, London: W. Heinemann, 1946, pp. 188.

S. Roodhouse Gloyne, *John Hunter*, Edinburgh: E. & S. Livingstone, 1950, pp. 104.

John Kobler, *The reluctant surgeon: a biography of John Hunter*, New York: Doubleday, 1960, pp. 359.

NOTES AND REFERENCES

1   V. Woolf, 'Sterne' in *Collected essays*, ed. L. Woolf, vol. 3, p. 86, London: Hogarth Press, 1967.

2   Sometimes the term 'scientific biography' is used to describe those biographies that emphasize the psycho-analytical treatment of the biographee. In this paper the term is used to designate those works written about men and women whose chief preoccupation or fame was derived from their scientific activity, without regard for whether or not the biographer used psycho-analytical insights. Such usage is in line with the designation 'literary biography' for those works about people whose great fame came from their writings, without raising the question of the literary merit of the biography.

3   Full citations for the biographies on which this essay is chiefly based are given in the Appendix, where they are listed in chronological order.

4　The history of scientific biography has not been studied exhaustively. A recent discussion is J. Z. Fullmer, 'Davy's biographers: notes on scientific biography', *Science* 1967, **155**, 285–91. A shorter paper is Harold I. Sharlin, 'The scientist in biography', *Bulletin of the Atomic Scientists*, Chicago 1963, **19**, 27–8. A. E. Rodin, 'The influence of biography on medical fame', *Canad. med. Assoc. J.* 1960, **83**, 1382–3, discusses some of the aims of a biographer, in conjunction with a book review of five biographies of different subjects.

Literary biography, in contrast, has been splendidly served by Richard D. Altick's *Lives and letters: a history of literary biography in England and America*, New York: A. A. Knopf, 1965. I have relied on his general interpretation. In addition Leon Edel's *Literary biography*, New York: Doubleday, 1959, and John A. Garraty, *The nature of biography*, New York: Vintage Press, 1964, were also of help. Edgar Johnson, *One mighty torrent: the drama of biography*, New York: Macmillan, 1955, offers a sampler and instructive guide to many great biographies.

5　J. Russell Reynolds, *The Harveian oration delivered at the Royal College of Physicians, London, on October 18, 1884*, London: J. and A. Churchill, 1884 [the work is unpaginated], pointed out that, 'There is a widely spread human struggle against allowing the bodies of those we have known, and reverenced, and loved, to merge into the common earth. We set up our barriers against it; we entomb, and we embalm;...and we utter a parable, as we do so, of our regard not only for the bodies, but for the lives of those individual men, as we tell of, or come to know them, in the thousand biographies, that surround us, each one of which is, in its very essence, "a feeble struggle with death" ' p. [3].

6　H. Nicholson, *The development of English biography*, pp. 17–19, London: Hogarth Press, 1959.

7　Part of the nineteenth-century biographical impetus for book-length study of Harvey may have been drawn off by the Harveian Orations, many of which embodied biographical material. W. J. Bishop and F. N. L. Poynter ('The Harveian orations, 1656–1947. A study in tradition', *Br. med. J.* 1947, **2**, 622–3) briefly review the works produced under the sponsorship of this venerable foundation. Close reading of all of them would doubtless provide an interesting survey of how fashions in biography and medical writing have changed. In the early part of the nineteenth century the Oration was in poor repute. *The Lancet*, 29 June 1833 (1832–1833, **2**, 452) complained that 'The Harveian Oration was delivered at the College of Physicians...by Dr. Paris...It consisted of the usual twaddle uttered on such occasions. The meeting ended in a jollification, and the proceedings have been duly recorded in the theatrical portion of the columns of the daily journals.' Eventually, however, the Orations reached a high standard. Some of those useful in connection with this study were as follows:

(*a*) Henry W. Acland, *The Harveian Oration 1865*, London: Macmillan, 1865, pp. 85.

(b) Arnold Chaplin, *The Harveian Oration on medicine in the century before Harvey delivered at the Royal College of Physicians of London, on October 18th, 1922*, London: J. Bale and Danielsson [n.d.], pp. 28.

(c) John William Ogle, *The Harveian Oration, 1880. Delivered June 25th*, London [no publisher given], 1881, pp. 209.

(d) George E. Paget, *The Harveian Oration 1866. Delivered June 26*, Cambridge: Deighton Bell & Co., 1866, pp. 49.

(e) Joseph Frank Payne, *Harvey and Galen. The Harveian Oration delivered before the Royal College of Physicians October 19, 1896*, London: Henry Froude, 1897, pp. 52.

(f) G. Owen Rees, *The Harveian Oration delivered at the Royal College of Physicians June 26, 1869*, London: Longmans, Green & Co., 1869, pp. 48.

(g) J. Russell Reynolds (1884), op. cit. (above, note 5) [unpaginated].

(h) George Rolleston, *The Harveian Oration of 1873*, London: Macmillan, 1873, pp. 90.

(i) Herbert R. Spencer, *William Harvey, obstetric physician and gynaecologist, being the Harveian Oration delivered at the Royal College of Physicians, October 18th, 1921*, London: Harrison, 1921, pp. 40.

8   William Harvey, *Exercitatio anatomica de motu cordis et sanguinis in animalibus*, Frankfurt: W. Fitzer, 1628. There are many editions of this work; Kenneth J. Franklin (*Movement of the heart and blood in animals...*, Oxford: Blackwell, 1957) provides both Latin and English texts.

9   William Harvey, *Exercitationes de generatione animalium*, Amsterdam: L. Elzevir, 1651. A convenient and useful edition is *Anatomical exercitations, concerning the generation of living creatures*: etc. [translator unknown], London: O. Pulleyn, 1653.

10 See in this connection Pagel (1966, see Appendix, p. 189) who documents (pp. 327–52) the careful studies that show Harvey to have written this work shortly after he published *De motu cordis*. See also C. Webster, 'Harvey's *De generatione*: its origins and relevance to the theory of circulation', *Br. J. Hist. Sci.* 1967, 3, 262–74.

11 Anon., 'Obituary of considerable persons; with biographical anecdotes', *Gent. Mag.* 1793, 63, 964–5.

12 A. E. Rodin (1960, op. cit., above, note 4) concluded that 'The best formula for medical immortality is the combination of a great doctor and an excellent contemporary biographer' (p. 1383).

13 Aubrey's *Brief Lives* was not published until 1813. Since then there have been many editions. A recent one is that edited by Oliver Lawson Dick, Ann Arbor: University of Michigan Press, 1957. The complete transcript of Aubrey's section on William Harvey is included as an appendix to Sir Geoffrey Keynes's *The Life of William Harvey* (see Appendix, p. 189), pp. 431–7. Obviously Aubrey could have little influence on biography while his work was unpublished. Even the first issue of the text was edited to a certain degree, but excision and textual modification could not rob the work of its charm, or of its penetrating biographical techniques.

14 He fictitiously styled himself Anthony-à-Wood, and was markedly un-

grateful for Aubrey's efforts on his behalf, calling him 'a shiftless person, roving and magotie-headed, and sometimes little better than crased'. Cited from Altick (1965, above, note 4), p. 24.

15 Perhaps it should be pointed out that the spectrum of Harvey biographies, by and large, is livelier than many another; John Aubrey's influence, however diluted by time, is perpetuated still.

16 Jessé Foot [the Elder] (1744–1826) wrote several other biographies, in addition to that of Hunter. One was devoted to his friend, a Bowdlerizer of *Hamlet*, Arthur Murphy; a second was devoted to a joint life of Andrew Robinson and his wife, the Countess of Strathmore. Robinson was a celebrated rapist and duellist. Because Foot had spent several years in the West Indies, he felt qualified to publish a popular pamphlet defending the way the West Indian planters treated their slaves. He also attacked Wilberforce and the abolition party. His greatest wrath, however, was always reserved for Hunter.

17 The work forms the introductory portion to the four-volume *The works of John Hunter F.R.S. with notes*, ed. James F. Palmer (see Appendix, p. 190).

18 Oppenheimer (1946, see Appendix, p. 190) covers this famous case in detail.

19 Adams (1818), see Appendix, p. 190.

20 Paget (1897), see Appendix, p. 190.

21 Willis (1878), see Appendix, p. 189.

22 Power (1897), see Appendix, p. 189.

23 There have been many editions of this work. *Father and son: a study of two temperaments* was first published anonymously in October 1907. A Penguin edition appeared in 1949.

24 Chauvois (1957), see Appendix, p. 189.

25 Kobler (1960), see Appendix, p. 190. In this discussion I have ignored Garet Rogers [pseud.], *Brother surgeons, a novel*, London: Putnam, 1957, a fictionalized story based on the lives of John and William Hunter. Since it is more fiction than biography it falls outside the general scope of this paper.

26 Keynes (1966), op. cit. (above, note 13).

27 Pagel (1967), see Appendix, p. 189.

11 The History of Scientific and Social Medicine

EDWIN CLARKE

The evolution of medical historiography is as fascinating a study as the history of medicine itself. Since the earliest-known contribution, contained in *On ancient medicine*,[1] written by one of the Hippocratic physicians, there have been variations in its purposes, aims, and techniques. Thus the author of this ancient Greek work, although sharing with the modern historian an interest in the past, was not concerned with ancient medical opinion *per se*. Rather he used the latter as a means of evaluating contemporary practice in the light of previous experience and so, hopefully, of improving it. Medicine itself manifests constant change and this, on a smaller scale, is also true of the historiography of it. It is, for example, reasonable to suggest that just as some of Osler's approaches to clinical medicine are now outmoded, some of his historical methodology is likewise out of date.

In view of this modification there is a need today to consider the form that the history of medicine as a discipline might take, so that whatever developments occur in the future will, it is hoped, be orderly and planned and in the direction of improvement. The history of medicine as presently constituted, however, is protean in its make-up. Medicine as a science and an art makes contact with most human activities, and thus to depict its history adequately, each must be represented. Yet at the same time it is usually accepted that a sprawling subject may lead to a dissipation of energy and resources and perhaps to the creation of unconnected groups of specialized workers.

The following paper explores the possibility of avoiding these hazards by defining one portion of medical history which might be thought of as its central theme and which could therefore receive most attention. As was pointed out by Georg Urdang in 1927 concerning the history of pharmacy, the most urgent problems pertaining to any branch of study are first the organization of the discipline and second the demarcation of subject-matter boundaries.[2] It is the second with which we shall be concerned.

II

The history of medicine as a modern teaching and research discipline did not appear until the late eighteenth century,[3] its origins, along with those of the general historical profession, being attributable mainly to romanticism and humanism. Its subsequent erratic career through the nineteenth century has been traced by Heischkel,[4] Rosen[5] and Miller[6] and during the first few decades the approach was often doxographical rather than historical. Moreover, as in the case of the Hippocratic writer, indulgence in it was likely to be pragmatic because the medical concepts of the first third of the century were often those of earlier centuries and thus a study of them would help to extend the physician's professional skill. At the same time, however, the study of medical history for its own sake was advocated throughout the nineteenth century, with disappointing results on the whole.[7]

The history of medicine as an academic department of learning, although fostered especially in Germany, Austria and France at the end of the nineteenth century, did not become wholly effective until 1905 when a chair in the subject was created in the University of Leipzig and Karl Sudhoff, the first incumbent, began to build up the Institut für die Geschichte der Medizin.[8] Further developments up to the second milestone, the appointment in 1932 of Henry E. Sigerist as Director of the Institute of the History of Medicine in the Johns Hopkins University, and then up to the Second World War, are recounted by Rosen.[9]

Throughout these periods and up to the present day, a campaign has been conducted to popularize the history of medicine, both as a subject to be represented in the medical school by teaching and research, and also as a study to be cultivated to some degree by all practitioners of medicine. Naturally enough a large body of literature, consisting of papers with titles such as 'The value of medical history', 'The present need for the study of…', has been generated.[10]

Agitation for the acceptance of the history of medicine as a respect-
able and rewarding topic which should engage the attentions of both
medical students and practitioners, continues to be made.[11] This
must necessarily indicate that in certain parts of the world, at least,
the unconvinced are still very much in evidence. Voluble and
plaintive attempts to vindicate a subject are themselves indicative
of the opposition it induces or the lack of enthusiasm for it. It may
also reveal the historian's own doubts and it may induce in the
minds of others, uncertainties and suspicions which did not previously exist. After all, no one has to justify the presence in the
medical curriculum of the essential scientific or clinical disciplines.
Better by far to proceed without repeated pleas and apologies, and
it is hoped that this book by suggesting new levels and topics of
scholarship may help to make this easier.

The status of medical history, of course, varies in each country,
due to a variety of local circumstances. The fact, however, that in
Britain the recent *Report* of the Royal Commission on Medical
Education,[12] whilst suggesting widespread and revolutionary
changes, makes no reference whatsoever to the history of medicine,
means that in this country at least the efforts of those who wish to
promote the discipline as a part of the system of medical education
or as a postgraduate study, have been largely in vain. That in this
Report, which is based on a wide sampling of opinion, medical history should not even be considered worthy of mention is a highly
significant and, for the historian of medicine, a disappointing
development. A similar problem, but not nearly so serious, seems to
exist to some extent in the United States where the place of history
in medical education was persuasively argued by Rosen twenty years
ago,[13] and by others both before him and since,[14] but it is still being
sought today.[15] In view of this disappointing state of affairs in
Britain, and perhaps elsewhere, it is essential to discover why it
exists. Although local factors must be kept in mind, the following
discussion will transcend national confines.

III

First of all, the basic thesis that a knowledge of the history of a
professional subject is of advantage to its practitioners can be
accepted here, even though there are many who would not be wholly

196

in agreement with it. In the case of medicine, they would probably point out that if all other factors are equal, it is difficult to prove that a physician or surgeon who has studied the history of medicine is necessarily more capable in his practice than his colleague who has not, when they are judged by the criterion of therapeutic achievement. It is not intended to deal with this argument here for it has been discussed over and over again in the many articles alluded to already.[16]

As pointed out above (p. vii) and elsewhere,[17] a problem which the history of medicine faces relates to its large size and its widespread boundaries. Although it may not have the dimensions of the history of science, it is one of the larger bodies of historical knowledge. Interpreted in its broadest sense, it encompasses everything that has ever taken place in medicine throughout the world. But it also includes the contacts medicine has made with art, bibliography, literature, philosophy, religion, science, technology and a host of other subjects. Furthermore, some would include within its capacious confines the histories of some of the life technologies such as nursing, pharmacy and veterinary medicine, or at least some parts of them. The end result is a diffuse, unwieldy mass of data which no one individual could ever encompass, even superficially. Although each component has a role to play somewhere in history, it is pertinent to ask if they should all be given equal emphasis.

A helpful and pertinent analogy can be made here with certain other branches of learning such as anthropology, archaeology, sociology or ethnology which began with wide confines but which have gradually consolidated or fragmented to produce more clearly defined entities; the same is true of certain medical sciences although the reverse is also operative, as for example the blurring of the boundaries between topics studied at the molecular level, and between anatomy and physiology, although here the separation was an artificial one, created for pedagogic purposes. It is therefore reasonable to suggest that a process of comparable consolidation might perhaps eventually take place in the case of the history of medicine. In most research, both scientific and scholarly, there is the frequent need for convergence upon a small area of knowledge, rather than a diffusion over a wide one with all the consequent evils. In the case of the history of medicine it might be advantageous for its practitioners to define more specifically an essential and limited portion, without, of course, either creating artificial or rigid boundaries, or entirely neglecting the remaining parts, or losing sight of medicine itself as a corporate body of knowledge. They could then concentrate their efforts upon it and leave the areas considered more peripheral, and therefore less essential, to the attention of others, or, should the need arise, study them in collaboration with experts from the particular overlapping field.

If it is agreed that it may be better to pay more attention to one part of the history of medicine than to others, the next consideration is to decide which this should be. The problem can best be tackled by inquiring which of the topics usually included under the term 'medical history' can, with advantage, be considered less essential.

(1) First of all, most will admit that although the life technologies are closely associated with the practice of medicine, they can be very readily excluded from its history. Thus the history of pharmacy, dentistry and of nursing are now autonomous branches of learning, closely linked however with the mother subject, medical history. In the case of pharmacy, overlap is bound to occur in the fields of materia medica, therapeutics and pharmacology but the more technical aspects of pharmacy require their own historical discipline; it is noteworthy that historians of pharmacy have recently been discussing the contents and boundaries of their discipline.[18] The history of technology itself is another young and developing branch of learning and as pointed out elsewhere (p. 167) the historian of medicine may learn from its organization and methodology.

(2) Medical bibliography is another technology to be discussed here. It is an important specialty, ancillary to the history of medicine, and in the past has often been considered part of it; the relationships of these two are discussed elsewhere in this volume (pp. 307–8). As it becomes an increasingly precise and more complex technique, however, it seems natural that bibliography should be left to those who specialize in it. The role of these experts in relation to the history of medicine is comparable to the relationship to clinical medicine of the pharmacologist who identifies, describes and classifies therapeutic agents and establishes standards of purity for them. The bibliographer does likewise for the historian of medicine, but with books.

(3) Medicine today is represented in most human activities and this was also the case in the past. Thus, the contacts made between

medicine and the fine arts, drama, law, literature, music, philosophy, religion, and other bodies of non-scientific knowledge have been many and various. For a balanced and overall view of medicine a consideration of them is essential in teaching and in research, even though only a small problem is being investigated; Sigerist's book on *Civilization and disease*[19] exemplifies this approach. However, the deeper historical excavation of some of these interdisciplinary areas is best undertaken by the person already an expert in them, working, if necessary, in collaboration with a medical historian or advised by him. Thus the most appropriate person to discuss the medical aspects of art history is an art historian,[20] aided where necessary by a person who can interpret the medical features. The same is true for the other subjects and the non-medical expert can often, if necessary, study the relevant medical subject in order to increase his appreciation of technical data and so assist his research. Although occasionally a medically qualified person may have sufficient skill to act as both the non-medical and the medical expert, the readily available evidence in the form of uninspired and inexpert books and periodical articles indicates the more frequent situation where, unknown perhaps to himself, the medical man is only the expert in medicine. The reverse also pertains and the non-medical person may investigate material he too is not equipped to handle. There is no doubt that the history of medicine has a place for a large variety of workers, medical and non-medical, but each must be aware of his limitations and must avoid problems for which he does not possess the requisite skills.

(4) Some of the special topics at present thought to be part of medical history may voluntarily move away from it. This is perhaps happening to palaeopathology which, although represented in this volume (Kerley, pp. 135–56), is now attracting the attention of the anthropologist more than in the past. Perhaps this is the type of specialty of which there may be several, where the professional of the future will have his basic training in the non-medical field but will also acquire experience in selected parts of medicine only, in this instance anatomy, pathology, radiology, etc. Likewise as the teaching of Greek and Latin declines in certain countries, it may be that detailed studies in Graeco-Roman medicine will be taken over completely by classicists collaborating with medical men.

(5) The problems relating to the diseases suffered by famous

individuals and the closely allied considerations of the effect of disease on historical events have always been popular with medical men. This type of theoretical or 'armchair' diagnosis often leads to unhistorical, unscientific and unwarranted speculation, although clearly it is an important part of the history of medicine as it brings the subject into direct contact with general history. Unfortunately many contributions to it by doctors have been characterized either by uncritical theorizing on disease or by an equally sinister lack of historical sense. On the other hand, this activity seems on rare occasions to have been successful;[21] this, however, is a notable exception. Once again collaboration between a general and medical historian is more likely to guarantee the respectability of the end result, rather than leaving this topic entirely within the confines of medical history.

(6) Finally there is the vast amount of uncritical, repetitive, biographical, institutional and anecdotal writing, the indulgence in what is often called the history of medicine but which is more accurately termed 'medical antiquarianism'. It is this portion of 'the history of medicine' which receives the greatest amount of criticism from historians and others, and justifiably so, if its products are published. The part-timer is mainly responsible for this, yet he will always have an important role to play and the discipline could not flourish without his support and enthusiasm. Furthermore he is often better able to write on the technical aspects of the history of his special field of medicine than the historian of medicine although he may not have enough general historical background knowledge of the scientific data he is handling. Perhaps some method of utilizing his interest more profitably, for example by collaboration with experts, would help, as well as a method of exerting a stricter control over his writings. Unfortunately, it is widely assumed that whereas only certain individuals can practise a scientific subject successfully because of the appropriate skills and training needed, anyone can study and write history without any formal tuition. It is mostly this naïve ignorance of the principles of historical method and of historiography that accounts for so much of the third-rate history of medicine produced today.

Concerning the publication of certain types of medical history, it is said that Sigerist believed a professional medical historian should be complimented not only for the books and articles he inspires others to write, but also for those he prevents from being printed. In branches of learning such as archaeology, general history, and in most of the humanities, the part-timer or amateur has found his place and makes a valuable contribution. No doubt the same will eventually pertain in the history of medicine, just as is now happening in the history of science, and this too will help to sharpen the 'image' of medical history. No one is barred and all are welcome, so long as the nature of the history of medicine as a discipline is understood, personal limitations are recognized if publication is contemplated and good history is achieved. The scheme of training for part-time participants in medical history provided by the Worshipful Society of Apothecaries of London may be an excellent method of bringing this about.

Medical antiques, medals, stamps and many other artifacts usually have little to offer the medical historian proper but their careful collection is essential if all aspects of medicine in the past are to be preserved.

IV

Having suggested that less emphasis might be placed upon a number of seemingly extraneous components of the popularly accepted constellation comprising 'the history of medicine', the essential core of the subject can be revealed. As all of medicine and its associated technologies are directed towards man in health and in disease, it would seem to follow naturally that the history of medicine should have the same nucleus. This in essence means that medical history proper should be compounded of all the scientific and social aspects of human health and of disease. It can be thought of as fundamentally the history of the medical sciences and of the history of medicine in society. There are thus two parts to consider.

(1) Concerning the history of the medical sciences, both preclinical and clinical subjects are envisaged, with the main emphasis being placed on the growth of scientific, medical thought. This is in keeping with developments in the sister discipline, the history of science, where increasing vigour and acceptability today is in part due to a concentration upon the evolution of scientific concepts. There seems every reason to suppose that a similar approach will add respectability and depth to the history of medicine where it is

needed. For the implementation of this orientation there are two inseparably interwoven parts of the topic to be taken into account: first, the history of medical science *per se*, and second, its multitudinous background. The first and foremost is the tracing by critical and penetrating analysis the genesis, evolution, and occasional decline, of scientific ideas in medicine. The second is the study of the economic, financial, philosophic, political, social, technological and other factors which have influenced this progression, or regression, and may be included under the generic term 'social' for want of a better collective word. Clearly these influences may be as important as the scientific advance itself and as medicine and science develop greater social significance and complexity, they will obviously become of increasing concern to the historian. This field has yet to be explored fully. It involves the investigation of the well-known 'interplay of social and internal factors' to which Shryock in particular has contributed so much[22] and it aims to produce Rosenberg's 'historical sociology of medical knowledge' (p. 31). Although the historiography of ideas will be the central theme, non-ideas such as individuals, epidemics and other events (Temkin, p. 1) naturally are included here.

One of the potential hazards in the study of the history of the medical sciences, as in the historical analysis of other sciences, is that workers will produce scholarly monographs which are related neither to each other nor to the many and varied associated events outside their chosen subject. The evil effects of the fragmentation of the medical sciences themselves which encourages the creation of closed intellectual groups must be avoided in the historical investigation of them. The 'social' aspects of the history of the medical sciences will help to avoid such an unsatisfactory outcome and to make sure that impeccable objective history, acceptable to the most critical general historian, is being produced by historians of medicine and not just an uncritical record of facts. They should also remind us to examine past achievements in terms of their contemporary ideas, concepts, and related problems, and not of ours today. And when investigating the accomplishments of an individual, historians of medicine must, like historians of science, first attempt to discover the meaning to this person of what he wrote. They should then, as Hall suggests, proceed to compare and generalize and thus, hopefully, to produce 'true history'.[23] In addition, some problems of historical interpretation and explanation may be analysable from points of view that Kuhn has discussed for the history of science.[24] He also points out that when the historian of science begins to think of historical rather than scientific problems, then the history of science becomes history; this can be the case in the history of medicine too.

(2) The portion of the central nucleus just discussed deals with medicine as a science. But medicine is also an art and unlike other sciences it is concerned primarily with human beings. The second portion therefore of the essential part of medical history, which is, of course, intimately associated with the above, deals with the multifarious aspects of the history of medicine in society; the history of human society in its struggle with disease; the maintenance of health; the history of the medical profession in society; the way in which medicine has reached its position and status in the complex social structure of today. Again, there is the interaction of the external and internal factors influencing medicine. This is also a very large area of the history of medicine in need of much deeper and varied study, some aspects of which are discussed elsewhere by Rosenberg (pp. 22–35), Roberts (pp. 36–56), and McKeown (pp. 57–74).

In many instances the practitioner of the history of medical science and of the history of medicine in society will be purveying intellectual history, for, like the historian of science, he too should be an intellectual historian. In addition to being concerned with the content and structure of ideas and concepts he will, as F. L. Baumer puts it, also 'study...their development and relation to each other in time, how and why they appear and spread at a particular time, and their effects on concrete historical situations'.[25] He will, in sum, wish to examine their *Zeitgeist*, their effects on the world at large, and their causation; and carry out '...a tough analysis...of both the process and dynamics of intellectual change within a relatively short period of history'.[26] Broad surveys are, of course, needed but it is the convergence, as with a microscope, upon a problem, as for example by the case history technique (pp. 211–32), together with comparative studies of related branches of thought, and external influences, especially social, which will be of the greatest value in helping to build the history of medicine into a discipline of solid scholarship.

As Baumer concludes, intellectual history gives '...insights into the historical process as a whole. And to see the whole, if only dimly, is, after all, the aim of education.'[27] This would seem to be a legitimate objective for the history of scientific and social ideas in medicine.

Having advocated the pruning of topics often judged to be part of medical history, in order to achieve greater compactness, it might be thought paradoxical to suggest the inclusion of more, as this book does, such as medical anthropology (Brothwell, pp. 114–34; Hackett, pp. 99–111) and historical demography (McKeown, pp. 57–74). But these and others are just the kinds of scientific, para-medical themes that the new history of medicine must cultivate. Its past has been mainly built on literary and bibliographical attachments and these although important in some aspects of the subject are not enough today. The more connections the history of medicine has with scientific disciplines, the more it is likely to prosper. It must, of course, also achieve close contact with the history of science, especially of biology, and with the history of technology, yet preserving its autonomy.

V

Here then is a suggested method of realigning the history of medicine: a concentration of talent and effort upon all parts of the history of the scientific and sociological aspects of man in health and in disease, which in practice implies a study of the history of the medical sciences and of medicine in society. It would be an advantage to have a term other than 'the history of medicine' or 'medical history' so that this activity could be more readily identified; to provide a discipline or a concept with a precise and descriptive name, gives it specificity and thrust. Such terms as 'historical medicine'[28] and 'the history and sociology of the medical sciences'[29] have been suggested but neither is entirely satisfactory. Perhaps 'the history of scientific and social thought in bio-medicine' is the most appropriate, although also the most cumbersome. Or, conversely, the epithets such as 'medical antiquarianism' or 'medico-historical journalism' should be employed more widely and 'the history of medicine' reserved for the activities outlined above.

It has been implied that such a realignment of medical history will benefit the subject in general and as an academic discipline in particular. There are however other advantages which are of varying magnitude:

(1) Studying the history of the medical sciences means that most attention will be given to the nineteenth and twentieth centuries. Furthermore as medical and scientific data accumulate at an ever-increasing rate, the closer the historian dares come to the present day the better. The hazards of so doing are well known but it can usefully demonstrate to disbelievers how an historical approach can make the appreciation of recent advances easier and, of greater significance, how it brings the medical historian closer to students and to his scientific colleagues.

(2) Medical scientists who are unable to accept the traditional 'history of medicine' because they consider it to be a hobby, or too esoteric, or too distant from present-day medicine, especially if the practitioner is not medically qualified, may perhaps be attracted to the history of the medical sciences. After all, as Temkin has pointed out,[30] they carry out an historical technique themselves when they review the preceding literature dealing with the topic upon which they are about to write. The historian of medical science is also doing this but in greater detail and with deeper penetration into the past. He is also bringing into evidence all the interacting scientific, technological and non-scientific factors in order to create accurate and comprehensive history.

(3) Students likewise are more attracted to a subject which deals with the evolution of the scientific and social material they are learning. The majority of them are exceedingly utilitarian and demand some helpful and measurable return from the subjects they have been exposed to. They can be shown that the history of scientific and social medicine introduces a new dimension to their studies. Just as a mathematical or a genetical approach to medical data is of increasing necessity, so an historical one can be equally essential and rewarding. It will assist students in the acquisition and understanding of factual information and give them the perspective and the wider horizon which they will need more and more as medicine progresses with ever-increasing acceleration and complexity. But it can, in addition, provide a method of understanding more readily certain topics in the medical sciences because historically one necessarily proceeds from the simplest to the more complex. Thus an account of the evolution of our present-day concept

of nerve transmission or of haemodynamics facilitates the student's and also the teacher's task. The essential difference in history between working back into time from a known present, and studying the past with no knowledge of the modern state of affairs is well recognized as an important factor in historical research but in teaching, the former technique has much to recommend it.

The sociological aspects of the history of medicine are of comparable value to the student and the arguments put forward by Sigerist, Rosen, Rosenberg (see p. 34), Shyrock and others to support this do not have to be cited here. We need only quote Rosen's revealing statement, made when reviewing the first volume of Sigerist's *A history of medicine* (1951), '...medicine is an activity whose development can be most fully understood only when considered in relation to the network of social interaction within which it occurs'.[31]

Fundamentally the history of medicine as regards its educational value should be nothing more nor less than a medical specialty coordinated with the student's scientific and social studies. At the same time it should indicate the unity of the diverse components of modern medical practice and, on the other hand, the role of medicine as an integral element of society. As both a research and a teaching activity, it must be integrated with contemporary medicine,[32] with clinical and pre-clinical research in the medical school, with many non-medical university disciplines, in particular with the history of science and general and social history, and with extramural experts. But the basic requirement is that the medical historian and his subject should be integrated in the medical school with its teachers, its students and its curriculum. One of the ways in which such an objective can be achieved is to reshape the history of medicine as a subject, to concentrate professional and part-time activity in the area of the history of scientific and social medicine and above all to increase the level of scholarship.

In view of the somewhat discouraging situation, present in certain countries, any reassessment and redeployment capable of habilitating the history of medicine is worthy of serious consideration. If this cannot increase the respectability and acceptance of the subject, then medical history, for the time being or for ever, will become an insignificant, somewhat esoteric, emasculated research discipline.

206

REFERENCES

1 W. H. S. Jones, *Philosophy and medicine in Ancient Greece: with an edition of Περὶ ἀρχαίης ἰητρικῆς*, Supplement 8 of *Bull. Hist. Med.* 1946, ch. 3 (pp. 67–8).
2 G. Urdang, *Wesen und Bedeutung der Geschichte der Pharmacie, Drei Vorträge*, p. 5, Berlin: J. Springer, 1927.
3 The history of medical historiography has been dealt with in particular by Professor Edith Heischkel: e.g., *Die Medizingeschichtschreibung von ihren Anfängen bis zum Beginn des 16. Jahrhunderts*, Berlin: E. Ebering, 1938; *Die Medizinhistoriographie im XVIII. Jahrhundert*, Leiden: E. J. Brill, 1931; and 'Die Geschichte der Medizingeschichtschreibung' in W. Artelt, *Einführung in die Medizinhistorik: ihr Wesen, ihre Arbeitsweise und ihre Hilfsmittel*, pp. 202–37, Stuttgart: F. Enke, 1949; see also 'An exhibit on the history of medical historiography', *Bull. Hist. Med.* 1952, 26, 277–87.
4 Edith Heischkel, 'Die deutsche Medizingeschichtschreibung in der ersten Hälfte des 19. Jahrhunderts', *Kl. Wchschr.* 1933, 12, 714–17; L. Edelstein, 'Medical historiography in 1847', *Bull. Hist. Med.* 1947, 21, 495–511.
5 G. Rosen, 'The place of history in medical education', *Bull. Hist. Med.* 1948, 22, 594–627.
6 G. Miller, 'Backgrounds of current activities in the history of science and medicine', *J. Hist. Med.* 1958, 13, 160–78.
7 The pleas of Corneille Boeckx of Belgium (*Discours sur l'utilité de l'histoire de la médecine*, Anvers: J. B. Heirstraeten, 1839) and by H. Kühnholtz of Montpellier ('Discours sur les avantages de l'histoire de la médecine' in *Cours de la médecine et de bibliographie médicale fait, en 1836, dans la Faculté de Montpellier*, Montpellier and Paris, 1837) are typical of those made early in the century.
8 Henry E. Sigerist, 'Forschungsinstitute für Geschichte der Medizin und der Naturwissenschaften' in Ludolph Brauer, Mendelssohn Bartholdy and Adolf Meyer (eds.), *Forschungsinstitute, ihre Geschichte, Organisation und Ziele*, vol. 1, pp. 391–405, Hamburg: P. Hartung, 1930.
9 Rosen, op. cit. (above, note 5), pp. 611–25.
10 The following are representatives of the extensive literature:
'Medical history. A neglected branch of medical education', *Assoc. Med. J.* 7 January 1853, p. 4, and subsequent comments on pp. 47–8, 97, 103–5, 137;
A. Castan, *De l'enseignement de l'histoire de la médecine: son caractère et son but*, Montpellier & Cette: Boehm, 1874, pp. 23;
C. Bouchard, *Utilité et objet de l'histoire de la médecine*, Paris: F. Savy, 1876, pp. 21;
D. C. C. Owen, 'On the value of the historical study of medicine', *Bgham. med. Rev.* 1889, 26, 1–16;
T. Puschmann, 'Die Bedeutung der Geschichte für die Medicin und die Naturwissenschaften', *D. med. Wschr.* 1889, 15, 817–20;

J. K. Proksch, *Die Nothwendigkeit des Geschichtsstudiums in der Medicin. Ein Mahnruf*, Bonn: P. Hanstein, 1901, pp. 34;

E. F. Cordell, 'The importance of the study of the history of medicine', *Trans. med. chir. Fac. Md.* 1904, pp. 19–35 [reprint only seen];

H. Magnus, 'Der Wert der Geschichte für die moderne induktive Natur-betrachtung und Medicin', *Abh. Gesch. Med.* Breslau, Heft 11, 1904, pp. 24;

B. Laufer, 'A plea for the study of the history of medicine and natural sciences', *Science* 1907, 25, 889–95;

R. E. Schlueter, 'The necessity for studying medical history', *J. Mo. med. Ass.* 1916, 13, 385–7;

P. Diepgen, 'Über Wert, Aufgabe und Methode des medizinhistorischen Unterrichtes', *Fortschr. Med.* 1920, 37, 517–20;

K. Sudhoff, 'Aims and value of medical history in self-development and professional life of the physician', *Med. Life* 1923, 30, 331–6;

A. O. Whipple, 'The history of medicine as an aid in the study of medicine', *Columbia Alumni News* 1924, 16, 42–4;

J. L. Miller, 'Has medical history any value?', *Sth. Med. Surg.* March 1929, pp. [9], [reprint only seen];

W. Szumowski, 'Sur la nécessité de rendre l'étude de l'histoire de la médecine obligatoire dans les universités', *Atti dell VIII° Congresso Internazionale di Storia della Medicina—Roma dal 22 al 27 Settembre 1930*, pp. 289–99, Pisa: V. Lischi and Figli, 1931;

J. H. Walsh, 'The pleasant pathway to medical wisdom through medical history', *Med. Life* 1930, 37, 345–60;

C. S. Burwell, 'The introduction of medical history into the general medical curriculum', *Sth. Med. J.* Birmingham, Alabama, 1932, 25, 427–30;

R. Caballero and R. d'Onofrio Botana, 'Necessidad de incorporar a los planes de estudios de medicina la historia de les doctrinas médicas', *Sem. méd. B. Aires* 1934, 2, 1433–9;

P. Diepgen, 'Die Bedeutung der Medizingeschichte für den praktischen Arzt', *Schering-Kahlbaum med. Mitt.* 1934, 6, 226–31;

St Clair Thomson, 'The present need for the study of the history of medicine', *Proc. R. Soc. Med.* 1934, 27, 1–4;

G. H. Lathrope, 'Why medical history for the medical librarian?', *Bull. med. Lib. Ass.* 1939–40, 28, 17–23;

O. Temkin, 'An essay on the usefulness of medical history for medicine', *Bull. Hist. Med.* 1946, 19, 9–47;

E. H. Ackerknecht, 'The role of medical history in medical education', *Bull. Hist. Med.* 1947, 21, 135–45;

G. Zilboorg, 'Medical history as a force in medical functioning' in *Victor Robinson Memorial Volume: essays on the history of medicine*, pp. 415–20, New York: Froben Press, 1948;

W. Pagel, 'Julius Pagel and the significance of medical history for medicine', *Bull. Hist. Med.* 1951, 25, 207–25;

H. E. Sigerist, 'The autonomy of the history of medicine and its place in the university', *Acta. med. scand.* 1952, Supplement 266, pp. 109–13;

H. E. Sigerist, 'Medical history in medical education', *Practitioner* 1953, 171, 188–94;

G. Rosen, 'Purposes and values of medical history' in I. Galdston (ed.), *On the utility of medical history*, pp. 11–19, New York: International Universities Press, 1957;

I. Galdston, 'On the utility of medical history' in ibid., pp. 3–9;

A. Feigenbaum, 'Why history of medicine and science?', *Acta med. Orient.* 1957, 16, 140–5;

W. C. Stout, 'The importance of dental history', *Tex. dent. J.* 1957, 75, 507–8;

J. Bostock, 'Medicine's need for history', *Med. J. Austral.* 1958, 2, 557–61;

K. D. Keele, 'The value of medical history to the doctor', *Conn. Med.* 1959, 23, 75–6;

J. Camacho Gamba, 'El valor de la historia en la medicina', *Rev. Colombia Pediat.* 1959, 18, 84–103;

D. Guthrie, 'The need for medical history', *The Scotsman*, 20 July 1959;

G. Rath, 'The history of medicine—a living force', *Ciba Symposium* 1960, 88, 104–9.

Anon., 'The value of medical history', *J. Nat. med. Ass.* 1960, 52, 365–6;

G. Rosen, 'Purposes and values of medical history', *J. A. Einstein Med. Cent.* 1962, 10, 92–7;

P. R. Fleming, 'The value of history of medicine', *The Broadway* 1963, R19, 40–1;

M. Sendrail, 'L'histoire de la médecine mérite-t-elle d'être enseignée', *Concours méd.* 1964, 86, 177–81;

O. H. Wangensteen, 'Role of medical history as incentive to scholarship and spur to interdisciplinary research', *Mayo Clin. Proc.* 1967, 42, 345–9;

W. Fraser-Moodie, 'It is good occasionally to unroll the pages of the past', *Br. J. oral Surg.* 1967, 5, 77–85.

11 D. Keele, 'Uses and abuses of medical history', *Br. Med. J.* 1966, 2, 1251–4; E. Clarke, 'Medical history: a neglected subject', *Murmer* (*Camb. Univ. med. J.*) Michaelmas 1966, pp. 1–5; F. N. L. Poynter, 'The value of medical history in both education and research', *Med. J. Austral.* 1967, 2, 871–5.

12 *Royal Commission on Medical Education 1965–68 Report*, London: Her Majesty's Stationery Office, [1968], pp. 404; known as the *Todd Report* after the Chairman of the Commission, the Rt. Hon. the Lord Todd.

13 Rosen, op. cit. (above, note 5).

14 There is no need to list all the pleas and arguments but as a representative proclamation, see the report of the Committee on the Teaching of Medical History of the American Association of the History of Medicine, R. H. Shryock (Chairman), I. Galdston, O. Temkin, 'Statement of the Editorial Sub-Committee', *Bull. Hist. Med.* 1951, 25, 571–7.

15 J. B. Blake (ed.), *Education in the history of medicine, Report of a Macy Conference...June 22–24, 1966*, New York: Hafner, 1968.

16 Op. cit. (above, note 10).

17 E. Clarke, 'Practical historical medicine', *Verhandlungen des XX. Internationalen Kongresses für Geschichte der Medizin Berlin, 22.–27. August 1966*, pp. 352–5, Hildesheim: G. Olms, 1968; and 'The history and sociology of the medical sciences', paper read at XIIth International Conference of the History of Science, Paris, 27 August 1968.

18 A. Berman (ed.), *Pharmaceutical historiography. Proceedings of a Colloquium ...January 22–23, 1966*, Madison: American Institute of the History of Pharmacy, 1967, pp. 145.

19 H. E. Sigerist, *Civilization and disease*, Chicago: University of Chicago Press (Phoenix book), 1962.

20 An excellent example of the masterly way in which an art historian, admittedly one of the most outstanding, handles contacts made between medicine and art is E. Panofsky, 'Artist, scientist, genius: notes on the "Renaissance—Dammerung" ' in *The Renaissance : six essays*, pp. 123–82, New York and Evanston: Harper and Row, 1962.

21 I. Macalpine and R. Hunter, *Porphyria—a royal malady*, London: B.M.A., 1968, and idem, *George III and the mad business*, London: Allen Lane the Penguin Press, 1969.

22 R. H. Shryock, 'The interplay of social and internal factors in the history of modern medicine', *The Scientific Monthly* 1953, 76, 221–30.

23 A. R. Hall, 'Can the history of science be history?', *Br. J. Hist. Sci.* 1969, 4, 207–20.

24 T. S. Kuhn, *The structure of scientific revolutions*, Chicago and London: University of Chicago Press (Phoenix book), 1962. But see L. S. King, *The road to medical enlightenment 1650–1659*, pp. 5–7, London: Macdonald, 1970.

25 F. L. Baumer, 'Intellectual history and its problems', *Journal of Modern History* 1949, 21, 191–203, see p. 191.

26 Ibid., p. 195.

27 Ibid., pp. 202–3.

28 Clarke, op. cit. (above, note 17).

29 Ibid.

30 O. Temkin, 'Scientific medicine and historical research', *Persp. Biol. Med.* 1959, 3, 70–85, see pp. 72–3.

31 G. Rosen, 'The new history of medicine: a review', *J. Hist. Med.* 1951, 6, 516–22, see pp. 519–20.

32 'We do not want to cultivate medical history as a mere search for antiquities, as a kind of hunt for curios, but rather as a vital, integral part of medicine', G. Rosen, 'What is past is prologue', *J. Hist. Med.* 1946, 1, 3–5, see p. 4.

12 The Case History Method in the Historiography of the Medical Sciences

FREDERIC L. HOLMES

The method of case histories has become increasingly popular in various fields of learning, including history itself; and the question is sometimes raised whether such an approach is an effective way to deal also with the history of science and the history of medicine. In this particular application, however, there is a special complication, for case histories are advocated not merely to understand the past, but also to introduce science or medicine itself to students who are not intending to be specialists in these activities. I will address myself here primarily to the question as it relates to the history of science, but most of the considerations are relevant as well to the history of medicine, especially to the history of the medical sciences.

A convenient starting-point for assessing the possibilities and limitations of this approach is the experience of the *Harvard Case Histories in experimental science*, published in 1957 under the editorship of James B. Conant and Leonard K. Nash. These two volumes, together with an undergraduate course at Harvard based on them, constituted an ambitious effort to impart to non-scientists '...an understanding both of the methods of experimental science and of the growth of scientific research as an organised activity of society'.[1] This simultaneous introduction to science and the history of science was intended primarily for students majoring in the humanities or social sciences, who might later in their lives as citizens, administrators, or journalists be called upon to make judgements concerning scientific research projects for which they could not be experts. Conant explained in an introduction why he thought that a study of cases drawn from the past could be especially useful for this purpose:

Modern science has become so complicated that today methods of research cannot be studied by looking over the shoulder of the scientist at work. If one could transport a visitor, however, to a laboratory where significant results were being obtained at an early stage in the history of a particular science, the situation would be far different. For when a science is in its infancy, and a new field is opened by a great pioneer, the relevant information of the past can be summed up in a relatively brief compass.[2]

'...such periods in the history of science', Conant acknowledged, 'are relatively few.'[2] The aim of the case histories was to recapture several such events in order that the non-scientific reader might in some sense share an experience of the way in which science has advanced.

Of the eight case histories, Conant edited four, Leonard Nash two, and Duane Roller two. They included 'Robert Boyle's experiments in pneumatics'; 'The overthrow of the phlogiston theory'; 'The early development of the concepts of temperature and heat'; 'The atomic-molecular theory'; 'Plants and the atmosphere'; 'Pasteur's study of fermentation'; 'Pasteur's and Tyndall's study of spontaneous generation'; and 'The development of the concept of electric charge'. These topics were well chosen for the objectives of the programme. Each dealt with a discovery of scientific concepts of fundamental and lasting importance, but which can be described without unduly complicated technical language. Long passages from the key writings of the scientists involved brought the reader into direct contact with their thoughts, while the editors added interpretations enabling the modern reader to follow the ideas more easily. After their publication these cases formed the basic reading for one of the natural science courses in the general education programme at Harvard University. Taught at first by Conant and afterwards by Nash, the course was intended as an optional replacement for ordinary introductory science courses in fulfilment of the science requirement for non-science majors.

II

Several years ago I participated briefly in this course as a graduate student discussion section leader, and have since then been engaged in teaching the history of science for its own sake. From the joint perspective of these experiences I have come to feel that the Harvard effort achieved some success, but that there were evident limitations inherent in the approach. Those who took the course seemed generally enthusiastic, but their response was probably to the high quality of Nash's teaching more than to the merits of the method. The individual cases in the published series are uneven in their capacity to fulfil their objectives. The outstanding case study is Nash's 'The atomic-molecular theory'.[3] It treats in detail John Dalton's conception of atoms, its reception and application to chemistry; Gay-Lussac's law of combining volumes of gases; Dalton's reasons for not accepting the significance of this discovery for his own atomic theory; and Avogadro's reconciliation of Gay-Lussac's results with Dalton's atomism. In more condensed form it summarizes the difficulties which prevented Avogadro's solution from being widely accepted and which restricted the influence of the atomic theory until 1858, when Cannizzaro resolved the crucial problems. Nash managed to give a lucid discussion of the historical problem and at the same time to teach some simple fundamentals of modern chemistry, such as the way in which reactions are portrayed in chemical equations, the calculations of atomic weights from combining proportions, the determination of molecular formulae, and the meaning of the laws of multiple and equivalent proportions. By patient, repeated explanation of the key ideas he helped readers without much prior scientific background to follow through a fairly complicated network of considerations. Not only did the case serve its function well, but it has been recognized as a very clear historical account in its own right, and is cited as a source by other histories of chemistry, although some details require revision in the light of more recent research.

Conant's 'Robert Boyle's experiments in pneumatics'[4] deals with a less complex situation. The study consists primarily of lengthy passages from Boyle's own accounts of his experiments with vacuum pumps, interspersed with relatively short explanatory comments and preceded by a succinct account of the prior contributions of Torricelli, Pascal, and Stevin to the concept of a 'sea of the air'. The topic is extraordinarily well chosen. It deals not only with a field in its infancy, but with a period in which experimental science itself was novel; consequently the brief discussion of background knowledge seems sufficient. Boyle's voluminous descriptions of his methods bring out characteristics of experimentation that in later stages of development would be taken for granted.

Nevertheless, from this work resulted Boyle's law, a simple relationship which is still of everyday utility in science, and which affords an opportunity for incisive comments on the importance of quantitative considerations in science as well as on the degree to which an 'empirical' law is inherent in the data or requires a mental construction. Thus this case seems to fulfil with economy the double objective which Conant set for the series.

In the second case by Conant, 'The overthrow of the phlogiston theory: the chemical revolution of 1775–1789',[5] the limitations of the general approach become more apparent. The case focuses on parts of key memoirs by Lavoisier and by Priestley which pinpoint the discovery of oxygen, Lavoisier's new interpretation of combustion, and the respective methods of the two chemists. Again the technical knowledge necessary to read the original sources is restricted enough to be explained by the editor as needed, and the events are of great import. The historical complexity of the chemical revolution, however, is not easily compatible with the simplicity and clarity demanded by the purposes of the case history programme. Contrary to many general historical accounts, chemistry was not a primitive science when Lavoisier entered it. There was already a large body of accumulated knowledge about the composition and reactions of many substances, and about methods of handling and investigating them. The events leading to the work of Lavoisier involved the contributions of numerous men. The view portrayed in this case is too narrow to give the reader a comprehension of the meaning of the chemical revolution, even though the case describes well a few key factors at the centre of the story. The discussion of the phlogiston theory, for example, does not make clear the breadth of explanation which that theory had offered, and by not sufficiently depicting its power is not able to present adequately the impact of its overthrow.

In one of the studies concerned with a later period, 'Pasteur's study of fermentation', Conant recognized the increasingly acute problem of background information by opening the case with a compact ten-page summary of elementary principles of biochemistry needed by the student in order to understand the situation.[6] Despite the clarity of this presentation, its brevity makes it hard for a reader unacquainted with chemistry to absorb all of the material compressed into it, and it does not distinguish between knowledge available to Pasteur when he did his work and knowledge acquired afterwards. Consequently the reader still does not have an adequate view of the historical context within which the investigations occupying the rest of the case occurred.

Some of the difficulties illustrated above might be alleviated by revisions and expansions of the cases, but I think that the problems could not easily be resolved, for they arise less from faulty execution than from a basic conflict between the dual requirements of interpreting historical events and of teaching something about modern science. Even 'the atomic-molecular theory', which I believe comes closest to reconciling these divergent aims, does not always escape the dilemmas. Nash sometimes introduces ambiguities, for example, when he states concepts of early nineteenth-century chemistry in modernized forms, either to make them clearer to readers of the present time or to teach a truth of the modern science. It is not always evident whether in so doing he has modified the original meanings and introduced into the discussion a precision visible only in retrospect. Even when he is careful to preface a statement with 'a modern statement of the law of multiple proportions might run:...',[7] the contemporary and the modern tend to merge; in other places there are similar shifts without such explicit indication.

More overt instances of modernizing past ideas occur in Roller's 'The early development of the concepts of temperature and heat: the rise and decline of the caloric theory'. In discussing Rumford's measurement of the heat produced by a cylinder revolving in a box immersed in water, Roller omits Rumford's own method of estimating the total quantity of heat generated; he says 'We here replace Rumford's description of his calculation by a somewhat more concise statement utilizing modern thermal units.'[8] The substitution serves the double purpose of simplicity and of imparting a little information about current usage of British thermal units, but it does not enhance the accuracy of the historical description.

The educational role envisioned for the case histories necessitates not only simplifications and modernizations, but also a sharp distinction between those ideas of the past which have proven to be correct and those which are 'now known' to have been erroneous. For if one is to introduce students to science through this method, it would appear irresponsible to allow them to believe unwittingly that old mistaken statements were true. Thus the purpose of the previously mentioned sketch of elementary biochemistry by Conant seems to have been not so much to aid the student to understand the relation of Pasteur's work to the state of science in his time as it was to alert the reader to '...see how his views must now be modified in the light of later work'.[9] Similarly the various studies carefully point out within the texts individual statements of a writer quoted which are incorrect. Erroneous views are included when they are essential to understand the logic of an ensuing outcome, but otherwise they are often omitted. Many historians of science have handled matters similarly even without the constraint of designing their accounts for the same educational use, so that the *Harvard Case Histories* are not in this respect conspicuous. Nevertheless historians have recently been trying to free themselves from such selectivity and retrospective judgements of the past in order to evaluate achievements more fairly within the framework of contemporary problems or standards. The special demands placed on these case histories therefore cause them to run counter to promising trends in the history of science.

A more fundamental weakness in the case history method for introducing students to the methods of science is that the selection necessary to find suitable cases imposes an unbalanced image both of science and of the history of science. For most of the time that the sciences have existed they have not been in their infancy, and they have not been simple; and it is probably misleading to say that the ways in which advances were made in each of them when it was just beginning were very similar to the ways in which they progress when they are more complex and well-developed. In *The structure of scientific revolutions* Thomas Kuhn argues persuasively that the manner in which scientists in a given field carry on their research changes substantially when that field has reached a certain stage of development which he defines as 'paradigmatic'. The activity begins to be more rigorous, demanding, and accessible only to experts, and the experts operate differently from their predecessors.[10] The use of case histories drawn only from the early phases of development of various fields would therefore not give a picture so applicable to typical modern sciences as Conant suggested. Moreover, the impression that science is relatively simple, which students not familiar with it through other exposure may absorb from these studies, has drawbacks. When I was associated with the course based on these cases it seemed to me that some of the students came to feel that they could master scientific thought handily, because they were not aware of how carefully the cases had been constructed to avoid the complications which would have baffled them. Such facile overconfidence may be just as undesirable as the awe of science that befalls those who have had no contact with it.

The pedagogical objective also results in the selection of cases which illustrate the establishment of knowledge of permanent value for later science, since the students are thereby able to pick up some useful scientific information even while they focus their attention on the historical developments. Thus Nash could conclude his discussion of the atomic-molecular theory with the statement that 'Its revival by Cannizzaro...rapidly swept this scheme to the prominent position among the concepts of science that it has continued to occupy with honor until the present day.'[11] Certainly such outcomes represent science at its most successful, and should be amply represented in any account of its past. The history of science, however, embraces many other kinds of events besides permanent acquisitions of knowledge. It includes ideas which once played significant roles but are since either disproven or forgotten; it includes searches which even in their own time went unfulfilled but which are not therefore less interesting historically; it includes the reactions of scientific communities to a variety of problems not restricted to discoveries. Case histories based on such stories would also illuminate the nature of scientific activity, but they are unlikely candidates for a programme which seeks to introduce people to science, because they are less likely to impart extant scientific content along with historical perspective.

The selective bias of the programme extends deeper than the exclusion only of cases which would not treat enduring discoveries describable in relatively simple language. Many historical situations which meet these conditions are still ill-adapted to the educational purpose because the historical pattern of events is itself so complicated that their recounting would tend to confuse the clarity for which the case studies must strive. Some cases may be handled by leaving out the infertile pathways of research, the setbacks and other factors which seem not to have been logically essential preconditions to the eventual result. This rationalization can be bought, however, only at the price of making science appear to advance more

217

methodically and economically than it actually does. Many historically important cases must be ruled out, because their events cannot be reduced to a simple enough pattern to be helpful as part of an introduction to the understanding of science. Nash found, for example, that when he tried to use as a case for his course the emergence of structural organic chemistry between 1830 and 1860, he could not avoid getting into an account of the historical situation so involved that it interfered with his effort to explain the scientific methods and reasoning exemplified. Consequently he gradually abandoned the attempt to depict the history realistically and began instead to present only the logical bases of the reasoning which chemists of the period typically utilized to build up their knowledge of organic molecules. One of the most impressive of the published cases in terms of its portrayal of a historical sequence of events is Nash's 'Plants and the atmosphere'.[12] Yet this case was soon dropped from his own course, because the historical rather than the scientific complexity made it too difficult to use.

The *Harvard Case Histories* were ably done, and their strengths and weaknesses provide a fair picture of what can be expected from the approach to science which they were intended to implement. The results suggest that the method can aid in explaining scientific activity to non-scientists, but that contradictions inherent in the aims of the method make it unlikely that it can succeed as the primary means for bringing students who are not otherwise pursuing the study of science into contact with it. The underlying difficulty is that whenever a historical account is made to sustain a burden external to the aims of history itself the account is easily distorted in the process. As a specialized form of history, the history of science is subject to the same problems that Herbert Butterfield has asserted befall general history when it is studied with an eye fastened too closely on the present. Butterfield pointed out in his well-known *The whig interpretation of history* that history can only illuminate the present if we do not from the start seize upon those aspects of previous times which are most analogous to modern times. 'It makes all the difference in the world', he wrote, 'whether we already assume the present at the beginning of our study of history and keep it as a basis of reference, or whether we wait and suspend our judgment until we discover it at the end.'[13] Only if we first immerse ourselves in the past for its own sake, taking seriously the assumption that the past is in many ways different from the present, can history provide a truer vision of ourselves. Arguments similar to Butterfield's can be applied to the history of science; if we are constrained to select material and to analyse the writings of earlier scientists in such a way as to illustrate certain features which we have decided in advance are characteristic of science present as well as past, we shall only confirm what we believed already and shall not learn anything new about the nature of scientific activities. The *Harvard Case Histories* suffer in varying degrees from this defect. Some are organized from the start to substantiate certain conceptions about scientific method. Others show less disposition to force events into predetermined patterns, but still cannot escape biases imposed by the task of having to embody 'lessons' too directly applicable to the understanding of modern science.

If one sought to profit from Butterfield's views by writing case histories without selecting the subject-matter or interpreting it with too close reference to their instructive purpose, the result would be improved histories, but they would be less suitable as an introduction to science; for Conant's objective was to find a way to present the subject simply, whereas Butterfield pointed out that true history does not provide simplicity. Far from it, he said, '...the more we examine the way in which things happen, the more we are driven from the simple to the complex'.[14]

If this view of history is reasonable, as I think it is, it is difficult to see how the case histories could fully achieve their aims. I believe that they should not be expected to. The history of science can, I believe, contribute significantly to non-scientists' understanding of science, but only if it is freed from the role of introducing science itself. The responsibility for teaching the sciences to students in such a manner that those who do not intend to concentrate in them can find interest and comprehension should belong to scientists themselves. For this purpose I do not think formal history of science is necessary. After a student has gained some acquaintance with the present state of a field of science he will be prepared to appreciate the added perspective that the history of the science can provide: that the knowledge he has been presented as a rational system is not static but has undergone a continuous process of change. The historical view will not make science appear simpler to him, as the *Harvard Case Histories* sought to make it, but will add to his sense of the complexity of science. For many humanist students accustomed to historical treatments of other subjects, this historical dimension may then make science more meaningful than the rational scientific approach alone. They would by this time be in no danger of confusing the history of the subject with the subject itself, as they may be if the history of science is allowed to be a substitute for instead of a supplement to an introductory science course.

III

A more promising role for case histories than their use as an introduction to science is as an approach to the history of science itself. Butterfield suggested that, 'It is only by...looking at some point in history through the microscope that we can really visualise the complicated movements that lie behind any historical change.'[15] Elting Morison has recently advocated that such a view could serve as a basis for teaching history. 'One of the most profitable ways to learn historical meaning', he suggested, 'is through the intensive examination of the small situation—what is usually called today the case study.' Morison illustrated his position by showing that if one studied fully such a seemingly simple situation as the appointment of a federal judge in New York in 1905 so as to include all of the complexities radiating from it, one could illuminate not only the process of Federal justice, but the whole political process in the United States.[16] Similar modes of inquiry and presentation ought to be particularly effective in the history of science. Whether or not one believes that science proceeds by the systematic application of a 'scientific method', there are undoubtedly regularities in the organization of scientific activity which render that activity especially amenable to the identification in a given historical situation of factors whose analysis would illuminate analogous situations.

In carrying out such a programme one must be careful not to fall into the same dilemma which confronted the Harvard case history effort: that is of starting out with predetermined generalizations about the history of science which the cases will be written to illustrate. If the initial objective is only to portray as far as is possible the numerous dimensions of a given historical situation and to allow the characteristics which may have more general applicability to emerge from the study as it goes, one may be able to achieve case studies which will be good specific histories and also broadly illustrative.

The possibilities in this kind of case history can perhaps best be suggested by illustrating how the ramifications of some particular past scientific investigation extended outward from the basic outline of the central events. A convenient example is the discovery of the glycogenic function of the liver by Claude Bernard. The result itself is quite uncomplicated to describe in comparison to the many facets of the historical circumstances that surrounded it; and the interest is enhanced by the fact that Bernard utilized some aspects of the discovery himself as brief case histories to support his views of scientific method.

In 1848 Bernard found that the blood and the liver tissue of a dog contained sugar, even when the animal had been kept on a diet excluding carbohydrates. He concluded, contrary to the current views of his time, that animals do not derive their sugar exclusively from nutrients, but that the liver produces it. He confirmed his view of the role of the liver by detecting sugar in the blood leaving that organ, but not in the blood passing from the intestines to the liver in the portal vein. In 1855 he observed that if he passed water through the blood vessels of an isolated liver until all of the sugar had been flushed out of the organ, within a few hours more sugar had formed in it. From this result he concluded that the source of the sugar ordinarily entering the bloodstream is an insoluble material stored in the liver. By 1857 he had isolated the insoluble material, which he named glycogen, characterized its chemical properties, and proven that it can be converted to glucose by ferments or acids.

Bernard devoted numerous articles, treatises, and hours of his yearly lecture courses to describing how he had reached these results. In his celebrated *Introduction to the study of experimental medicine*, however, he managed to compress into a few paragraphs what he regarded as the crucial steps in his research that had produced the discoveries. He had, he said, from the beginning of his career attempted to determine what becomes of alimentary substances when they pass into the body.

...I conceived the hypothesis that sugar introduced into the blood through nutrition might be destroyed in the lungs or in the general capillaries. The theory, indeed, which then prevailed and which was naturally my proper starting point, assumed that the sugar present in animals came exclusively from foods, and that it was destroyed in animal organisms by the phenomena of combustion, i.e., of respiration...But I was immediately led to see that the theory...was false. As a result of the experiments which I shall describe further on, I was not indeed led to find an organ for destroying sugar, but, on the contrary, I discovered an organ for making it, and I found that all animal blood contains sugar even when they do not eat it.[17]

Bernard emphasized these leading ideas without detailing his technical procedures, because the purpose of his account was to justify a general principle of experimental science. A scientist must never believe absolutely in theories, he maintained, for they are only hypotheses, useful in suggesting new experiments. One should always be prepared to abandon a theory whenever he encounters a fact in opposition to it. When in a later section Bernard described briefly the experiments by which he had shown that an animal produces rather than merely destroys sugar, he did so because the nature of the proof could in itself be depicted as an illustration of a rule for good experimentation. After finding sugar in the hepatic veins of a dog fed sugar, he automatically followed the procedure of counterproof, testing similarly an animal which had not eaten any sugar. It was then unexpectedly, and because of his scrupulous observance of this practice, he claimed, that he found sugar also present when it could not be derived from nutrients.[18] Bernard recalled a later stage in the investigation as an illustration of still another precept for the experimentalist. Intending to make duplicate estimates of the quantity of sugar in the tissue of a liver, he did the first determination immediately after the death of the animal, but was by chance delayed in making the second until the next day. Once again he was surprised, for he found a considerably larger proportion of sugar by the second analysis. Further investigations to seek the cause of the difference led him to the washing experiments by which he proved that there is a material in the liver which is convertible to sugar. The point of this account in the *Introduction* was to support Bernard's argument that when a scientist encounters discordant results he must not discount one of them, or take an average, but must search out the cause of the discrepancy in the differing conditions of the respective experiments.[19]

These and other examples from his research which Bernard discussed in his *Introduction* illustrated elegantly his conception of the methods of experimental science. They were, however, far from literal historical descriptions of his discoveries, even though he said of the preceding account that he had '...just very briefly told how these facts were discovered...'[20] He had been highly selective in focusing on those moments out of long years of work which embodied dramatically the generalizations he wished to establish. Furthermore, the drastic foreshortening condensed into a few concentrated episodes sequences of reasoning which had actually developed in more gradual stages from accumulations of evidence of which only the most striking were described. Bernard's intention clearly was to use his experiences as sources of 'lessons' about science, not to provide a balanced and accurate history of his investigations.

A more realistic account of the stages in Bernard's glycogen research can be reconstructed from his published research papers and lectures. J. M. D. Olmsted, F. G. Young, and Nikolaus Mani are a few of the historians who have given very good treatments based on these sources.[21] The resulting narratives are more complicated than that in the *Introduction*, but still show a tight logical progression of hypothesis or probing question, discovery, further question, further discovery, so that Bernard's final case seems constructed from a chain of essential links.

Recently M. G. Grmek has shown from a study of the laboratory notebooks left by Bernard that his pathway was more meandering than the published documents reveal. The interplay of hypothesis and experiment did not always lead so smoothly to positive results, and Bernard sometimes persisted in following ideas which were leading him nowhere. Grmek points out that Bernard's own recapitulation in the *Introduction* is misleading. The statement from the passage previously quoted, 'But I was immediately led to see that the theory...was false', skips over the fact that while Bernard sought the pathway of sugar in the organism he continued for several years to accept that theory, until his chance discovery of 1848 set him on the successful track. Grmek shows also that Bernard did not always follow his own precepts about experimentation. When confronted with a finding by Louis Figuier that, contrary to his own results, the portal blood contains sugar, Bernard did not try to find the reasons for the differences in the results, but simply maintained the validity of his own in opposition to those of his challenger.[22]

Grmek's forty-page treatment probably comes as close to describing the actual sequence of events in Bernard's glycogen research as the surviving records will allow. Although Bernard's progress appears more uneven, it is no less impressive. The account begins to convey the complexity of such a historical process while still depicting a pattern of scientific activity which can serve as an illustrative case study. Grmek also provides a succinct description of the contemporary knowledge of sugar in the organism which formed the starting-point for Bernard's work. But these factors are only the first steps towards a full explanation of what Bernard did.

Some additional factors are treated in a stimulating book by Joseph Schiller, entitled *Claude Bernard et les problèmes scientifiques de son temps*. Schiller compares the general methodology embodied in Bernard's work with that of his contemporaries and predecessors. The glycogen research, according to Schiller, represented an important departure in the whole problem of nutrition, for Bernard was the first to combine vivisection with chemical analysis in such a way as to follow the chemical evolution of organic molecules in their pathways within the body. To bear out this claim, which Bernard had often made himself, Schiller contrasts the approach of chemists such as Liebig and Dumas, who sought answers to analogous questions on the basis of chemical analyses alone;[23] and of previous biologists whose conceptions of nutrition derived partly from tradition, partly from anatomical and histological considerations.[24] He traces the sources of both the physiological and chemical components of Bernard's approach to the influence of men in his scientific milieu. Magendie served as Bernard's principal scientific mentor, while he learned in the laboratory of Jules Pelouze how to apply the new chemical methods available for handling organic materials.[25] Schiller also assesses some of the broader consequences of the discovery of the glycogen function of the liver, such as the disproof of a supposed fundamental distinction between the processes of vegetable and of animal life; the weakening of vitalism; and the provision of foundations for chemical histology and chemical embryology.[26] Each of these topics, which Schiller discusses succinctly, could be expanded into detailed expositions of the complexity of interactions between the achievements of one scientist and the work of numerous contemporaries.

I have dealt briefly with certain of these interactions in a study of the reaction of Bernard to the animal chemistry of Liebig and of Dumas.[27] To understand the approach Bernard took in his research on the nutritional role of sugar in 1848 and afterwards, as well as to appreciate his general statements concerning the role of chemistry in physiology, one must examine the situation in which he found himself at the beginning of his career in 1842. Trained by a physiologist who stressed above all the importance of vivisection, he encountered immediately the formidable impact of the theories of nutrition proposed by these eminent chemists, each of whom based his views primarily upon knowledge of the chemical composition of organic materials rather than on physiological experimentation. The differences between the theories of the German and the French chemists were being debated in the Academy of Sciences, and a new physiologist interested in nutrition could hardly afford to ignore them. Yet Bernard was from the start sceptical, and he sought deliberately for ways to demonstrate that chemical theories must be subjected to the critique of physiological experiments if one were to determine what actually takes place in the body rather than what might possibly occur. For several years he could find only subordinate issues on which to raise his challenge, and he undoubtedly exerted less influence upon the chemists than they did on him. He continued for this period to assume the basic meaning of nutrition outlined in Dumas's scheme, and tried therefore to ascertain where in the body the disappearance of nutritional sugar that Dumas postulated actually took place. When finally he discovered that sugar is instead formed in the body, he immediately saw the central importance of the result as proof of his contention that '...chemistry must never adventure alone in the examination of animal functions'.[28] This conclusion was not due solely to the unexpected contradiction of a central tenet of the chemical theory, as he later recounted the story in his *Introduction*, but also to the fact that the result fulfilled the objective he had long before set for himself of finding occasions to demonstrate the inadequacy of the methods of the chemists.

The need to come to terms with the ideas of Liebig and Dumas thus exerted an especially striking influence on Bernard, but it would be necessary to examine the interactions with the work of many other people as well in order to account fully for the course of his work on the glycogen function. These interactions should not be presented only from the point of view of their effects on Bernard, however, but also from the perspective of the other scientists themselves. Otherwise the efforts of the others may appear as mere foils to bring out the advantages of his achievements. The chemists whose approach he opposed actually made a significant contribution to defining the problem of metabolism, a significance Bernard was not able fully to appreciate, even as he saw the shortcomings of which they were not aware. One of the objectives of a historical case study would be to illustrate the way in which each scientist sharing in the investigation of some general problem has a limited, partial view of that problem depending upon his previous experience, individual idiosyncrasies, and the particular portion of the problem which is his central concern.

As important to the understanding of a given scientific investigation as the influence of the work of other scientists on it is the impact of that work itself on the subsequent efforts of others. Here also one should not only view the interaction from the standpoint of the role of the work and its author, but should also try to see what meaning it had for those who related it to their own interests. A particularly revealing example in Bernard's case is the way in which the German chemist C. G. Lehmann treated the discovery of 1848 that sugar forms in the liver. Bernard often pointed out, in later years when his conclusions came under question, that Lehmann had confirmed his finding that there is a considerable quantity of sugar in the hepatic veins and little or none in the portal vein. Lehmann had done this, and reported it in a paper published in 1850,[29] but it is surprising, in view of the importance of the observations to Bernard, how small a part the verification of these results played in Lehmann's article. The comparison of the sugar content of the portal and hepatic veins was just one of a series of analyses; Lehmann indicated only briefly in a short paragraph (p. 140) and again in his summary (p. 162) that his investigations confirmed Bernard's hypothesis that sugar is formed in the liver. The reason that Lehmann did not focus more on this phenomenon is that he was attempting a complete comparative analysis of the blood before and after it traverses the liver, to detect all of the transformations its constituents undergo. He apparently hoped that by determining which substances disappeared or were diminished during the passage he could infer which materials in the blood are the sources from which the constituents of the bile are produced. Finding that fibrin disappears, he concluded that it might be used up in the formation of bile and perhaps of sugar.[29] By thus treating the appearance of sugar as merely one of a number of transformations resulting from processes that serve principally the secretion of bile, Lehmann may seem to have overlooked the true significance of Bernard's conclusions, for Bernard himself considered his discovery to be of a completely new function of the liver, independent of the production of bile. Lehmann's interpretation, however, is quite natural in view of the way in which Bernard's analyses could be fitted into his own research problem. It is also reasonable that he would regard bile formation as the central problem, even though it was not a novel one. Although this function of the liver had been known since ancient times, very little was yet understood of the chemical processes involved. In just these years chemists and physiologists were greatly interested in applying the recent advances in methods of analysis of organic fluids to open a fresh attack on the old but still mysterious problem. Another prominent physiologist, F. T. Frerichs, incorporated Bernard's discovery more explicitly than Lehmann did into a theory of the chemical processes in the liver which produce bile.[30] Bernard had not seen his result as part of this problem, because he had not set out to investigate the function of the liver, but to trace the fate of the sugar in the blood. Thus the same observations had rather different significances to these men because they placed them in the context of different phenomena. Only by viewing the situation from the perspective of each person involved can one see that a scientific discovery has not a single face for everyone, but various meanings for different individuals according to the connections which the new information makes with their own work.

The most vivid interactions and differences of perspective arise, of course, when a scientific conclusion becomes the subject of controversy, and it is then also that it is most essential to attempt to understand the standpoint of each of the disputants. Bernard's theory that the liver produces sugar ran into a heavy barrage of criticism in 1855, when he had completed his research on the blood entering and leaving the liver but did not yet have the confirming evidence of his liver-washing experiment. Louis Figuier, Bernard's leading critic, had found sugar in the portal blood, and argued that this discovery disproved Bernard's views. F. A. Longet joined in the attack with additional experiments and observations. Lehmann, Poggiale, and others produced results supporting Bernard, who vigorously defended his own cause. Physicians and newspaper editors entered the debate, and at one time the weekly *Le Moniteur des Hôpitaux* claimed that 'M. Bernard will be fortunate if he traverses safely and soundly the cross-fire that at this moment is being directed at him.'[31]

The opposition to Bernard ranged from valid experimental objections and defence of Dumas's chemical theories to medical conservatism, and probably some harassment born of professional rivalry. On each side there were misunderstandings of the positions of the other or the mistaking of verbal differences for contradictory conceptions, and an inability to consider that two explanations posed as alternatives might be complementary. Each participant had a different approach and understanding of the problem. Only a careful account of the direction from which each came to the problem, his previous experience and concerns, and his objectives could lead to a historical understanding of the dispute and to enlightenment about the role such affairs play in the movement of science. Even though Bernard dominated the question of the glycogen function and held the initiative for most of the time, his critics were not merely negative. Sometimes they were right, and he did not see the whole problem; when they were wrong they still forced him to modify and strengthen his foundations. The view of the glycogenic function eventually accepted was neither that which Bernard defended at the time nor that of his opponents, but incorporated some of the ideas of each.

The controversy also affords glimpses of the way in which the social positions of individuals within the scientific community may affect the handling of the issue, and of the mechanisms a particular scientific community may utilize to control such situations. The Academy of Sciences appointed a commission to judge between the claims of Figuier and of Bernard. This commission decided completely in favour of Bernard, but as has been pointed out,[32] their opinion seems not to have been impartial. The commissioners repeated the crucial experiments of Figuier using Bernard's methods of analysis and did not bother to try Figuier's own methods. One might ask the reason for this bias. In an apparent gesture of fairness, Bernard, who was entitled to sit on the commission, vacated his place; but the remaining members, Dumas, Pelouze, and Rayer, were all friends of his. Furthermore, as a member of the Academy, recently appointed to teach at the Sorbonne and to succeed Magendie at the Collège de France, Bernard had just completed his rise into the inner circle of the rather tight scientific establishment in Paris. Figuier, on the other hand, was clearly regarded as an outsider. When discussing his claims Bernard and other commentators sometimes made pointed allusions to Figuier's inexperience in experimental physiology and implied that he did not yet understand how research should be done.[33] In his first papers Figuier was vulnerable and seemed easily disposed of; but he did not give up easily in the face of official dismissal of his position. He met the criticisms of his methods by further refinements and remained convinced that the portal blood contained sugar. His later protestations were increasingly ignored, until long afterwards Bernard found to his chagrin that Figuier's results were right. Such slighting of important work can be partially explained by technical obstacles at the time to a definitive investigation of the problem, but a full explanation is possible only if the historian also takes into account the apparatus of authority in the scientific community. The situation appears to be a prominent example of a characteristic of nineteenth-century French science which Maurice Crosland has elucidated in his study of the Society of Arcueil: the very strong tendency of those men who belonged to the powerful circles of established scientists in Paris to advance the cause of their own associates at the expense of all others.[34] In other settings the social structure of science has often been more open to the claims of newcomers, but there always is a structure of some sort whose features exert an influence on the course of research and thought.

The scientific establishment was not the same as the medical establishment in Paris. For the latter Bernard's views posed different problems. From the start Bernard made clear the significance of his discoveries concerning the production of sugar for understanding diabetes. Consequently his results were of vital importance to physicians, which probably explains the excitement the controversies of 1855 aroused. In the medical literature, case descriptions influenced by Bernard's work had already begun to appear.[35] To some medical men Bernard's conclusions may have appeared to have a destructive effect upon practice. Bouchardat and other physicians had at this time been having some success in controlling diabetics by diets which eliminated carbohydrates. Bernard's view that the appearance of sugar in the body is independent of alimentation would seem to imply that such treatment is futile, and to leave physicians with no way to handle the illness. Because of the overlap between the concerns of medicine and of physiology the scientific debate was coloured in sometimes obvious, sometimes undoubtedly subtle ways by the knowledge of the practical consequences of the outcome.

Accounts of Bernard's discovery ordinarily emphasize its novelty, the break with the ideas and methods of the past that it represented. Historians of science tend to be concerned most often with change. But in any scientific situation there are equally important elements of continuity, which one should also describe if one is to achieve a balanced case study. Bernard's discovery of the glycogen function was only part of a broader investigation of the whole process of nutrition that he was attempting. In this objective, and in the approach he brought to it, he was carrying on a physiological tradition which had begun a century earlier with the studies of digestion by Réaumur. Many people, including Spallanzani, William Beaumont, J. N. Eberle, Theodor Schwann, Friedrich Tiedemann and Leopold Gmelin, had contributed to the development of this tradition. A close examination of their work would show that Bernard shared many of their assumptions and methods of analysis, and that he was taking a long stride along the same path they had been following.

IV

I have enumerated only a few of the most obvious historical factors attending Bernard's discovery, factors typical of the kinds of considerations that are relevant to a full understanding of many comparable situations in the history of science. It is easy to foresee that such a historical account of an investigation whose essential technical results can be summarized in a few pages would occupy a sizeable volume. Such a study would therefore not conform to the

230

aim of the *Harvard Case Histories* of presenting the essential background information in brief compass, and would not furnish a
simple way to understand science. In a broader sense, however, it
would meet Conant's goal of teaching something about science as
well as about the past development of science. Relieved of the task
of providing a total initial image of science, such case studies could
help students to appreciate that all sciences are historical processes
as well as bodies of knowledge. This particular case would be
successful if from it they might come to understand that the historical circumstances under which discoveries are made are at least
as complex and interesting as the new knowledge itself.

REFERENCES AND NOTES

1 J. B. Conant, 'Introduction' to J. B. Conant and L. K. Nash (eds.), *Harvard Case Histories in experimental science*, 2 vols., 1, p. vii, Cambridge,
   Mass.: Harvard University Press, 1957.
2 Ibid., 1, viii.
3 Ibid., 1, 215–321.
4 Ibid., 1, 1–63.
5 Ibid., 1, 65–115.
6 Ibid., 11, 440–50.
7 Ibid., 1, 243.
8 Ibid., 1, 184.
9 Ibid., 11, 450.
10 T. B. Kuhn, *The structure of scientific revolutions*, pp. 10–22 (vol. 11, no. 2
   of *International encyclopedia of unified science*), Chicago: University of
   Chicago Press, 1962.
11 *Harvard Case Histories*, 1957, op. cit. (above, note 1), 1, 319.
12 Ibid., 11, 323–436.
13 H. Butterfield, *The whig interpretation of history*, pp. 62–3, London: G.
   Bell, 1951.
14 Ibid., p. 21.
15 Ibid.
16 E. E. Morison, 'On teaching history', *Ventures: Magazine of the Yale
   Graduate School* (Yale University Press) Fall 1966, 6, No. 2, 42–3 [num-
   bers individually paginated].
17 Claude Bernard, *An introduction to the study of experimental medicine*, transl.
   H. C. Greene, p. 163, New York: Dover, 1957.
18 Ibid., pp. 181–2.
19 Ibid., pp. 165–7.
20 Ibid., p. 167.
21 J. M. D. Olmsted, 'Chapter twelve. The glycogenic function of the liver'

in *Claude Bernard. Physiologist*, pp. 156–74, New York and London: Harper, 1938;

F. G. Young, 'Claude Bernard and the theory of the glycogenic function of the liver', *Ann. Sci.* 1937, **2**, 47–83;

N. Mani, 'Die Entdeckung des Glykogens durch Claude Bernard', *Z. klin. Chemie* 1964, **2**, 97–104.

22 M. D. Grmek, 'La glycogénèse et le diabète dans l'œuvre de Claude Bernard' in Claude Bernard, *Leçon sur le diabète*, pp. 187–234, Paris: Cercle du livre Précieux, 1968.

23 J. Schiller, *Claude Bernard et les problèmes scientifiques de son temps*, pp. 71–90, Paris: Editions du Cèdre, 1967.

24 Ibid., 'La nutrition et la méthode experimentale', pp. 91–104.

25 Ibid., pp. 59–70.

26 Ibid., 'Les conséquences de la découverte de la glycogénèse hépatique', pp. 111–17.

27 F. L. Holmes, 'Claude Bernard and animal chemistry', paper read to a colloquium of historians of biology in Cambridge, Mass., April 1966. I am now completing a longer treatment of these events.

28 Claude Bernard, 'De l'origine du sucre dans l'économie animale', *C. r. Séanc. Soc. Biol.*, 1849 [published 1850], **1**, 121–33, see p. 132 [second of two paginations].

29 C. G. Lehmann, 'Einige vergleichende Analysen des Blutes der Pfortader der Lebervenen', *Ber. sächs. Ges. (Akad.) Wiss. Math.-Phys. Cl.* Leipzig 1850, pp. 131–64; Sitzung den 30. November 1850. This discussion applies only to Lehmann's view in 1850. In 1855 he was drawn into a fuller investigation of the specific question of the production of sugar as Bernard's results came under attack.

30 F. T. Frerichs, 'Die Verdauung' in R. Wagner (ed.), *Handwörterbuch der Physiologie*, Band 3, 1. Abt., pp. 830–2, Braunschweig: Vieweg, 1846.

31 H. de Castelnau, 'Le sucre et le foie—le pancreas et les corps gras', *Le Moniteur des Hôpitaux* Paris 1855, **3**, 145–6, see p. 145. Many of the key articles produced by this debate were republished in this journal between February and November 1855, together with frequent editorial comments by Castelnau.

32 Olmsted, 1938, op. cit. (above, note 21), pp. 168–71; Grmek, 1968, op. cit. (above, note 22), pp. 221–4.

33 P. Lorain, 'Sucre dans la chair musculaire', *Le Moniteur des Hôpitaux* Paris 1855, **3**, 144 [letter to H. de Castelnau]; C. Bernard, 'De la fonction glucogénique du foie', ibid., pp. 154–6.

34 M. Crosland, *The Society of Arcueil: a view of French science at the time of Napoleon I*, p. 474, London: Heinemann, 1967.

35 See, for example, [G.] Andral, 'De quelques faits pathologiques propres à éclairer la question de la production du sucre dans l'économie animale', *Le Moniteur des Hôpitaux* Paris 1855, **3**, 731–2, and M. Semmola, 'Note sur une nouvelle maladie glucogénique (éphidrose sucrée) et sur la glucogénie en général', ibid., pp. 940–1.

13 Editing and Translating a Galenic Text

PHILLIP DE LACY

The study of Greek medical texts must necessarily be a cooperative enterprise. For one thing, these texts often include much that is not primarily medical. Galen, at least, finds opportunities to discuss language, logic and literature, to mention political, social and religious institutions, and to introduce a wide variety of historical and philosophical problems in the course of his presentation of his views on psychology, physiology, anatomy, and other matters more directly relevant to medicine. Besides this range of subject-matter in medical treatises, there are the usual problems encountered in the study of any ancient text: reconstructing the original, tracing its sources and its history, and determining its precise meaning. Still a third reason for cooperation is the sheer bulk of the material to be studied. It is a major investment of time merely to read the Hippocratic corpus and the surviving works of Galen, and of course they by no means exhaust the list of extant medical writings. One can only conclude that it would be foolhardy for any one person to undertake the task of editing and translating a major work of Galen.[1]

Yet this is exactly what I did back in 1961, when I agreed to edit and translate Galen's *De placitis Hippocratis et Platonis* for the Corpus Medicorum Graecorum. I was attracted to the work because of its importance for the history of Greek Philosophy, especially Stoicism; it is in fact more philosophical than medical. But it was obvious from the start that I would need help of many kinds, and especially in the biological and medical areas, where I have no professional competence whatever.

It is gratifying to report that the persons and organizations whose help I have sought have been uniformly responsive. Financial support was obtained in the form of a four-year research grant

(1962–66) from the National Institutes of Health. Colleagues, physicians, research assistants, librarians and others have given assistance on a great variety of problems. But unfortunately assistance cannot be sought until meaningful questions have been formulated, and even meaningful questions must not be asked of others until one's own resources for answering them have been exhausted. Consultation with others has therefore been limited more by the difficulty of asking questions than of finding persons ready and able to answer them. The most successful procedure, in my opinion, has been to go ahead with the preparation of text and translation, giving tentative solutions to the problems encountered, then to submit copies to readers of diverse backgrounds—philologists, philosophers, biologists, etc.—and to make revisions in the light of their comments. In this way many errors have been detected and removed.

The first step in the preparation of text and translation was purely philological: the construction of a provisional Greek text of the nine books of the treatise. The best available printed text was that of I. Müller published in 1874.[2] The best manuscript, beginning in the middle of Book II and extending through most of Book IX, was identified some ten years after Müller's edition appeared. It is known as H (Hamilton 270) and resides in the Deutsche Staatsbibliothek in Berlin.[3] The next most important manuscript, one part of which is in Cambridge (Cantabr. 47) and the other in Florence (Laur. 74, 22), was known to Müller. It contains all that remains of Book I, all of Book II, most of Book V, and parts of Books III, IV and VI. All other Greek manuscripts and editions derive ultimately from H and are useful only where H is now defective or where they have attempted to correct errors in H. When the evidence for the Greek text had been assembled from these and other sources, but especially from H, Müller's printed text was revised and emended.

The next step was to type a working copy of the revised Greek text. Here I was fortunate indeed in having two graduate assistants able to type Greek with speed and accuracy. They made the pages short, most of them less than ten lines long, in order to leave room for notes and to facilitate further revision. The total number of pages was 1389; these were arranged in nine loose-leaf notebooks, each page of Greek facing a blank page on which a translation would eventually appear.

As soon as the provisional text was completed my assistant and I put it on IBM cards and with the cooperation of the Computer Center of Northwestern University we obtained a complete concordance, listing alphabetically every occurrence of every word in its context. The total number of entries in the concordance is about 93 000. It has been a major instrument in the work of editing and translating. For one thing, it facilitates the study of Galen's language and style and thus provides guidelines for correcting scribal errors in the manuscripts, testing one's own attempts at emendation, and rejecting erroneous readings proposed by editors and commentators. An example of this last is the reading ἀφανής, proposed by Kalb-fleisch[4] at p. 606.12 of Müller's edition, where manuscript H is damaged. This reading was accepted into the provisional text, but the concordance immediately revealed that the word ἀφανής occurs nowhere else in the treatise. I therefore re-examined the damaged portion of H, detected a few traces of the lost letters, and with the help of B. Einarson, Professor of Greek at the University of Chicago, recovered the correct reading, ἀζυγής.

The concordance has also made it much easier to find one's way in this large mass of Greek, to bring together similar passages that may be several hundred pages apart, to determine the precise meaning of some technical word or phrase by locating and examining every instance of its use, and even to recapture passages that one vaguely remembers.

Translation is the ultimate test of one's understanding of a text. It is a sobering experience. There is an almost irresistible temptation to be vague and imprecise when one encounters an obscure passage in the original. Then, if ever, one needs the help of honest friends. Often enough, the attempt to make the translation clear and precise leads to the detection of an error in the Greek text, or sends one in search of parallels in Galen's other writings, or necessitates background reading in Hippocrates or Aristotle. Some of the most difficult passages in the treatise are quotations from the lost works of Chrysippus *On the soul* and *On the affections*; they take for granted a familiarity with Stoic jargon and with the Stoic doctrines of *pneuma*, *tonos*, and the like. Thus editing, translating and annotating advanced *pari passu*, to the point where all of the nine books are now equipped with tentative texts, translations, and notes. One book, the eighth, was studied by my capable assistant, Mr Frederick

Rusch, as his doctoral dissertation. Two others have reached the stage where they can be xeroxed entire and submitted to readers. The process of revision is in itself endless, but it must soon be called to an arbitrary halt, so that the edition can be published. Then it will be up to others to continue the inquiry.

In a complex problem such as this perhaps the most important methodological problem is that of fluidity. It is not possible to complete work on page one before beginning page two, but every page is subject to revision whenever new insights are gained and new evidence appears. Here the mechanical aids are a hindrance rather than a help. A xerox copy made six months ago is now obsolete and ought to be destroyed. The IBM concordance was based on a provisional text that has been altered in hundreds of places, so that the concordance now contains an abundance of ghosts and can no longer be trusted to give a reliable account of the text. This threat of obsolescence makes communication difficult; one hesitates to submit to others for comment a passage that may be altered before their answer is received; and one is reluctant to place in their hands a document that contains uncorrected errors.

In this connection I believe that machine indexes, if improperly used, could do great harm. A machine index, by its very usefulness, comes between the scholar and the text. It enables him to exploit far more texts than he could possibly find time to read. The next generation of scholars will have machine indexes of many major Greek writers, perhaps even of Hippocrates and Galen, and no doubt they will lead to significant advances in knowledge. But the indexes themselves will be no better than the texts on which they are based; those that are based on poor texts will only perpetuate their errors. The writings of Galen are an excellent example. A complete index to all of Galen would be of tremendous help to persons working in Greek medicine; but so much of Galen has not yet been properly edited that such an index, if made today, would be even more defective than my concordance has come to be. It is imperative that some means be found whereby the instruments of progress may themselves keep step with the advances that they make possible.

To sum up, the basic methods used in editing Galen's *De placitis Hippocratis et Platonis* have been wholly traditional. The work has been facilitated by the assistance received from others and by cer-

tain mechanical aids; the latter, however, have certain disadvantages
which set a limit to their usefulness.

NOTES AND REFERENCES

1 In spite of the difficulties, considerable work is now being done on the
   text of Galen. See especially the bibliography compiled by K. Schubring
   and published in vol. xx of the reprint of Kühn (*Opera omnia*. Editionem
   curavit C. G. Kühn, Leipzig: Cnobloch, 1821–33, 20 vols. in 22: reprint,
   Hildesheim: Olms, 1965); and J. Kollesch, 'Das Corpus Medicorum
   Graecorum—Konzeption und Durchführung', *Medizinhistorisches Journal*
   1968, 3, 68–73.
2 *Claudii Galeni de placitis Hippocratis et Platonis libri novem*, Recensuit et
   explanavit Iwanus Mueller [with Latin translation], Leipzig: B. G.
   Teubner, 1874.
3 First identified by E. Wellmann, 'Codex Hamilton 329 (Galenos)', *Rhein.
   Mus.* 1885, 40, 30–7. Subsequently it was the subject of two dissertations:
   J. Petersen, *In Galeni de placitis Hippocratis et Platonis libros quaestiones
   criticae*, Göttingen, 1888; and C. Kalbfleisch, *In Galeni de placitis Hippocratis et Platonis libros observationes criticae*, Berlin, 1892. An excellent
   description of the manuscript in its present damaged state may be
   found in C. De Boer, *Die Handschriften-Verzeichnisse der Königlichen
   Bibliothek zu Berlin*: vol. xi, *Verzeichnis der gr. Handschriften*, ii (Berlin,
   1897), pp. 231f.
4 Op. cit., p. 7.

14 Statistical Methods applied to Ancient Medical Writings

WILLIAM C. WAKE

The ancient medical writings which have survived seem to be those which were at one time grouped together in libraries but many now exist without dates, places of composition or authorship recorded. Moreover they frequently survived in part only and have joined with other fragments of doubtful relevance. To use these works as source material for historical studies it is desirable to know when they were written, the author and the extent to which they are homogeneous. Traditional approaches to these problems involve internal and external evidence, the former being compounded of subject-matter and style. We are concerned here almost entirely with style and with a particular way of measuring aspects of it. Judgements of stylistic similarity have had in the past a subjective dependence on the believed recognition of complex elements of rhythm, vocabulary and syntax. The one element of style which may be thought to have a numerical basis is the *hapax legomenon*, the singular occurrence of a word otherwise unknown or at least very rare.

In the late nineteenth century it was realized[1,2] that some elements of style could be expressed quantitatively but this was not exploited until rediscovered in 1938.[3] The rise during the twentieth century of the statistics appropriate to small samples and the significance of differences opened the opportunity for investigation for anyone with the patience to count and record stylistic features. The era of counting 'by hand' for statistical purposes lasted only twenty years before computers took over. It is now possible to sort, tabulate, count and perform mathematical and logical operations rapidly on complete literary texts. The pioneer in this use of computers, at least in Britain, has been A. Q. Morton[4] but American workers have used computers for literary analysis and Ellegård in Sweden was early in the field with his use of a computer for handling vast quantities of data in the solution of the eighteenth-century historico-literary problem of the Junius letters.[5]

Statistical nature of writing

Writing involves the frequent repetition of some words and the occasional use of many more. Statistics deals with assemblages or populations and the more examples we have the more precise our information about the population. It follows that frequently occurring features are, in general, of greater statistical interest than rare ones. The lengths of sentences measured in words or syllables, or letters in a word, can be expressed as distributions, the number of occurrences being distributed over the variable quantity of length. Occurrences of words or word forms can be expressed as simple ratios such as occurrences per sentence or per line or again expressed as a distribution, for example, the proportion of sentences (or lines) containing 0, 1, 2, 3,...n, occurrences of the word specified.

There is no acceptable way of dealing with very rare words: infrequent words can be classified in terms of the distance between successive occurrences but, obviously, this fails when a word occurs only once or twice in a work.

Choice of method

The nature of the data to be collected and the method of analysis to be employed will depend on the problem to be studied. Ancient texts, however, impose severe limitations on method. Ellegård's examination of the Junius problem depended on the comparison of texts involving a million words from known contemporary literature and of 127 000 words from the letters of Junius. Texts of this size are not available from the ancient world, they do not exist now and never existed on this scale. Methods for use with ancient texts must be able to deal with short samples and limited vocabularies.

The major problem is always the integrity of the text. A possible method for detecting discontinuities was suggested by the writer in 1964 (Cusum technique, see pp. 251–4) but there is urgent need for some other means of knowing when some change takes place in style. This change may be a complete break due to the juxtaposition of two works which have at some time become fused and copied as though continuous, or a brief change from the incorporation of a gloss. There is also the possibility of such interpolation influencing the values of parameters describing distributions.

The choice of method should also be influenced by the audience to whom the work is addressed. Advanced statistical techniques should only be used when no simpler means will serve. It will then be necessary to explain what the technique does and why; how, can be relegated to an appendix. In general, limited results with very simple arithmetical techniques will command the greatest support from classicists.

Examination of the results of analysis

It is too frequently assumed that causal connections can be established by statistical methods. This is rarely so. The typical statistical hypothesis is expressed in a 'null' form which states that no difference exists between two samples or sample and population. This hypothesis is tested and if the probability of its truth is less than 1 in 20, or 1 in 100, or even 1 in 1000, it is considered unlikely or extremely unlikely. The choice of the odds used in the judgment is, of course, quite arbitrary.

Evidence offered by statistical methods has to be weighed with other evidence obtained by classical scholarship. It is perhaps easier to weigh as it has a numeric basis. It is also true that traditional methods have been accorded a weight based on the emotions of the scholar rather than anything else; but it must be emphasized that statistical methods cannot *replace* traditional ones nor can it be assumed where conflict exists that the numeric method is right. Statistics are only as reliable as the data on which they are based and their interpretation relies on an understanding of that data as well as on the correct use of statistical method.

II

THE COLLECTION OF DATA

The extent and nature of the data will determine the mode of collection. If an exhaustive statistical exercise is mounted, it will probably be quicker and more accurate to arrange for the text to be transcribed on to a tape for computer operation but if a more limited programme is planned, simple enumeration will produce the data required more quickly than preparing a tape. Sentence lengths can be counted, particles or prepositions underlined and then counted very rapidly without appreciable error. If parts of speech such as nouns, adjectives, adverbs or verbs are to be recorded rather than specific words, there is no alternative to marking the text by hand and then counting. Computer programs are easily written to identify and list occurrences of specific words but not grammatical parts other than particles and the like which can be individually programed. A number of classical texts are now available on tape and the list is gradually extending.[6,7] Although quotation is made in this article from work which is computer based, the Hippocratic data quoted were all obtained by simple counting and shows clearly that as a tool for research it is adequate to answer many questions. Where a large-scale survey is contemplated, for example a search of the Galenic *Corpus*, the computer is more appropriate though transcription of this *Corpus* on to tape would at present prices cost several thousand pounds. In the following survey a modern text is assumed and, if not available, would have to be prepared. Incunabulae and sixteenth-century printed texts contain all the scribal abbreviations and ligatures, as instance the Foes' text of Hippocrates[8] which uses punctuation almost at random and requires transliteration unless one is accustomed to scribal texts.[9]

III

THE NATURE OF STATISTICAL PROBLEMS

There are three problems associated with the length of the text.

(i) *The question of chance variation*

If writing were merely a random collection of words arranged in sentences by some chance process we could easily calculate the variability expected from a given sample and how this would alter with length. Certain features of the text do occur randomly but others, such as sentence lengths, do not. An author tends to use groups of short sentences perhaps to give emphasis or raise the emotional tone and, between these groups, longer sentences range. For random features the mean rate of occurrence will be subject to variation measured by the *standard error of the mean* and inversely proportional to the square root of the length of the text.

(ii) *Minimum adequate size*

For sentence lengths and other features not randomly used, the variability behaves in a standard manner only for samples in excess of certain minimum lengths which vary from author to author.

(iii) *Features not proportional to text length*

Whereas the occurrence of nouns in the Hippocratic work *Prognostic* is 15 per 100 words and within the sampling error is the same for any consecutive 100 words of the text, the frequency of recurrence of nouns is a complex function of the textual length. Thus the number of nouns that occur x times, where x is taken successively as 1, 2, 3, 4,... etc., is not proportional to the textual length. Tables of frequency distributed over occurrences have been suggested to measure the richness of an author's vocabulary. Much ingenuity has been involved in devising parameters that convey in a single number the information given in the frequency table. Such are Yule's *Characteristic*[10] and Williams's *Index of Diversity*.[11] The situation is illustrated in Table 1.[12]

In the first half of the text there are 455 occurrences of nouns and in the whole text 858 occurrences; occurrences naturally being proportional to the length of text. However, the number of nouns which occur at given frequencies are not proportional to length, the second half producing much less than the first. The number of nouns occurring once in the whole text but which actually appear in the second half is not (151–120) because some of the 120 nouns which occur once in the first half occur again in the second and hence move into the class of twice-occurring nouns when the sample size is doubled. Only nouns which occur very frequently vary in number of occurrences directly proportionally to sample size.

After preliminary work by Yule[3] and the writer,[12] the statistical examination of textual features which, like nouns, are not proportional to length of text has been avoided by those interested in problems of authorship although linguistic studies have been made of the way individual words of a vocabulary are distributed.[13]

TABLE 1. Noun occurrences in the Hippocratic book, *Regimen in acute diseases* (effect of sample size)

Occurrences	Sample		Whole text	
	Number of nouns	Total of occurrences	Number of nouns	Total of occurrences
1	120	120	151	151
2	29	58	44	88
3	15	45	19	57
4	10	40	10	40
5	5	25	10	50
6	1	6	6	36
7	3	21	3	21
8	2	16	4	32
9	1	9	1	9
10	2	20	1	10
11	1	11	3	33
12	1	12	4	48
13	1	13	–	–
14	3	42	3	42
15	–	–	–	–
16	–	–	3	48
17	1	17	4	68
18			1	18
19			1	19
20			–	–
21			1	21
31			1	31
36			1	36
Totals	195	455	271	858

IV

REPETITIVE ELEMENTS AND DISTRIBUTIONS

The most fruitful work on the study of the authorship of ancient texts has used frequency distributions or the rate of occurrence of repetitive elements of the text. The earliest though abortive attempt to use repetitive elements in Plato was that of Lutoslawski.[2] Wake[14] reported on sentence-length distributions of the Pauline Epistles in 1948 and in 1957 generally on problems of sentence length in ancient texts.[15] The simple repetitive elements afforded by the particles and particularly by *kai* were first used by Morton[16] with the Pauline Epistles but later on with a very wide range of Greek texts.[17]

From these surveys it appears that the ancient author was a man who wrote in periods in which the proportion of short, medium and long sentences remained remarkably constant as do also the frequency with which he used *kai* and *de*. The establishment of these simple facts rests on attested works compared with others ascribed but now rejected by a consensus of scholars. A non-controversial example is provided by Xenophon. The mean sentence length of accepted and spurious works shows easy differentiation.

TABLE 2. Mean sentence lengths of genuine and spurious works of Xenophon

Work	Mean length words	Work	Mean length words
Hero	18.9	*Sparta*	17.5
Agesilaus	20.0	*On Horses*	81.1
Ways and Means	19.2	*Cynegeticus:*	
Hipparchicus	19.6	Part 1	15.4
		Part 2	14.6

The *Cynegeticus* is known to be spurious. Two points must be emphasized. The sentence-length distribution cannot be completely characterized by its mean; distributions which are very different may have indistinguishable means. Secondly, there is no reason why two authors should not show in their writings the *same* sentence-length distribution, but two writings with different distributions are very unlikely to be the work of one author.

V

HOMOGENEITY AND SAMPLE SIZE

Although a minimum length of text from which to collect data may seem a trivial requirement it is, in fact, a major handicap. Ancient texts have been repeatedly glossed with the glosses incorporated into the text. Scholars have spent much effort eliminating these but medical texts have not been worked through to the same extent as others of more general interest. Obviously, the text used must be free from glosses, lacunae and other textual uncertainties. Textual emendments which help the meaning and are justified thereby are generally inadmissible in statistical data. An example concerns Aristotle's *De generatione* where, after Book 1, Peck's edition[18] shows 6 to 7 per cent of the sentences to be involved in textual uncertainties, sufficient to render the later books unsuitable for statistical purposes.

A minimum length of text is required so that the standard errors of the statistics used are reasonably small; otherwise differentiation of one author from another becomes impossible. There is real need for a numeric method capable of indicating the occurrence of glosses but, as these are usually limited to a single sentence, there is little hope of being able to achieve this by statistical methods.

Quotations present difficulties; the first is the obvious one that if one writer quotes another, the quotation, even in reported speech, is not an example of the style of the first writer and should therefore be omitted. The extent to which quotation distorts the surrounding sentences is not usually important as frank quotations, except in Hellenistic works, are rare. The second problem is then one of deciding whether a given sequence of words is a quotation of another sequence of not quite identical words. Morton[19] has looked at this in the context of the early Christian Fathers quoting from the New Testament as known today. He concluded from an examination of word frequency and word patterns that most of the quotations regarded by New Testament scholars as definite had only a moderate probability and those felt to be very likely are statistically very unlikely.

VI

PARAMETERS AND DISTRIBUTIONS

Sentence-length distributions

It is convenient to group sentences as is done in Table 3 and to calculate the required parameters from the grouped data using linear interpolation within the group. Fig. 1 shows smoothed curves making clear how very different the two distributious are. For most purposes it suffices to calculate the mean, the first quartile Q_1 as a measure of the short sentences and the ninth decile D_9 as a measure of the long sentences. If x is the length of the mid-point of a sentence

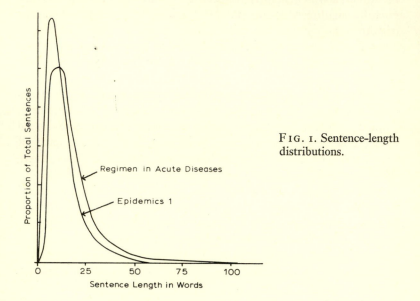

FIG. 1. Sentence-length distributions.

group and f the frequency of occurrence in that group, and n the total number of sentences in the sample, $\Sigma f = n$ and the mean, $m = \Sigma f x / n$ where the summations denoted by Σ are over all groups. Q_1 is obtained as a sentence length below which lie one-quarter of the sentences and D_9 as the length above which only one-tenth of the sentences lie. These are calculated by taking the groups together until the further addition of another group would exceed the required number. The position of these percentiles within the group is then calculated by taking the required proportion of the group interval.

246

TABLE 3. Linear sentence-length distributions of two Hippocratic works

Sentence length in words	Regimen in acute diseases	Epidemics I
1–5	23	52
6–10	84	89
11–15	91	61
16–20	59	30
21–25	45	21
26–30	22	9
31–35	9	9
36–40	7	3
41–45	6	4
46–50	3	–
51–55	2	1
56–60	–	–
61–65	1	–
66–70	–	–
71–75	1	–
81–85	1	–
86–90	–	–
91–95	1	–
111–115	–	1
Totals	355	278

The group intervals are taken as 0.5 to 5.5, 5.5 to 10.5, and so on. Q_1 for *Regimen in acute diseases* is 9.4. There are 355 sentences in the work (see Table 3) and Q_1 occurs in the cumulative distribution after 88 sentences. There are 23 sentences in the first group so that 64 sentences have to be supplied from the sentence group of 84 sentences.

The quartile therefore occurs at a length of $5.5 + \left(\dfrac{65}{84} \times 5 \right)$, i.e., $5.5 + 3.9 = 9.4$ words.

Table 4 shows these constants for a group of three Hippocratic works.

The similarities and differences are here obvious but in general these are to be judged against the calculated standard error for the constants used, that for the mean being (*standard deviation*/$\sqrt{n}$); the others can be obtained from standard books.

An alternative involves recasting the data in logarithmic form as

TABLE 4. Constants of sentence-length distributions for three Hippocratic works

Constant of distribution	Prognostic	Regimen in acute diseases	Epidemics I
Mean	17.7	17.0	12.8
Q_1	10.5	9.4	6.5
D_9	31.3	29.5	25.5
Size of work (number of sentences)	286	355	278

sentence-length distributions then show the well-known symmetrical normal distribution[20] instead of being skew. A convenient allocation of sentence lengths to logarithmic groups is given in Table 5 which can be compared with Table 3; similarly the histogram of the data from Table 5 is shown in Fig. 2 together with the theoretical curve for a normal distribution fitted to this data and can be compared with Fig. 1.

Binomial distributions

Where an event can occur in alternative ways—heads or tails for example—the relative frequency of occurrence on n occasions is given by the binomial theorem from which the mean number of occurrences can be calculated and, more importantly, a standard error which can be used to judge the significance of departures from expected frequencies. Table 6 gives the number of occurrences of the conjunction *kai* and the total number of words in the first five works of Isocrates[17] followed by the percentage occurrence of *kai*. Whilst one might conclude without calculation that the first work differs from the others, as is in fact the case for it is known to be spurious, one might wish to consider whether work 3 differs significantly from works 2, 4 and 5. The theory of binomial distributions can be applied, regarding each word as '*kai*' or 'not *kai*' in a total of 3737 occasions in work 3 and 6539 in work 4. The standard error is $p(100 - p)\left(\dfrac{1}{n_1} + \dfrac{1}{n_2}\right)^{\frac{1}{2}}$ where p is weighted mean percentage for the two works 5.10, and n_1 and n_2 the total work occurrences of

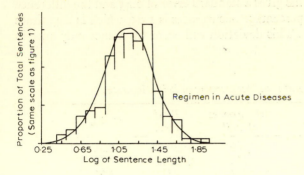

FIG. 2. Log-normal distribution of sentences.

TABLE 5. Logarithmic distribution of sentence lengths for *Regimen in acute diseases*

Sentence length	Mean log length	Number of words
2	0.35	1
3	0.45	4
4	0.55	6
5	0.65	12
6	0.75	15
7	0.85	17
8–10*	0.95	41
10–12*	1.05	50
13–15	1.15	52
16–19	1.25	48
20–25	1.35	56
26–31	1.45	24
32–39	1.55	12
40–50	1.65	11
51–63	1.75	2
64–79	1.85	2
80–100	1.95	2
Total		355
Mean		1.150
Standard deviation		0.257

*Sentences of exactly 10 words are arbitrarily divided equally between these two groups.

249

3737 and 6539. This gives a standard error of 0.45 and the difference between the two percentage occurrences is 1.05, which is 2.33 times its standard error. This deviation will occur by chance only once in 100 times.

TABLE 6. Occurrences of *kai* in Isocrates

Work	Occurrences of 'kai'	Total words	% 'kai'
1	69	2903	2.38
2	140	3006	4.67
3	213	3737	5.71
4	311	6539	4.76
5	250	5352	4.67

Poisson distributions

This is another important distribution related to the binomial distribution. Whereas simple reckoning of words like *kai, de, mē, ou, en* as proportions of the total number of words present gives the easiest means of characterizing texts and, as Morton has shown,[17] is as informative as any method if the results are to be expressed by a single figure, it can be argued that the way in which these words occur should contain additional information throwing light on the way a particular author uses these small, habit-forming words. In fact the data can be presented in the form of a distribution which is frequently Poissonian. Thus, if we consider the number of occurrences in each sentence or if we wish to avoid sentence structure in groups of a few lines of the text, Table 7 is obtained. The data are again taken from Morton[17] and refer to the occurrences of *kai* in a typical work of Demosthenes.

Occurrences of such words in sentences instead of groups of words tend to conform to a negative binomial rather than a Poisson distribution. However this may be, the point is that by characterizing the distribution as well as the mean number of occurrences, further information has become available which may prove important where differentiation is difficult or indicate parts of a text which may have scribal errors such as repetition triggered by one of these words (dittography) which could show a deviation from expected frequency of sentences or sections containing the higher frequencies of three or more occurrences.

TABLE 7. Occurrences of *kai* in 20 word samples

	Number of occurrences observed	Expected for Poisson distribution
None	35	34.0
One	38	37.2
Two	18	20.5
Three	9	7.6
Four	1	2.1
Five	1	0.6
Number of samples	102	102
Total number of occurrences	110	

VII

EXISTENCE AND POSITION OF TEXTUAL DISCONTINUITIES

In most statistical work the independent opinion of the textual critic has been used in deciding the location of samples from which statistical data are required. Displacement of passages is more common in ancient texts than would be expected by the layman and a typical example of the confused text is provided by the Hippocratic books, *Fractures*, *Joints* and *Mochlicon* [instruments for reducing dislocations).* If there is a known or obvious discontinuity, samples of the homogeneous text on both sides of the discontinuity can be examined and compared. The statistical problem is to provide some way of examining serial data which will indicate when a change has taken place. Such methods are needed for detecting glosses and change of style—thereby suggesting but not proving change of author—when the subject-matter apparently flows freely forward. The only suggestion which can be offered for this purpose is the statistical technique known as Cumulative Sum analysis, or Cusum.[21] In this technique a mean is found and then departures from this

* These are abbreviated to F, J, and M.

mean are added serially and the varying result plotted. Unlike purely random series of numbers, the Cusum plot for sentence lengths shows with the literary texts a more or less regular pattern of peaks and troughs which, it was hoped, would prove characteristic of a given author. When a discontinuity occurred and the level altered, it was expected that the plot would run out of control by continuously increasing or decreasing from the exact point of the discontinuity. The use of the computer program to plot Cusum has made this function easy to examine but has shown that interpretation is often ambiguous.

The matter will be much clearer with an actual example taken from the F-J-M group of Hippocratic works. Using Withington's text in the Loeb edition[22] we find M VII–XIX is a verbal repetition of J XVIII–XXIX and these chapters are derived from F XXXVIII–XLVII and elsewhere. Withington suggests an epitome of F was made for M and that this has at some time been transferred to J to fill a gap caused by manuscript damage or loss. He gives scholarly reasons for this based on peculiarities of vocabulary and construction. It may be reasonably assumed that M is by a different hand, just as it is usually assumed that J and F are parts of one book. Withington's suggestion amounts to a discontinuity between J XVI and J XVII. Continuity of subject during J XIII–XVI suggests that this passage is examined and run on into the passage which starts with J XVII and continues to J XXIX. The method will be clear from Table 8, which gives only the beginning of the Cusum series for log sentence length which is plotted complete in Fig. 3.

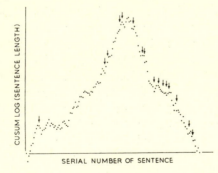

FIG. 3. Serial Cusum for log (sentence-length) of *Joints* XIII to XXIX.

Logs have been used here mainly for scaling convenience; actual sentence lengths could equally well have been used.

TABLE 8. Cusum series for J XIII onwards. Mean of all log (sentence length) from J XII to J XXIX, 1.087

Sentence numbered from start of passage	Sentence length in words	Log sentence length	Deviation from mean	Sum of deviations
1	13	1.114	0.027	0.027
2	10	1.000	− 0.087	− 0.060
3	10	1.000	− 0.087	− 0.147
4	29	1.462	0.375	0.229
*	*	*	*	*
*	*	*	*	*
*	*	*	*	*
138	23	1.362	0.275	0.388
139	5	0.699	− 0.388	0.000

It will be appreciated that a run of sentences approximating to the mean used will appear generally horizontal as, for example, sentences 17 to 34. The steady increase from sentences 35 to 47 and 52 to 77 imply runs of sentences of similar mean length but above the overall mean. The diagram finishes at zero because the overall deviations from an overall mean must, by definition, be zero. The last sentence of each chapter is marked with an arrow to assist location. (The chapters are, of course, a late subdivision of the text determined by subject-matter.)

Now the major discontinuity shown at the top of the diagram is caused by the change postulated by Withington but is only apparent 7 sentences later due to the general variability. However, a second feature which does not appear in Withington's analysis is clear from the diagram. The steady upward trend showing sentences longer than the overall mean and typical of the passage before the major discontinuity is interrupted between sentences 12 and, say, 34. This corresponds to the start of chapter XIV and about halfway through. The end of chapter XIII and the sentence in chapter XIV starting: '*ắlloi d'aû tinés eisin, hoi tines katamathóntes toûto...*' we find continuity of subject-matter. Chapter XIII discusses damage to the shoulder and recommends mechanical treatment but also dressing. 'The projecting part however should be forced down, the bulk of the compresses placed over it and the strongest pressure made here.'

Ending with 'The acromion becomes painless in a few days, if it is properly bandaged', and the other end of the discontinuity starts '(Again),* there are (certain) others, who, recognizing a tendency to slip in these dressings...' The preceding sentences are repetitious. Examination of the text supports the idea of interpolation at this point.

It will be realized that not all statistically demonstrated discontinuities can be accepted as real in the textual sense. Cusum analysis is a sensitive tool and the reasons for the patterned nature of the plots obtained lie in the field of spectral analysis and have not yet been explored in this context. However, Cusum plot can easily be run on a computer, programs already exist and attention can quickly be focused on uncertain passages as in the instance which has been discussed. It is, undoubtedly, a valuable tool the results from which ought to be considered whenever discontinuities are invoked or suspected. The 22 sentences unexpectedly picked out of chapter XIV represent a fairly short passage and there is hope that combinations of methods may enable the one- or two-sentence gloss to be 'indicated' even though 'proved' may always be too strong a word.

VIII

COMPARISON OF VOCABULARY

It was at one time hoped that a comparison of vocabulary, a measure may be of its richness, would be useful in identifying an author.[10] It is now generally accepted that vocabulary, as has been demonstrated for nouns,[12] is determined substantially by subject-matter and that it is the small inconsequential words and phrases which provide in their frequency of use hallmarks of a given author. This has been shown on a substantial scale for English texts by Ellegård[5] and by Mosteller and Wallace,[23] and Morton[17] has provided a mass of data from the corpus of Greek literary works. It is useful to examine, therefore, whether the classical methods used by scholars can be sharpened by statistical handling of the same type of data. We may consider the use in Hippocratic writings of two words for 'pain', *odunē*, occurring frequently in the *Iliad* but only rarely in the

* 'Again' is the translation of *de* inserted to meet the needs of the context and would not necessarily have been used.

Odyssey, and *ponos* which has the primary meaning of toil, hard or dangerous work in Homer generally and secondarily in the tragedies and in Hippocrates of 'pain'. Their occurrences in certain works are given in the first two lines of Table 9.

TABLE 9. Comparison of occurrences for words translated 'pain'

		Regimen in acute diseases	Prognostic	Epidemics I
Observed	*odunē*	14	21	5
occurrences	*ponos*	9	11	7
Adjusted to equal	*odunē*	14	25.0	8.5
length of text	*ponos*	9	13.1	11.9
Expected occurrences	*odunē*	13.4	22.2	11.8
for random allocation	*ponos*	9.9	15.8	8.5

The observed occurrences seem to show a pattern in which *Regimen in acute diseases* and *Prognostic* differ from *Epidemics* I as indeed they almost certainly do. It is tempting therefore to submit this as another piece of evidence to support this conclusion. However, even the non-mathematical might wish to adjust the figures on the argument that different lengths of text are involved and that occurrences might be expected to be proportional to length. This has been done from known figures for the number of words in the text and is given in the third and fourth lines of the table. When so adjusted, if the impression persists that real differences are there then either the original data or those adjusted to equal text length should be examined by calculating the expected occurrences for chance random allocation. In lines 5 and 6 of the table the 81.5 occurrences of lines 3 and 4 have been allocated in the most probable manner. The expected number of occurrences of *odunē* in *Regimen in acute diseases* is given by the proportion $a.b/n$ where a is the total occurrences of the word in all works, b the total occurrences of both words in *Regimen in acute diseases*, and n the total of both words in all works. Similarly for the other expectations. The well-known χ^2 distribution, for which tables are available showing the value at different levels of probability, may be written

$$\chi^2 = \Sigma \text{ (Deviation from Expectation)}^2/\text{Expectation,}$$

255

where Σ implies summation. In this example χ^2 involves the summation of 6 terms and has a value of 3.07. Tables show that this result has a probability of about 20 per cent and is therefore quite likely to occur by chance. In spite of the seeming pattern of differences, particularly between *Prognostic* and *Epidemics* I, these figures could occur by chance and do not support the idea that the usages of these two words differ in these two works.

In fact, certain other words having a general meaning in this field are used by the author of *Regimen in acute diseases*. The words are *algēdōn* and *algēma*. The first is used only once, and is therefore in this context an *hapax legomenon*, and the second, three times. At this level of use their non-occurrence in other works is not surprising as will be realized from the variations of the other words shown to be no greater than chance expectation. The one feature of scholarly practice which the statistician can legitimately criticize is the placing of undue weight on words of low frequency with the *hapax legomenon* featuring most and in reality having the least significance.

IX

CHOICE OF PROBLEM

The posing of the statistical problem is secondary to the historico-medical or literary one for it is here assumed that one wishes to solve a statistical problem in order to throw light on the primary study. The real problem is likely to be one of the following types, all of which have the possibility of being visualized in statistical terms.

(i) The matching problem. To which of two known authors is a given text to be assigned? This is the problem of the Federalist Papers.[23] This is rare in ancient literature; too much knowledge is required and usually quite a lot of text.

(ii) Is there a core of works of common authorship? (The Hippocratic Problem.)

(iii) Are there spurious works in a corpus of writings known to be substantially by one author? (The Galenic Problem.)

(iv) What is the relation between two or more overlapping works? (This problem may be illustrated by the three Aristotelian *Ethics* with books common to the *Nicomachean* and *Eudemian ethics* or the relation of *Joints, Fractures* and *Mochlicon*.

(v) Does the text exhibit change of author at a given place?

(vi) Does a text contain hitherto unrecognized discontinuities?

(vii) Can the family line of given differing readings of a text be established in order to establish priorities and hence preferred readings? (This is the problem of the Italian and German texts of *De imitatione Christi*.[24])

The statistical problem should be chosen economically both from the standpoint of the work involved and the presentation of the evidence to an appropriate audience. It must also be concerned with texts from which adequate data can be extracted for statistics is concerned with numbers and the precision of the conclusions increases with increasing number of occurrences of the facts which provide its raw material. It is, for example, difficult to formulate a statistical problem involving authorship of the Hippocratic Oath because the text is too short; it comprises—depending on the text used—about 250 words in 11 sentences and in any case there are only fragments of other texts of similar date. The texts must be in fairly good condition so that data collected are not modified by the unconscious inclusion of scribal mistakes or editorial glosses. This tends to limit the problems chosen to those involving texts already well known and therefore to statistical attempts at problems which have been inconclusively tackled by traditional methods over the years. The authorship and integrity of Plato's seventh letter can well stand as a challenge in this respect.

Problems most capable of statistical handling are those involving frequencies of occurrence of single classes such as given words, or sentence lengths rather than multiple classes such as word forms (nouns or verbs, etc.). Statistical studies of vocabulary, though of importance in linguistics, do not seem helpful in the problem we have here except in a very limited sense.

X

There is already in being a body of experience and technique which enable statistical reasoning to be used in problems associated with ancient texts. The theory of reasoning (by Bayesian inference) from the occurrences of word features in samples of known and unknown authorship to conclusions about authorship is not discussed. It has been considered by Mosteller and Wallace[23] and it may be considered a logical conclusion to a statistical argument to advance

257

figures for the probability of the correctness of those conclusions. What is here presented is a variety of simple methods from which additional tools can be chosen as occasion suggests and with the proviso that the evidence offered must be weighed with other evidence. There is no royal road to proof. The identification of books with a possible common author is a major matter; the identification of a discontinuity in a text is by comparison a minor one but circumstance could be such that this identification could have a greater impact on historical studies.

ACKNOWLEDGEMENT

It is a pleasant duty to record my indebtedness to the Rev. A. Q. Morton for many exchanges of ideas in this field of study.

REFERENCES

1   T. C. Mendenhall, 'The characteristic curves of composition', *Science* 1887, 9 (214, supplement), 237–49. Cited by C. B. Williams, 'Studies in the history of probability and statistics IV. A note on an early statistical study of literary style', *Biometrika* 1956, 43, 248–56.

2   W. Lutoslawsky, *Growth of Plato's logic, with an account of Plato's style and of the chronology of his writings*, London: Longmans & Co., 1897.

3   G. Udny Yule, 'On sentence-length as a statistical characteristic of style in prose: with application to two cases of disputed authorship', *Biometrika* 1939, 30, 363–90.

4   A. Q. Morton dealt with this in a paper written in 1961 and which appeared in *Report on use of computers*, the 1961–63 Report of Carnegie Research Scholars. It was later published as the article cited in note 16.

5   H. A. Ellegård, *A statistical method for determining authorship. The Junius Letters, 1769–1772*, Göteborg, 1962 (Gothenburg Studies in English, No. 13).

6   *Calculi* is a mimeographed loose-leaf information sheet published and distributed (at present without charge) by the Department of Classics, Dartmouth College, Hanover, New Hampshire 03755, U.S.A.

7   The British Academy, Burlington Gardens, London w.1, has set up a Committee on the Use of Computers in Textual Criticism.

8   A. Foes, *Magni Hippocratis medicorum omnium facile principis, opera omnia quae extant*, etc., 2 vols., Geneva: S. Chouët, 1557–62.

9   A convenient reference for ligatures is W. Wallace, 'An index of Greek ligatures and contractions', *J. Hellenic Studies* 1923, 43, 183–93.

10 G. Udny Yule, *The statistical study of literary vocabulary*, Cambridge: The University Press, 1944.
11 C. B. Williams, 'Yule's "characteristic" and the Index of Diversity', *Nature, Lond.* 1946, **157**, 482.
12 W. C. Wake, *The Corpus Hippocraticum*, Ph.D. Thesis, London University, 1951.
13 G. Herdan, *Type-token mathematics. A textbook of mathematical linguistics*, 's-Gravenhage: Mouton & Co., 1960.
14 W. C. Wake, 'The authenticity of the Pauline Epistles. A contribution from statistical analysis', *Hibbert J.* 1948, **47**, 50–5.
15 W. C. Wake, 'Sentence-length distributions of Greek authors', *Jl. R. statist. Soc.* 1957, A **120**, 331–46.
16 A. Q. Morton, Chapter IX, 'The authorship of the Pauline Corpus. A study of the occurrence of *kai* in Greek prose' in H. Anderson and W. Barclay (eds.), *The New Testament in historical and contemporary perspective. Essays in memory of G. H. C. Macgregor*, pp. 209–35, Oxford: Blackwell, 1965.
17 A. Q. Morton, 'The authorship of Greek prose', *Jl. R. statist. Soc.* 1965, A **128**, 169–233.
18 Aristotle, *Aristotle: Generation of animals*, with an English translation by A. L. Peck, London: W. Heinemann, 1943 (The Loeb Classical Library).
19 A. Q. Morton, *The chance generation of verbal coincidences in Greek prose*, Lecture delivered in Faculty of Divinity, Glasgow University. To be published, Edinburgh: Oliver & Boyd.
20 'A note on the statistical analysis of sentence-length as a criterion of literary style', *Biometrika* 1939, **31**, 356–61.
21 D. Goldsmith (ed.), *Cumulative sum techniques*, Edinburgh: Oliver & Boyd, 1964 (Imperial Chemical Industries Monograph 3).
22 *Hippocrates*, with an English translation by Dr E. T. Withington, vol. III, London: W. Heinemann, 1927 (The Loeb Classical Library).
23 Frederick Mosteller and David L. Wallace, 'Inference in an authorship problem. A comparative study of discrimination methods applied to the authorship of the disputed *Federalist* papers', *J. Am. statist. Ass.* 1963, **58**, 275–309.
24 G. Udny Yule, 'Cumulative sampling: a speculation as to what happens in copying manuscripts', *Jl. R. statist. Soc.* 1946, **109**, 44–52.

Since the completion of this article the following important monographs have become available:

C. B. Williams, *Style and vocabulary: numerical studies*, London: Griffin, 1970.
L. Doležel and R. W. Bailey (eds.), *Statistics and style*, New York: Elsevier, 1969.

15 Automation and the Control of Historical Sources: Problems and Possibilities

JOHN B. BLAKE

The bibliographical control of historical source material has been one of the major functions of libraries since antiquity, for whatever is written or published becomes part of the past and, if it is preserved, a potential source of information about the past. With the explosive growth of publication in recent years, especially in science and technology, ever more sophisticated methods are being urged and developed to make it possible to find the information in these publications rapidly and efficiently. Nearly all these new systems make use of some form of automated equipment, most commonly computers. It is the purpose of this paper to examine some aspects of the growing use of automation for bibliographical control as it relates to original sources and secondary works in the history of medicine.

II

Before examining particular applications, it may be well to review briefly some of the characteristics of modern data-processing equipment. The computer is not the only one, and in some instances may not even be the best. Optical coincidence systems such as Termatrex, for example, provide a capability for post-coordinate indexing and have been used enthusiastically in certain applications where the body of material to be indexed is reasonably small, where relatively a very modest expenditure and simplicity of operation are essential, and where a printed product is not required.[1] The more familiar 80-column punch card or tab card can also be used without a computer for sorting, selecting, collating, and other tasks useful in preparing indexes and other bibliographic controls.

Computers, however, can carry out these operations more accurately and with incredible speed. They can carry out tasks that are much more complex, and they can print data, once it has been entered into the machine's store, rapidly, as often as needed, and in a variety of formats without the necessity of repeated keyboarding. The computer can store large amounts of data in a small space, its store can easily be duplicated, and selected parts of the store can be retrieved at will, provided proper provision was made initially for this task. The computer is a highly efficient tool for the composition and printing of lists (especially those that change frequently, such as library serial holdings), for the preparation and printing of name indexes, catalogue cards, and book catalogues, for the preparation and printing of KWIC ('Key Word In Context') and KWOC ('Key Word Out of Context') indexes, and for searching files for index terms stored with a citation or abstract of a document. In one form or another all these virtues are useful and have been applied in systems for information retrieval, in libraries and elsewhere.[2]

Computers do have certain disadvantages, however. The typical limited fount of upper-case letters only found in most printers is linguistically and aesthetically unsatisfying. However, upper and lower case, and even diacritical marks, are now available and presumably will be coming into increasing use. More important, both the physical equipment and the intellectual preparation necessary to use it—the programming—are expensive. As Charles P. Bourne has pointed out, this makes them most profitable for information searching when (1) there is need for an exhaustive search of a large file; (2) there is need for a rapid response and the computer is available on demand; (3) the questions asked, or the material filed, are especially complex; (4) large numbers of searches must be carried out; and (5) the field covered lacks good bibliographical control in a conventional form and does not readily lend itself to such control.[3] Because of its cost and the necessity of using the equipment in the most efficient manner possible, most large-scale operations have provided for batch processing, leading to delays and inconvenience in access. The necessity, in most systems, for the ultimate user to work through a search specialist rather than by direct interaction with the machine has also tended at times to increase the delays. Time-sharing on-line computer systems can overcome these difficulties—at still greater expense.

Though many experiments in direct computer abstracting and indexing are going forward, computers cannot yet create an index language for information retrieval systems, although they can help through such means as the preparation of word counts. Computers cannot yet perform the conceptual analysis necessary for assigning index terms to a book, journal article, or manuscript, or for deciding what terms to use, and in what combinations, when the file is to be searched. In short, as F. W. Lancaster writes, they cannot solve the central problem of information retrieval.[4]

III

The sources of medical history are many and various. They include published monographs, journals and other serials, congress proceedings and other composite volumes. They include medieval codices and modern correspondence, diaries, drafts, and other manuscript records, personal, institutional, and governmental. Sources may also include pictures ranging from Pompeian murals to laboratory photographs, and the instruments and equipment of the researcher or physician—including, for future historians, computers themselves and data stored on magnetic tapes. While documents or objects related specifically to medicine form the chief source material for medical historians, those whose interest extends to the social, humanistic, philosophical, or economic aspects of medicine broadly conceived may find sources in almost any area of human activity.

The total amount of potential original source material for the history of medicine is vast. The National Library of Medicine alone holds in the neighbourhood of 1 500 000 items of published literature—monographs, serial volumes, pamphlets, theses, government documents, and so on. In the first three series of the *Index-Catalogue* alone, 1 760 269 journal articles are indexed by subject. The amount of non-medical material of interest to medical historians is virtually unlimited. Obviously the progress of bibliographical controls for medical history must continue to depend in large measure on the improvement of bibliographical controls for all research libraries, particularly in those broader fields within which its interest chiefly lies: medicine and history.

IV

There is probably no aspect of bibliographical control of historical sources which is more advanced, at least in the United States, than the author approach to monographs. Over the past century or more, standards of bibliographical description have been developed by the library profession and accepted so widely that a reasonably intelligent and experienced user with citation in hand can walk into almost any well-organized library in the country and with at most a few minutes' orientation to institutional peculiarities determine for himself by examining the card catalogue whether that library has the book he wants. This splendid record of interlibrary cooperation has also made possible the compilation of the National Union Catalog on cards in the Library of Congress, now scheduled for publication in some 600 volumes. This lists by author and with locations literally millions of books in research libraries throughout the United States; it is in constant use by scholars in search of a particular book. Other countries have the catalogues of their great national libraries, like the British Museum and the Bibliothèque Nationale, as well as national bibliographies of varying degrees of completeness. In addition, medicine is fortunate in having a number of catalogues published by large special libraries, such as the *Index-catalogue of the Library of the Surgeon General's Office*, the *Catalogue of sixteenth century printed books in the National Library of Medicine*, and the *Catalogue of printed books in the Wellcome Historical Medical Library*, as well as those for special collections like the Osler, Cushing, and Waller. In addition, many specialized non-medical bibliographies, such as the short-title catalogues of Pollard and Redgrave and Wing, include medical works and list locations.

These tools may be used not only to find out where a book is located but also to find citations relating to particular persons, topics, places, and periods. A wealth of additional indexes and bibliographies, arranged or indexed by author, subject, or both, is also available. Many of them also provide an approach by time and/or place, the latter often through the use of indexes to printers. For historians the older bibliographies sometimes gain added usefulness by virtue of their date of publication. In searching the well-known *Literatura medica digesta* of Wilhelm G. Ploucquet, for example, those interested in the eighteenth century or earlier are automatically relieved of the necessity of wading through anything issued since 1813. The list of such older general medical bibliographies in Estelle Brodman's *The development of medical bibliography* is impressive in its number. In addition to general bibliographies and general medical bibliographies, many specialized works, which Brodman does not list, such as Heinrich Laehr's *Die Literatur der Psychiatrie, Neurologie und Psychologie von 1459–1799* (Berlin: Reimer, 1900), S. H. de Vigiliis von Creutzenfeld's *Bibliotheca Chirurgica* (Vienna: Trattner, 1781), and *A bibliography of infantile paralysis, 1789–1949* (Philadelphia: Lippincott, 1951), prepared under the direction of the National Foundation, provide guides to particular topics. Others, ranging from Richard J. Durling's informative census of Galen imprints[5] to the elaborate bibliographies of Sir Geoffrey Keynes, provide information on the works of particular authors. In fact, the number of existing bibliographies and guides in which one may search for citations to the medical literature seems inexhaustible.

Yet it is undoubtedly true that additional bibliographies and indexes could usefully be prepared. It is still difficult to track down all the writings of many authors, particularly those in periodical publications; many subjects lack adequate comprehensive bibliographies, and relatively few indexes provide for a satisfactory approach by time and place. Unquestionably, computers can be useful in the compilation of additional bibliographies of the older literature, just as they are for the current. Of particular value for historians would be the relative ease with which additional indexes or approaches to the material in the bibliographies could be prepared.

In this connection, we may note the so-called 'Apple Pie' project at the Newcastle University Library, an experimental system set up for cataloguing two collections of old books, including one—the Pybus collection—of about 2000 old medical books. The study was, however, managed from the viewpoint of the historian of books and not of medicine: it sought to demonstrate the feasibility of using a computer to provide indexes of such characteristics as printers and publishers, place of publication, bindings, and former owners, but omitted subject indexing altogether on grounds of difficulty. The author of the project realized that it was too small to be worth while by itself—the same job could have been done more cheaply by

264

hand. He was aiming ultimately for a master union catalogue of old books in machine-readable form.[6] While the indexing goals of this particular study were perhaps not those of greatest interest to historians of medicine, there can be no doubt that it is technically feasible to prepare machine-readable catalogue records of old books as well as of new ones.

In many ways, a more attractive scheme than the creation of new, limited, specialized bibliographies would be to prepare in machine-readable form for retrieval from a computer store some of the huge amounts of data already existing in scattered form in the multitude of published bibliographies and other reference sources, including unpublished library catalogues, so that specialized bibliographies and lists of subjects, persons, places, periods, languages, and publishers in whatever combination or arrangement where desired could be prepared and printed on demand. What can be done by the conversion of existing data has been shown in a limited way by the project to automate the shelf-list of Widener Library at Harvard. Entering the existing shelf-list data into a computer has made it possible for the Harvard University Press to publish what are in effect classified catalogues of broad subject areas of the library's holdings. The books in each catalogue are also listed alphabetically by author and chronologically by date of publication. Harvard is the first to point out the limitations of the catalogues, but they have nevertheless provided bibliographic tools that may be of great value to those who are unable to use the facilities of Widener in person. Unfortunately none of the catalogues, as yet, covers monographs in medicine.

A somewhat similar project is the *Periodicals in the Countway Library*, which lists some 17 889 different serials alphabetically by title, as they are arranged on the library's shelves. Unlike most such computerized lists, it includes all holdings, not just those currently received. In November 1968, the Library of Congress announced the receipt of a grant from the Council on Library Resources to support a three-month project to determine the feasibility of converting its retrospective cataloguing records into machine-readable form.[7] Should this prove feasible, it will open up new possibilities for controlling, new ways of indexing important historical materials. It will not replace existing specialized bibliographies of the older medical literature. The intellectual labour and cost of editing the

millions of citations which they contain for consistency of bibliographic description and subject indexing, so that they could be
entered into and retrieved from a computer file, even if there were
enough people who could and would do it, stagger the imagination.
Even if it is technically possible, this reviewer cannot foresee the
day when it will ever be economically justifiable to construct such a
grand scheme for information retrieval from the early literature of
medicine.

V

In the control of manuscript sources, the use of automation would
appear to offer particularly significant opportunities. Computers
are already being widely used in the investigation of early manuscripts and texts, particularly for concordances and other word
studies.[8] Less appears to have been done in the area of cataloguing,
although the computer would seem ideally suited for the preparation of lists of incipits and similar data. The existence of such
excellent guides as the Thorndike-Kibre *Catalogue of incipits* may
make the question of bibliographic control seem less urgent. Even
so, one suspects that a union catalogue of early manuscripts compiled from existing catalogues of individual libraries might be
greeted with joy by those working in the medieval field. If new
collections—whether of original material or microfilm copies—are to
be catalogued *in extenso*, the advantages of the computer's sorting
ability for providing author, incipit, provenance, period, subject,
and perhaps other special files should be kept in mind.

Because medieval manuscripts have long been treasured by
libraries and studied by scholars, the existing bibliographic apparatus is extensive. Manuscripts of the last century or two, however,
have received much less attention until quite recent decades. A Conference on Science Manuscripts, called by the History of Science
Society in 1960, gave emphasis to this trend and has been published
in *Isis*.[9] More recently a committee on scientific and technological
manuscripts has been established in the Society of American
Archivists, which devoted a session of its 1967 annual meeting to
this area.

Despite this growing interest—and a much longer standing interest among general historians in the manuscripts of political figures—

the control of modern manuscript material deposited in our libraries and archives is in no sense comparable to the existing controls on books. Relatively few libraries have published separate catalogues. The *National Union Catalog of manuscript collections* (NUCMC), started by the Library of Congress in 1959, has published reported holdings to date in six fat volumes. The data already existing on cards in the National Union Catalog of books will be published in some six hundred. There are obvious reasons for this difference. Manuscripts are more difficult to control and index. The forms of documents and subjects covered in a single collection of papers may be quite diverse and unrelated, one to another. Collections when acquired are often haphazard in arrangement, and the repository itself has to impose an order which the author provides for a book. Each manuscript collection is unique, so that centralized cataloguing, except to the limited extent provided by NUCMC, is impossible. Moreover, if a particular copy of a rare book is not recorded in the National Union Catalog or other sources, some other copy in most cases will be. A particular manuscript collection, obviously, will not. Printed books are used by a great many more people than manuscripts, and much more attention has quite properly been given to their control. Standards and techniques for cataloguing manuscripts have been developed much more slowly, and although there is a growing consensus on the basic elements and procedures in the description of modern manuscript collections, resulting in part from the institution of NUCMC and from the examples set by the archival profession, the rules are by no means as precise and rigid or as universally accepted as those for cataloguing books. Individual manuscript collections often are very large, especially government archives, and, where inventories or registers are prepared for particular collections, it is generally not practicable to interfile descriptions from several registers by manual methods. The more abbreviated descriptions in NUCMC or such admirable works as *A guide to archives and manuscripts in the United States*, compiled by Philip Hamer, are not able to index in depth the collections they briefly describe. Additional guides to and indexes of manuscript collections have been identified by a number of persons doing research in the history of medicine and science as one of the prime desiderata in the control of historical sources.

In some cases, attempts have been made to provide users with

267

more detailed information by indexing every item in a collection. The largest such project is no doubt the programme for item indexing the Presidential Papers in the Library of Congress. Each letter is indexed for the names of correspondents and date; there is no subject index. Work was started with punch cards and tabulating machines for sorting and printing, and moved later to a computer sorter, which proved to be much quicker and more accurate. The Library anticipates still further advantages from this automation when it is able to tie in with the electronic composing system at the United States Government Printing Office. From the Library's tapes, it is expected, the Printing Office will be able to compose the 244 000 entries in the Theodore Roosevelt index—equivalent to three 500-page volumes—in a day. As the Library has pointed out, this is a data-processing programme—the indexes, not the tapes, are used for the retrieval of information. In the last two years, the overall cost per item for arranging, indexing, editing, filming—the collections are available for purchase on microfilm—and publishing, has been a little over four shillings and two pence.[10] A similar project has been started more recently in connection with planned catalogues of the papers of the Prime Ministers of Canada. Managers of this programme, however, have concluded that a subject approach to the papers was also necessary and that a standardized subject heading list was essential.[11]

During the past year, the Washington University School of Medicine Library in St Louis has completed and published an item index to its collection of the papers of William Beaumont. Each item was indexed for author, recipient(s), and other personal names; place of origin, destination(s), and other place names; date of document and other dates in document; subjects; document type; and document location. A separate punch card was prepared for each index line (e.g., one card for the author including also the recipient's name, and one card for the recipient showing also the author's name). Subject headings appear to have been chosen on an *ad hoc* basis as indexing progressed rather than from a standard list. Indexes of names, places, dates, and subjects together with a shelflist giving all the indexing data for each document were printed and published as a book of 165 pages, including 24 pages of introduction, with more than 17 000 line entries. According to the report of the librarian, the acting archivist spent full time from September to

April indexing the collection, and the machine costs plus printing and binding were approximately £1125. At this rate, allowing a modest salary for the indexer, the overall cost for processing the 643 documents in the collection must have been over £4. 3. 4. per item.[12] There has been no other comparable project in the field of medical history.

The head of the Presidential Papers Section of the Manuscript Division of the Library of Congress has argued that to justify automated item indexing of manuscripts, '(1) the collections should be of major importance and should have a sustained high subject quality; (2) the collections, for maximum technical efficiency, should be fairly extensive so that the project can include enough items to make it a production job rather than a custom job; and (3) the collections should be related to one another in some way to increase efficiency in standardization of indexing techniques'.[13] As of two years ago, the Library had sold more than 40 000 reels of microfilm of Presidential Papers. It is unlikely, however, that many medical history collections will be of the nature, size, and use to meet these criteria. I think it fair to say that the index to the Beaumont collection, while an interesting experiment, does not offer a practicable methodology for controlling manuscript sources.

Other efforts to control manuscript collections have led to experimentation with systems calling for more detailed information retrieval possibilities than the NUCMC offers without the prohibitive cost of item indexing. Perhaps the most interesting work along this line has been undertaken by Frank G. Burke, first at the Library of Congress Manuscripts Division and now at the National Archives. Originally conceived and inaugurated on a small scale with punch cards and tabulators in order to improve administrative controls over the Library's holdings, which total some 30 000 000 items in some 3000 collections, the system as first developed consisted of a master record for each collection including elements such as name and occupation(s) of the person with whom the collection was principally identified, the source, shelving location, whether a finding aid existed, whether reported to NUCMC, and so on. Even these data, selected, sorted, and printed out by computer in various formats, have proved useful in answering questions as well as in internal administration. However, the information provided did not include subjects or names other than

269

main entry. The Library next experimented with a programme to provide additional information without reindexing, rearranging, or redescribing collections that had already been processed. This was done by entering into a computer the information on container lists in existing registers and subjecting it to a modified KWIC programme, which has been given the new acronym SPINDEX (Selective Permutation INDEXing); it is, in fact, a form of Key-Word-Out-of-Context index.

The latter programme appeared to be of sufficient promise for the Council on Library Resources to support a two-year project for its further development in cooperation with other institutions, and the investigation is now being pursued by Mr Burke at the National Archives, with the collaboration of nine other major repositories. The system, labelled SPINDEX II, as it is developing is both more flexible and more complex than its immediate predecessor. It is intended to provide a comprehensive capability for administrative control, information retrieval, and publication. It retains the KWOC concept for subject indexing rather than an authority list of terms and use of existing records. The principal investigator is eloquent and enthusiastic in describing what he foresees as the potential for an information network throughout the National Archives, including regional centres and Presidential libraries, with eventual ties to university computer centres as well. According to a recent survey, only seven archives and manuscript collections in the United States were using computers in the management of their collections. However, 45 respondents (out of a total of 510) were developing or considering plans for their use. Undoubtedly they will be watching with great interest for the report on SPINDEX II.[14] There seems no reason to doubt that computers and other, less sophisticated automation equipment will come into increasing use in large manuscript collections—whether with the SPINDEX system or another remains to be seen—and that they will greatly enhance our ability to find the particular material that individual historians may be seeking.

VI

Turning now to modern literature on the history of medicine, we may note that the use of automation in the control of library materials has advanced furthest in connection with recent publications. At the National Library of Medicine, for example, all modern monographs and journal titles catalogued are entered into MEDLARS (MEDical Literature Analysis and Retrieval System) on magnetic tape and used with computer-driven photo-composing equipment for the preparation of catalogue cards and, more importantly, for the publication of *Current Catalog*, a bi-weekly with quarterly and annual cumulations. In this case, the chief benefit from the automated equipment has come from its ability to publish quickly and cumulate readily. Under the previous programme at the Library, cataloguing data created during one year was published well along in the next. With *Current Catalog*, cataloguing data for current literature are ordinarily published within a few weeks of receipt (cataloguing data for material more than two years old are published only in the cumulations). At present, the tapes containing the data cannot be used for information retrieval purposes at the National Library of Medicine. With the implementation of MEDLARS II, now under development, this and other improvements in control, of benefit to both library administrators and users, will become available.

Of broader scope is the Library of Congress MARC (MAchine Readable Cataloging) programme, designed to provide cataloging data on magnetic tape to the Library of Congress and to other subscribing libraries through the country. Distribution is expected to begin in 1969. In order to make the benefits of these systems as widespread as possible, the three national libraries—the Library of Congress, the National Library of Medicine, and the National Agricultural Library—are engaged in joint efforts to ensure compatibility of their various systems. All of these are directed at the control of current literature. They benefit the history of medicine by improving controls in this field along with others.

Another cooperative effort between the three national libraries is the programme to establish a national serials data bank, which would supplement and keep up to date the kind of information to be found in the *Union list of serials*. This, too, could redound to the benefit of medical history as to other fields of research.

By far the more difficult problem in the control of current literature is adequate means of retrieval of articles in journals and other composite publications. From a technical standpoint, an automated system for the history of medicine could no doubt be set up. MEDLARS has been functioning as a computer-based system since 1964, after a long period of development. Medical literature specialists at the National Library of Medicine (or elsewhere through contract) index some 2300 journals containing some 180 000 or more articles per year. The indexers assign subject headings from an authority list (MESH—MEdical Subject Headings). Their work, entered into the computer, is used as a basis for the publication of *Index Medicus* and a number of specialized recurring bibliographies and also for carrying out demand searches of the file in answer to specific questions. Not all of the original objectives have been met, but most have; and the experience gained is a vital aid in the planning of a more advanced system to be introduced early in the 1970's.[15]

MEDLARS is a large and expensive system, intended to handle nearly 200 000 citations a year. Its store will soon be up to 1 000 000 citations. The history of medicine is a small field, the total production of which is about 3000 to 4000 citations a year, including monographs. A five-year cumulation of citations for the history of medicine will be the equivalent of about one month's input to *Index Medicus*. No one is going to build a MEDLARS, or anything like it, just to handle 3000 citations a year in the history of medicine.

However, it is possible for our area of interest to gain some benefit from the activity. For purposes of retrieval the indexers assign many more subject headings to each article than appear in *Index Medicus*. A number of these are so-called 'check tags' for particular groups or other special features that are always noted when present. All historical articles indexed are specifically tagged as such, and, when appropriate, they are also tagged with chronological and geographical descriptors in addition to appropriate subject headings. A special monthly 'recurring demand search' retrieves these entries, which are used (along with material retrieved manually from other sources) in the preparation of the Library's *Bibliography of the history of medicine*. MEDLARS thus serves medical history as a screening and indexing device for a very large body of medical literature.

This arrangement is not without its problems. The subject heading system is designed for a very large body of data. The historical articles in *Index Medicus*, if one omits obituaries and current biographies, amount to less than one per cent of the total. The specificity required for efficient retrieval of current citations in all fields of medicine necessitates a subject heading list that becomes inordinately large for historical bibliography. Using 6000 subject headings to index 180 000 articles is by no means unreasonable. Using 6000 headings to index 3000 articles—or even a five-year cumulation of 15 000 articles—makes no sense at all.

The problem is where to draw the line. Recent evaluative studies of MEDLARS and other information retrieval systems have shown the important relationship between specificity of subject headings and the efficiency of a system. This has been measured in terms of 'recall', which is defined as the number of relevant citations on any given subject retrieved from a system in response to a search, divided by the number of relevant citations in the system, multiplied by 100; and 'precision', which is defined as the number of relevant citations retrieved divided by the total number retrieved, times 100. Increasing specificity has been shown to improve precision: a higher percentage of the citations retrieved will, in general, be relevant to the needs of the requester; he will have less useless material to wade through and sift out for himself. On the other hand, increasing specificity tends to lower recall; the searcher is likely to miss a higher percentage of relevant citations in the system. Construction of a subject heading list should, therefore, depend at least in part on the goals of the system. Those searching 'a few good articles' on a subject will prefer greater specificity. Those who want a comprehensive search as the basis of further research will generally be better served by a less specific system.[16]

It seems clear that a subject heading system designed for one very large automated system is not likely to be satisfactory in a small one used only in a published index. Certainly, in this writer's opinion, it was desirable greatly to reduce the specificity of MESH when using it for indexing historical articles, and this practice has been followed in the preparation of the *Bibliography of the history of medicine*.

VII

The history of medicine is a discipline with ties to two quite different fields of learning: medicine and history. MEDLARS, with some extensions, provides a means to index the occasional historical articles found in medical journals. Unfortunately the historical profession is not as well organized for the dissemination of current bibliographical data as are scientific and technological groups—which is hardly surprising, since history does not provide the same immediate payoff in what society perceives as urgent goals, industrial production, improved medical care, and national defence. A measure of the current distress is the fact that *Writings on American history*, long the major annual bibliography in its field, is now ten years behind in its coverage of recent literature and has never filled in the gap for the years of World War II.

A number of historians in the United States have seen the need and attempted to do something about it. Sponsored by a joint committee of the American Historical Association and the Organization of American Historians, a conference at Belmont in 1967 reviewed the present state of historical bibliography and explored means to improve it. On one point, at least, there was a consensus: in any future bibliographical reform computers would of necessity play an important role. The Association has appointed a Standing Committee on Bibliographical Services to History, but to date it has been unable to obtain support for a staff to begin full-time study and development of a programme. Meanwhile the American Council of Learned Societies is urging concerted action for bibliographical control of the social sciences and humanities.[17]

In history, the most up-to-date American system now available—other than lists of articles in the *American Historical Review* and similar journals—is the abstracting journals of Erich Boehm and the American Bibliographical Center in Santa Barbara, California: *Historical Abstracts*, covering world history since 1775, and *America : History and Life*, covering the history of the United States. By the use of a mnemonic 'cue' system the abstracts are themselves indexed for subject, period, name and place. These data are used to compile an index by computer.[18] The index is organized primarily by geography, and the subject index tags for an abstract on a particular subject in a particular area must be searched for under the place name. To find all articles on the history of medicine, therefore, one must search under all the geographical headings. While this may serve the regular historian reasonably well, it makes the service very difficult to use for a particular topic. It would seem that the compilers of the index are not taking proper full advantage of the computer's ability to permute terms; they could provide a more comprehensive index without additional intellectual effort.

The further development of bibliographical controls for current literature in history, the social sciences, and the humanities, all of which carry occasional articles of medical interest, would be a boon to medical historians as well as to the professions for which they would be more specifically designed. Unfortunately, at this point there is no clear indication that the necessary organization and resources capable of carrying out such a programme will be soon forthcoming.

The use of automation for the control of the current literature of medical history, especially the serial literature, offers intriguing possibilities for the production of more complete and useful bibliographies and for other techniques of information retrieval. But the field is too small to 'go it alone'. In practice to date, automation—MEDLARS—is providing pertinent basic material for the construction of bibliographies from a very substantial proportion of the total medical literature with an ease and efficiency that was impossible before the computerization of *Index Medicus*. We may hope for a system of historical bibliography in the future. Medical historians will have to design any system of their own to be compatible, in so far as possible, with both the scientific and the humanistic ways of controlling the literature.

NOTES AND REFERENCES

1 E. I. Wood, *Report on Project History Retrieval; texts and demonstrations of an optic-coincidence system of information retrieval for historical materials*, Philadelphia: Drexel Institute of Technology, 1966, pp. xiii, 123. In the optical coincidence system there is a card for each term (e.g., subject heading, place of origin, period, material, or whatever). Each term card has spaces representing particular numbers (say, from 1 to 10 000). Each item to be indexed is assigned a particular number, and the location for that number is punched in each term card having an applicable heading. If one wishes to determine to what items a set of one or more terms applies, the corresponding term cards are placed on a light table, and all the numbers which have those terms in common will then be visible as points of light. Appropriate specialized equipment is used for punching and reading the numbers.

2 The literature on automation, libraries and information retrieval is voluminous. I have found the following especially helpful: C. P. Bourne,

Methods of information handling, New York: Wiley, 1963, pp. xiv, 241; F. W. Lancaster, *Information retrieval systems: characteristics, testing, and evaluation*, New York: Wiley, 1968, pp. xiv, 222.

3 Bourne, op. cit. (above, note 2), p. 169.

4 Lancaster, op. cit. (above, note 2), p. 48.

5 R. J. Durling, 'A chronological census of Renaissance editions and translations of Galen', *Journal of the Warburg and Courtauld Institutes* 1961, 24, 230–305.

6 C. J. Hunt, 'The computer production of catalogues of old books' in N. S. M. Cox and M. W. Grose (eds.), *Organization and handling of bibliographic records by computer*, pp. 137–49, Newcastle upon Tyne: Oriel Press, 1967.

7 Library of Congress, *Information Bulletin* 1968, 27, 689–90.

8 'Directory of scholars active', *Computers and the Humanities* 1967, 1, 178–241, 2, 71–93; 1968, 2, 223–50, 3, 105–18. On pp. 231–7 of the present book, De Lacy discusses the use of computers in the editing and translation of a Greek medical text. Wake on pp. 238–59 deals with the use of statistical methods in the identification of authors of anonymous ancient medical writings.

9 'The conference on science manuscripts', *Isis* 1962, 53, 5–154.

10 R. M. Smith, 'Item indexing by automated processes', *American Archivist* 1967, 30, 295–302.

11 J. Atherton, 'Mechanization of the manuscript catalogue at the Public Archives of Canada', *American Archivist* 1967, 30, 303–9.

12 P. A. Cassidy and R. S. Sokol (comps.), *Index to the Wm. Beaumont, M.D. (1785–1853) manuscript collection*, St. Louis: Washington University School of Medicine, 1968, pp. 165; Washington University, School of Medicine, *Annual report of the library 1967–1968* [St. Louis, 1968] p. 19.

13 Smith, op. cit. (above, note 10), p. 302.

14 F. G. Burke, 'The application of automated techniques in the management and control of source materials', *American Archivist* 1967, 30, 255–78; F. G. Burke, 'Automation in bibliographical control of archives and manuscript collections' in D. H. Perman (ed.), *Bibliography and the historian: the conference at Belmont of the Joint Committee on Bibliographical Services to History, May 1967*, pp. 96–102, Santa Barbara: Clio, 1968; F. G. Burke, 'Report on a survey of automation activities in archives and manuscript repositories in the United States and Canada', *American Archivist* 1968, 31, 208–10.

15 *The Medlars story at the National Library of Medicine*, Bethesda: U.S. Public Health Service, 1963, pp. vii, 74; C. J. Austin, *Medlars, 1963–1967*, Bethesda: National Library of Medicine, 1968, pp. viii, 76 (Public Health Service Publication No. 1823).

16 Lancaster, op. cit. (above, note 2), pp. 54–74, 152–4.

17 Perman, 1968, op. cit. (above, note 14), pp. viii, 176.

18 E. H. Boehm, *The cue system for bibliography and indexing*, Santa Barbara: ABC-Clio, 1967, pp. 45 (Bibliography and Reference Series No. 7).

16 A Classification Scheme for Library Material in the History of Medicine

EDWIN CLARKE

One of the most difficult tasks facing the custodian of a library devoted to the history of medicine is the selection of a satisfactory method of arranging his books on the shelves, and of classifying other medico-historical materials. In a praiseworthy attempt to cope with the varied needs of many readers, both medical and non-medical, he may find that he completely satisfies none. Some librarians pay less attention to this matter, believing with some justification that the approach to a library's holdings should be by way of the catalogue and not by way of the shelves. Unfortunately some users, although realizing that it is often a time-wasting procedure, elect to go immediately to the books themselves, if access is permitted and if the classification system allows it. Scholars belong most commonly to this group and it would seem reasonable therefore that if their demands are to be met the classification and availability of library materials dealing with the history of medicine should be orientated towards their needs.

II

There are a number of methods of classifying books on the history of medicine used in various parts of the world, but none is entirely satisfactory. The difficulties encountered usually relate to the fact that general classification systems such as the Dewey method and that employed by the Library of Congress when applied to medico-historical holdings are unable to encompass adequately such a diverse and specialized subject. In some instances those caring for large medico-historical collections have devised their own system

277

of classification and this is true of the Wellcome Historical Medical Library.[1]

A closely related problem is the provision of a classification scheme for references to the secondary literature which are recorded either on index cards or as entries in a printed book, and for the arrangement of a reprint collection. Recent developments in this area have provided two new schemes. The first concerns the proposed cumulative edition of the annual bibliographies of the history of science which have appeared in *Isis*.[2] The Editor of this project has discussed[3] the various schemes available as well as the one that has been selected for the forthcoming *Isis cumulative bibliography*.[4] Although this relates in particular to the history of science, the history of medicine is included under the title, 'HS 26 Medicine and the medical sciences'. The second new scheme is provided by the *Bibliography of the history of medicine* and of related professions, issued annually by the National Library of Medicine;[5] it has introduced a further system, which in the section of 'Special topics' is alphabetical by subject. E. Gaskell, Librarian of the Wellcome Historical Medical Library, has described the subject headings used in his library,[6] pointing out that they are similar to those listed in the 1960 *Subject heading authority list* of the National Library of Medicine. Altogether there is a considerable literature on this topic, with special reference more recently to the assistance given by mechanical aids (see pp. 260–76).

III

It would seem essential to devise, if possible, a single scheme of subject classification which could be applied not only to books on shelves, but also to index cards in filing cabinets, reprints, pamphlets etc., or to entries in a published bibliography of secondary literature on the history of medicine. It can first of all be accepted however that a method universally appropriate and acceptable will be difficult to contrive. Yet certain criteria must be adhered to if this ideal is to be approached. Whatever the system, it must be simple, flexible, consistent and integrative. An attempt to discover the most suitable form of classification for the Library of the Sub-Department of the History of Medicine in University College London has resulted in the following arrangement, only the outlines of which

278

can be described here. Particular reference will be made to its use in the handling of printed sources, both primary and secondary, but it can also be applied to other medico-historical literary materials.

The so-called Garside Library Classification[7] is now employed in University College London and it seems to possess the four essential standards enumerated above; it has simplicity, flexibility and consistency and libraries on different academic subjects can be integrated within it. The shelf mark of each book has four basic classificatory elements:

(1) The name of the subject library. In the case of the Library of the Sub-Department of the History of Medicine this is 'Hist. Med.'

(2) One or two capital letters denoting the main sections Thus 'Anatomy' is C and 'Histology' is CM.

(3) A number, either a single digit having 'form' significance (for example '5' indicates textbooks[8]) or double figures representing the topic which is a subdivision of a main section. 'Histological Stains' is therefore denoted by CM 84.

(4) The first three letters of the word which will determine alphabetically the exact shelf place alongside items on the same topic. This is usually the author's or editor's name.

In a subject catalogue, guide-cards of distinctive colours can, if necessary, distinguish the categories, and these together with other refinements and details are dealt with by Garside.[7] On the shelves it is usually convenient to store folios and quartos separately and the size of the book, if larger than octavo, can be indicated in the notation. The scheme also provides a series of numbers to be used in place of the name of the subject library, enabling first the compilation in order of a complete subject catalogue of the whole College library and secondly, the arrangement, in the same order, of all books removed to a general library store. The medical part of the scheme is the work of Mr C. F. A. Marmoy, F.L.A., Librarian of the Thane Library of the Medical Sciences.

The Sub-Department of the History of Medicine in University College London is located in the Faculty of Medical Sciences and it is devoted mainly, although by no means exclusively, to the study of the history of the medical sciences. It would therefore seem appropriate that the classification system of its collection of books should be as similar as possible to that of the general library which serves the whole Faculty. This would mean that a highly specialized

historical library could be integrated not only with the overall
College scheme of classification, the Garside method, but also with
that of the medical library. In the case of the latter it is a special
advantage to have a system which users of the scientific library will
recognize and be able to follow readily when consulting the historical collection. But more important by far is the fact that just
as the history of medicine as an academic subject should be integrated with the medical school, so must its working materials be
associated as closely as possible with other medical school activities
and occupants. This is only possible if the existing classification
system is adopted, rather than encouraging isolationism by the
invention of a new one relating solely to the history of medicine
and not to medicine itself.

With these ideals in mind the following scheme has been constructed and is now in use. It is divided into ten sequences:

AA   Reference and Bibliography
AH   History, general
AS   Science, general
AX   Medicine, general
A–V   Medical sciences
W   Historical periods
WZ   Location by country
X   Medicine in art, literature, drama, music, religion,
      travel, etc.
Y   Biography
Z   Early and/or precious primary sources.

Under 'History, general' (Sequence AH) come general history,
historiography, philosophy of history, etc. In 'Science, general'
(Sequence AS) are included books on general science, philosophy of
science, education in science, conflict with religion, instruments,
museums, societies, collected papers or addresses, and other topics;
then come the history of science with general works first, followed
by histories of specific subjects (i.e. mathematics and physical
sciences only) arranged alphabetically, and finally the history of
technology. 'Medicine, general' (Sequence AX) contains much the
same as Sequence AS except that the sub-section on history of
medicine has only the general textbooks, collected papers, *Fest-
schriften*, congress proceedings, etc., and books on medical historiography, museums, and so forth. In each instance the sequence letters

follow 'Hist. Med.', and their subjects can be arranged alphabetic-ally or by the form numbers.[8]

Sequence A–V, 'Medical sciences', is the main portion of the scheme because it includes material on all medical subjects, clinical and pre-clinical. This is the part that follows almost exactly the classification used in the medical library of the Faculty which is itself a part of the Garside system; it ranges from A 'medical sciences generally' to V 'forensic medicine'. The main headings are: 'Medical sciences generally'; general biology; general anatomy, including histology and embryology; general physiology and bio-physics; biochemistry; systems of the body (each subdivided into anatomy, comparative anatomy, histology, embryology, physiology and disorders); pharmacology, materia medica and therapeutics; pathology, bacteriology, immunology and parasitology; general clinical medicine, diagnosis, geriatrics, infectious diseases, tropical medicine; surgery; gynaecology, obstetrics; paediatrics; armed forces medicine; preventive medicine including hygiene, public health, epidemiology, statistics, social medicine (the profession, finances, the patient, etc.), hospitals, nursing; forensic medicine.

Into this scheme can be fitted both primary and secondary material. The secondary historical works come first and in the case of some subjects such as the history of dentistry, pharmacy or of surgery, further classification will have to be planned, should the collections be large. The Garside system does not yet provide sub-divisions for some of the clinical topics but using the general prin-ciples of the scheme they can be devised. Only selected primary works will be included and among them will be modern standard textbooks for it is essential that they should be available in a depart-ment of medical history in order to emphasize its contact with the present. Moreover, it often happens that useful historical surveys are contained in these technical treatises. Valuable primary sources, however, if they are in the collection, must be arranged separately in an alphabetical author sequence (Sequence Z) without classification. It would be ideal to have all the primary and secondary material completely integrated but for reasons of security this unfortunately can never be achieved. In any case it would be difficult to fit much of the earlier material into a modern pattern with which it has little in common.

An example of this method of classification would be the notation for a book on the history of the role of acetylcholine in nervous transmission:

Hist. Med.   which indicates subject
A–V   'Medical sciences' Sequence
JN   which signifies 'Nervous system, Neurology'
64   The sequence leading to this number is: physiology (50), experimental (52), conduction of nerve impulse (56), chemical—humoral transmission (62), acetylcholine (64)

The complete identification, therefore, is 'Hist. Med. A–V JN 64 SMI', if the author's name is Smith.

Another example, a monograph say on Galen's surgery, would be distinguished by the symbols 'Hist. Med. A–V P GAL', where 'P' indicates 'Surgery'. The simplicity in this instance is evident.

The other Sequences, W, WZ, X, and Y, are self-explanatory. Thus 'Historical periods' (Sequence W) proceeds from prehistory (archaeology, palaeontology, palaeopathology, etc.) to primitive medicine (palaeo-medicine, folklore, magic, superstitions, astrology, etc.), to antiquity in general, non-Western civilizations (China, India, etc.), Mesopotamia, Egypt, Ancient Hebrews, Graeco-Roman antiquity, Middle Ages, etc. Items dealing primarily with non-medical aspects of these periods are arranged after those on specific medical topics. In this sequence and in the next (Sequence WZ, 'Location by country'), only general works are included. Those dealing with special subjects, as in the example cited above of Galen's surgery, should go with that special subject. Similarly a history of nutrition in the eighteenth century would be placed with 'Nutrition' and a book on the evolution of surgery in France will also be found with 'Surgery'. The consistency here is to place as many books as possible in the central part of the library, Sequence A–V 'Medical Sciences', and if necessary provide cross-references on the shelves as well as, of course, in the catalogue.

On the other hand, it could be argued that just as medicine up to the time of the Renaissance was a compact body of knowledge, so all historical material dealing with antiquity and the medieval period should be kept together in Sequence W. But in a department which is dealing mostly with the total, longitudinal growth of a scientific or social idea in medicine, the material should, as far as is feasible, be arranged according to medical and social subjects and their concepts. Other workers may hold more store by the overall content of medical knowledge in a given historical period, in which case Sequence W can be expanded according to their requirements. This merely illustrates the versatility and adaptability of the system. When Sequences W and WZ are combined in a title, as for example, 'The history of medicine in seventeenth-century England', the item should be placed in W (Historical periods).

Classification within Sequence W need only be alphabetical by author within the time periods as it will, on the whole, be relatively small in content. In the case of Sequence WZ, 'Location by country', the geographical numbers of the Garside scheme are used.[9] If it is considered more in keeping with individual needs to expand the sections on historical periods and locations, the subject listing of Sequence A–V can be applied. The subdivisions of Sequence X (art, literature, drama, music, religion, travel, etc.) can be denoted by the first three letters of the topic and of the author.

In the section on biography (Sequence Y), general and complete composite biographies precede those dealing with individuals, and books on non-medical and non-scientific individuals are included. Works on 'famous patients' should also go here, rather than in Sequence X.

The above considerations have dealt with books, but a card index of secondary references can be subjected to the same classification with excellent results. Reprints may also be organized in this way, for it is a great convenience to have immediately to hand all the available articles on a given subject. Alternatively, there is a persuasive argument in favour of storing them alphabetically by author and using a card index to reach their subject content; the card catalogue, however, will use the classification described above. In either case the catalogue card would indicate that the item was a pamphlet; thus [Pamph.] as used by Garside can be added to the notation.

IV

In common with all other schemes for the classification of library materials, this one is by no means perfect. Taken all in all, however, it seems to cope adequately with all types of medico-historical literary data, despite the diversity of this field of knowledge. Fewer difficulties seem to arise from its use than with other systems and, moreover, it conforms closely to the four obligatory criteria; it is simple, it is flexible, it is consistent throughout and it is integrative in several ways. What is equally important is that the plan, like that of the Wellcome Historical Medical Library, is conceived with the user's needs primarily in mind, whereas some classification systems have been created for the convenience of the librarian. In a diverse discipline like the history of medicine where many books are difficult to handle because of overlapping contents the choice of the precise classification of a book must be a group activity so that its place within the collections can be decided by departmental discussions and not governed by a librarian's rigid system of classification. No doubt considerable emendations will be necessary in the future but flexibility will allow these to be carried out; many difficult problems such as obsolete terminology and other matters not mentioned here have been discussed by Gaskell.[10]

It would seem appropriate to recommend this system in its as yet incomplete form, with the hope that if others adopt it and find it useful then librarians will be able to remove many of its present technical defects and disadvantages. As with the other contributions to this book a suggestion for further research is put forward which may or may not lead to further advances. This University College System is orientated fundamentally to a specific conception of the history of medicine as a subject that deals with the evolution of scientific and social thought in medicine (see pp. 194–210). It follows naturally that if an academic discipline is considered to possess a certain form or image, the materials which it uses and upon which it is based should be arranged so that they can take on the same conformation.

REFERENCES

1   The Library provides an unpublished document, 'Arrangement of books in the library reading room', pp. 4. The scheme is an adaptation of the Barnard classification; C. A. Barnard, *A classification for medical and veterinary libraries*, London: H. K. Lewis, 1955, pp. 279.
2   The latest number is 'Ninety-second critical bibliography of the history of science and its cultural influence (to 1 January 1967)', *Isis* 1967, vol. 58, No. 5, pp. 143.

3   M. Whitrow, 'Classification schemes for the history of science. A comparison', *J. Document.* 1964, **20**, 120–36.

4   The first portion (M. Whitrow (ed.), *Isis cumulative bibliography. A bibliography of the history of science formed from Isis critical bibliographies 1–90 1913–65*, Part I. Personalities and institutions) has been announced.

5   *Bibliography of the history of medicine*, Bethesda, Md.: National Library of Medicine, No. 1, 1965 and No. 2, 1966.

6   E. Gaskell, 'Subject headings in the Wellcome Historical Medical Library', *Bull. med. Lib. Ass.* 1964, **52**, 337–44. The Wellcome subject headings are also used in the exceedingly useful quarterly, *Current work in the history of medicine*, with only minor modifications.

7   K. Garside, 'The basic principles of the new library classification at University College, London', *J. Document.* 1954, **10**, 169–92.

8   Ibid., Table I, pp. 185–7. The 'form' numbers are: 1. Bibliographies. 2. Reference works. 3. Periodicals and serials. 4. Sources. 5. Textbooks. 6. Miscellanies. 7. Monographs. 8. History of the study of the subject. 9. Methodology.

9   Garside, ibid., Table II, pp. 187–91.

10 Gaskell, op. cit. (above, note 6).

17 Oral History. A Personal View

SAUL BENISON

There is a story that, when Robert Louis Stevenson was a boy, he turned to his mother while at play one day, and said, 'Look, Mama, I have drawed a man, now I am going to draw his soul.' There are many who, because of the probing interview techniques used by oral historians, look upon oral history as an attempt to draw men's souls. In fact the purpose of oral history is much more modest. It is to collect the memoirs of contemporaries for the use of future historians. It is done out of the philosophical conviction that the details of an individual human life will serve to illuminate and help differentiate for the future historian those vast forces which in our own time, ironically, assault the identity of the individual. The following chapter presents a survey of this recently popularized addition to historical methodology.

II

Learning about the individual has particular relevance for the history of medicine and science. A number of years ago the late, distinguished historian of science, George Sarton, made a special plea for such a point of view.

The history of science, and in particular the history of medicine (we can not repeat it too often) is not simply an account of discoveries. Its purpose is to explain the development of the scientific spirit, the history of man's reactions to truth, the history of the gradual liberation of our minds from darkness and prejudice. Discoveries are evanescent, for they are soon replaced by better ones. The historian must try not only to describe these evanescent discoveries but to find in science that which is timeless. When he does that he comes very close to the historian of art. To put it in other words, a man's name may be immortalized by his discoveries. Perhaps there was nothing else in him deserving of remembrance? He may have been a poor sort of man, a man whose mind was as sharp and narrow as a knife-edge? Or else the historian betrayed him? In so far as a scientist is also an artist, his personality can survive, otherwise not. It is the historian's main duty to revive the personalities, rather than enumerate their scientific excrescences. Discoveries may be important, but personalities are infinitely more so.[1]

Although one may quarrel with parts of Sarton's argument, its thrust cannot easily be denied. It matters not one whit that historians have yet to define with precision the individual's role in shaping history. What does matter is that there is such a problem. It exists because the individual cannot be banished from history. The oral historian gathering the memoirs of contemporaries is in the Sarton tradition. Indeed, one of the joys and burdens of his labour is that he is almost constantly beset by the problem of assessing the role of the individual in history. In a deep sense that problem is central to his inquiries. There are others.

Some look at oral history as a recent phenomenon. Its technology, the tape recorder and television camera, is certainly new. However, its major component, autobiography, has been a continuing facet of western historiography since Greek and Roman times. During the Renaissance, for example, many humanists used Greek and Roman autobiographies as models in developing their own art of self-portrayal. By the time of the Enlightenment, the demand for the 'confessions of outstanding men' was so great that entire collections were printed. Politicians, theologians, poets, philosophers, and historians all practised the art of autobiography. By the end of the eighteenth century, such writing had become so fixed a part of intellectual activity that the philosophers Herder and Goethe both urged that autobiographies from different countries and ages be collected, so that light could be thrown on the process of the liberation of the human personality. In the nineteenth century, and in our own time, autobiography has maintained its value and vitality as history.[2] A little more than forty years ago Dr L. R. Grote of Halle gathered the autobiographies of contemporary physicians in an effort to delineate the growth of modern medicine.[3] During this same period in the United States, Professor Carl Murchison assiduously collected the autobiographies of pioneers in psychology, in order to chart the development of the history of that discipline. In 1930 he published them in three volumes under the title *A history of psychology in autobiography*.[4] Its usefulness is attested to by the fact that the work still goes on; in recent years two more volumes have been published.[5]

Not all of oral history stems from autobiography. Some of its antecedents are rooted in the activities of anthropologists and folklorists who have long been engaged in collecting and analysing the oral traditions of man and most notably those of pre-literate societies.[6] One cannot easily differentiate the purposes of this happy and inquisitive company from those of individuals who engage in oral history today. The account of the efforts of the anthropologist George Bird Grinnell to collect the history of the Pawnee Indians in 1888 is a case in point.

Last spring I visited the Pawnee Agency in the Indian Territory. On the day after my arrival, I rode over to the house of Eagle Chief, whom...I had known for many years...we sat down and filled the pipe and talked. Through all our talk I could see that he was curious to know the object of my visit. At last he said, 'My son, I am glad that you have come to us once more. My mind is big when I look at you and talk to you...Why have you come again to the Pawnee village? What brings you here at this time?'

I answered, 'Father, we have come down here to visit the people and to talk to them; to ask them how things used to be in the olden times, to hear their stories, to get their history, and then to put all these things down in a book, so that in the years to come, after the tribe have all become like white people, the old things of the Pawnees shall not be forgotten.'

The chief meditated for a while and then said, 'It is good and it is time. Already the old things are being lost, and those who knew the secrets are many of them dead. If we had known how to write, we would have put all these things down, and they would not have been forgotten, but we could not write, and these stories were handed down from one to another. The old men told their grandchildren, and they told their grandchildren, and so the secrets and the stories and the doings of long ago have been handed down. It may be that they have changed as they passed from father to son, and it is well that they should be put down, so that our children, when they are like the white people, can know what were their fathers' ways.'[7]

Recent activities in oral history in the United States stem from

288

yet another source. In 1938 Professor Allan Nevins, in his hand-book of historiography, *The gateway to history*,[8] urged his fellow historians to form an organization which would undertake a system-atic attempt to obtain from the lips and papers of living Americans an extensive personal record of the part they had played in the political, economic, and cultural life of the nation. These proposals, however, evoked little enthusiasm in Nevins's contemporaries. Some had reservations concerning the wisdom of allowing historians to collect memoirs from the living. They were of the opinion that such a technique would necessarily endanger the historians' objectivity and lead in the end to the production of self-orientated, partisan accounts of recent events. Others felt that historians possessed neither the skills nor the funds needed to obtain verbatim auto-biographical interviews. In spite of these and other objections, Nevins continued to campaign for his technique. In 1948, when the tape recorder had lately been perfected for commercial purposes, he received funds from several sources and so was able to establish an oral history research office at Columbia University that could carry out the plans he had proposed a decade earlier. Nevins's persistence not only demonstrated a vindication of his original vision and pur-pose, it also reflected the growing need of those working in the field of contemporary history to discover a way of coping with some of the complexities created by modern technology for historical research.

Historians agree that modern, industrial society rests in part on the foundations of printing and the making of paper. These are im-portant not only because they are amongst the oldest of modern industrial and technological procedures, but also because they act as catalysts to human thought. 'It was printing', the historian George Renard once wrote, 'which gave wings to human thought and allowed it to spread far and wide and to reproduce itself un-ceasingly...'[9] Newspapers, magazines, books and a vast mechanically produced correspondence testify to the pervasiveness of print and paper communication in all parts of our public and private daily lives. The one constant end-result of business, government, and science seems to be the production of new records. In a little over twenty years the Atomic Energy Commission has created well over one million linear feet of records. In New York, advertisers advise radio listeners on the importance of storing private and business

289

papers in specially constructed vaults. In Washington, D.C., record-collecting agencies such as the National Archives, the Library of Congress, and the Smithsonian Institution, vie with one another for the space and the privilege of storing government and private records. In the last 25 years a new business known as 'records management' has made its appearance; its major function is to advise business firms how best to preserve and maintain their ever-growing records.

If historians who work in contemporary history bid fair to be overwhelmed by a superabundance of records, it must be remembered that this same technology paradoxically conspires to starve him of a great deal of the detail and variety inherent in the process of events. Much of what used to be put to paper is today lost because of superior methods of communication. Why write a letter for two hours, when a fifteen-minute telephone call serves the same purpose? A medical problem that might have resulted in a month's correspondence between two physicians 75 years ago, is today resolved by an airplane trip and a face-to-face meeting. The revolution in communication has not only made the world smaller, it has in addition changed the nature and uses of time. A little more than a hundred years ago, a handful of merchants and intellectuals interested in formulating a policy concerning Africa, met in the rooms of the American Geographical Society in New York to listen to a letter sent months before by David Livingstone from the banks of the Zambesi River. Today, a speech by Jomo Kenyatta in Kenya is almost immediately available to inhabitants in New York by means of radio and television and the subject of discussion and debate at the United Nations. The tempo of living makes claims on individual time and understanding that were unthought of fifty years ago. Under this pressure, previous habits such as keeping diaries and journals are discarded, with the consequent disappearance of these valuable manuscripts from the record. It is this paradox of simultaneous plenty and scarcity in contemporary records that in large measure defines the tasks of those who work in oral history.

The late Harold Innis once noted that the flexibility of the alphabet and its adaptation to mechanization facilitated an approximation of the printed word to the oral tradition. And that while it at first strengthened the written tradition by its emphasis on manuscripts, by the end of the sixteenth century printing helped make vernacular language an effective basis of literature in Europe.[10] One might add here that the tape recorder and television camera have made possible a new union of oral and written traditions.

III

In an important sense, oral history is misnamed. While it is true the oral historian helps to gather an oral memoir, it is equally true that this account is based on a written record. It is precisely this record which ultimately determines the course and content of his work. There are four parts of this work. Once a subject has been selected for interview, the oral historian, like any other historian, must prepare himself with a study of extant primary and secondary source material in order to identify and define relevant historical relationships and problems. Second, armed with a tape recorder, he must so befit himself and his preparatory work that he spurs the chosen subject's memory of the past. Third, he must collect from his subject, and from other people, supporting documents of contemporary demonstration, both as a check on the unreliability of memory and to supplement the account obtained. Fourth, he must edit, or help the subject to edit, the final preparation of the memoir so that it presents what the subject wants it to present.

The memoir that emerges as a result of this process is a new type of historical document. It has been produced by a participant in past events, but it is also the creation of the historian interviewer who has in fact helped to determine the historical problems and relationships to be investigated. This mutual product contributes to both the strength and the weakness inherent in oral history memoirs. Although such memoirs may contain unique and new information, in no sense are they exclusive historical sources; rather they are corroborative sources and guides. Actually they stand as first interpretations of recent history, filtered through particular individual experience at a particular moment of time. They therefore mark a beginning of interpretation not an end. They also mark the first ordering of a mass of primary and secondary material germane to a given individual's life or a series of historical problems.[11]

I have often been asked, 'How do you know you are getting the truth in your oral history interviews?' The answer is, 'I don't know.' At best, memory is a slender reed, and even well-intentioned people often misremember. Sometimes they lie. At other times, their prejudices recast events in such a manner as to make a professional propagandist blush. All of this all men do. It should be clearly understood that none of these memoirs will be given to the future historian with the notion that they contain the final and most accurate word on a given subject. In the end they will be received as but one of many documents. The future historian will in fact use, weigh, and examine them in relation to other extant documents. There can be little doubt that his evaluation of these records will be keener than our own, because time will furnish him with still more evidence and new perspective.[12]

What about the person who speaks from limited knowledge, or tells half-truths, or creates a myth? This is not the horror it appears to be, because such a person is also unwittingly giving us a psychologically revealing portrait of himself. Actually the collection of half-truths, myths, and prejudices is as valuable for history as pristine truth if they are appreciated and evaluated adequately. Often they lead to contradictions. In fact it is the contradictions that emerge from such material which pose the nicest historical problems. I would like here to give an example from my own experience.

A number of years ago I became interested in the changing techniques of treating various fevers, and more especially typhoid fever. When I interviewed physicians in New York, all agreed that the change in treatment of typhoid fever occurred after Eugene DuBois's and Warren Coleman's notable experiments on the basal metabolism of typhoid patients in the years between 1909 and 1915.[13] Boston physicians gave me another story. They maintained that Dr Fred Shattuck at the Massachusetts General Hospital switched from the traditional starvation to a high-caloric diet at least a decade before the investigations of DuBois and Coleman. Who was right? In the strictest sense, all were telling the truth as they knew it. As a matter of record, Shattuck's case histories revealed that he did indeed use a high-caloric diet at least a decade before DuBois and Coleman's experiments. The problem of priority is an uninteresting one. All too often it ends inquiry. If the focus is changed somewhat, and the problem of what led to a change in treatment in the first decade of the twentieth century is faced, the beautiful diversity that exists in history becomes apparent. Clearly different factors played a role in Boston and New York.

Vital statistics show that beginning in 1890, there was a marked and progressive decline of typhoid in Boston due largely to strict inspection of milk and water supplies,[14] and manifested by the number of patients admitted to hospital. This decline allowed Shattuck, a superb clinician trained in the French school of pathological anatomy, to observe his patients more carefully and by clinical and pathological observations to conclude empirically that starvation resulted in death but a high-caloric diet did not.[15] The factors in New York were quite different. Although New York produced many important public health figures at the beginning of the twentieth century, public health practice was inadequate. As late as 1909, terrible epidemics of typhoid fever raged in New York because of milk contamination. Only in 1910 did the Board of Health resolve that all milk drunk should be properly pasteurized.[16] Admissions to hospitals were constantly high, and during epidemics, physicians could do little but make their patients comfortable. DuBois's training was markedly different from Shattuck's. Educated at Columbia's College of Physicians and Surgeons in New York, after interning he turned to physiology and took postgraduate training in it in Magnus-Levy's laboratory, and in Kraus's clinic in the Charité in Berlin, under Theodore Brugsch. In Berlin, he learned in particular of the Pettenkofer-Voit chamber for studying basal metabolism and met a fellow New Yorker, Graham Lusk, the distinguished pioneer nutritionalist. Back in New York, he worked with Lusk who urged him and Coleman to study basal metabolism in typhoid fever.[17]

If memoirs are in future to act as catalysts for new inquiry, care must be taken in choosing subjects, as well as in preparing for interviews. All too frequently people are chosen to participate in oral history programmes because they have made a significant contribution to art, science, politics or letters, or, as is equally likely, on the basis of public fame or notoriety. I do not mean by this that people who have made significant contributions should not be interviewed. Far from it. I do suggest, however, that significance or importance is not always self-evident.

In his own time in the late nineteenth and early twentieth centuries, Sir William Osler was one of the most distinguished names in medicine, both in the United States and in Britain. His fame as a clinician and teacher was well deserved. His textbook, *Principles and*

293

practice of medicine, schooled generations of students and practitioners. Now one of his contemporaries at Oxford was Dr Archibald Garrod. I wonder how many oral historians called upon to make a choice between interviewing Osler or Garrod in 1910 would have chosen Garrod? Although Garrod was recognized as an unusual clinician and investigator, the implications of his work *Inborn errors of metabolism* were not well understood by his generation. Actually it was not appreciated until the rapid development of biochemical genetics in the late 1950's. In 1963 that appreciation finally dictated a reprinting of his pioneer work, some fifty-three years after it first saw the light of day.[18] The example is perhaps extreme, but it illuminates two points I wish to make. First, that what is important or significant is not always self-evident. Second, that it is a conceit to concentrate on obtaining the memoirs of people only on a basis of significant achievement. The history of medicine and science that concentrates on success or achievement is but half a history. Attention must also be given to those who failed, or never achieved a signal success, or perhaps laboured in areas that are not deemed important by contemporary judgement.

In the United States, most oral history programmes in medicine and science concentrate their efforts on obtaining the memoirs of those physicians and scientists who have retired or who are close to retirement age. There is good reason for such choice. The older physician or scientist is apt to have more time to give for historical purposes than a younger man still actively engaged in the clinic, laboratory, or classroom. Further, his age gives him a wide experience to draw on. Often he is a link to events that occurred fifty and sixty years before. Unfortunately, however, age does not always serve as the best criterion for choosing a subject. I have interviewed medical scientists at the age of 92 who were still actively engaged in research and capable of productive work. By the same token, I have interviewed others, who, although considerably younger men, were beginning to fail. Very often pressure is brought to bear on oral historians to interview famous people who are failing, on the grounds that their past eminence and achievement merit attention. It is neither a service nor a kindness to spend time with such a person. The person who has begun to senesce is often aware of his diminishing powers, and it is a cruelty to hold up a mirror to his condition by asking him to remember. If there is any rule that the

oral historian should adhere to, it is that the subject being interviewed must be mentally competent.

In addition to interviewing older individuals, I believe oral historians can with profit interview younger men. There are many
advantages to such a procedure. Although the younger man cannot
draw on as wide a range of historical experience as the older person,
his reminiscences are apt to be richer in detail and more disciplined.
If the younger man lives out his days, the oral historian can always
return for additions to the memoir as well as for re-examinations of
particular historical problems. The latter is most important. Man
continually rewrites his history. His views change. The opportunity
to re-examine historical problems at different time periods can
create a guide to those events and experiences that contribute to the
physician's or scientist's reinterpretation of the history of his
discipline.

Most historians agree that oral history requires research. There is,
however, a broad area of disagreement on the amount of research
necessary to conduct useful interviews. Some oral history programmes because of financial exigencies require little research. In
such programmes the oral historian is looked upon as an historical
Moses, who merely has to know how to tap his subject's memory in
order to have historical experience come gushing forth. Oral history
is not instant history, nor is the oral historian a magician. Actually
oral history requires very careful preparation. In my own work, I
allow between twenty and thirty hours of research for each hour of
interview. While this figure at first blush seems large, it is by no
means rigid. As one interviews subjects in the same field, this figure
drops because the interviewer is able to utilize the primary and
secondary data he has previously used with other subjects. It is for
this reason I believe that oral history programmes should be planned
to cover specific areas or problems rather than to choose notable
figures at random. Although the number of memoirs that emerge
from well-researched interviews is small, if the problem areas and
subjects are judiciously chosen, one can in a relatively brief period of
time produce a sufficient number of memoirs to give a good overall
view of contemporary historical developments in a given field of
medicine or science.

There is another aspect of research which should be mentioned.
Most oral historians make no attempt to integrate the research they

have done in preparation for their interviews with the memoir which is finally produced. As a result, it is difficult for the reader to evaluate the material put before him. To aid the reader, the oral historian should prepare a detailed guide to the primary and secondary materials which were used in the preparation of particular interviews. In so doing, he will enable the reader to understand that the questions asked, as well as the responses given, were not only based on the understanding of the historian, and the memory of the subject being interviewed, but were also dependent on a particular documentary record. That record in fact delineates the limits of the validity of the memoir which is gathered. In future, such material can also serve as a base for the re-evaluation and reinterpretation of the memoir, particularly as new sources become available.

In recent years there has been sharp debate among those who work in oral history on the problem of the depth of the interview. Unfortunately, there is no general rule which can be used as a guide for the number of hours to be spent with any given subject. That number depends on a variety of factors, the personality of the subject being interviewed, the primary and secondary data available for research, the amount of money which can be devoted to a given project, and the philosophy of the oral historian.[19]

Some historians and sociologists have concentrated their efforts on collecting interviews around a specific or special historical problem. These interviews are usually brief, and range in time from one to ten hours. Dr Harriet Zuckerman, a young sociologist at Columbia University, for example, has collected the reminiscences of Nobel Laureates in science, concentrating on the development of that aspect of their research which culminated in their winning a Nobel Prize.[20] The project on Sources for the History of Quantum Physics, jointly sponsored by the American Physical Society and the American Philosophical Society, and directed by Professor Thomas Kuhn, has used similar techniques in gathering material for a history of quantum physics.[21] Dr Richard Hewlett and Dr Oscar Anderson have done the same in preparing their history of the Atomic Energy Commission,[22] as has Dr Redmond C. Cochrane in his recent history of the National Bureau of Standards.[23] Although these interviews have been admirably researched, they will in future be of little use to the historian unless he happens to be interested in these particular problems. They are also wasteful. It may be all well and good to interview a scientist like Dr Max Delbrück for his contribution to quantum physics, but to cut him off at this point, and not examine his subsequent development as a biophysicist, is simply to miss an opportunity to examine an important facet of the growth of molecular biology.

My own belief is that oral history should be devoted to complete autobiographical explorations. By doing this, the historian not only has a chance to examine the genetic development of ideas in medicine and science, he also has the opportunity to explore the human and social aspects of a particular life-family relationship, education, political activity, and belief, and a wide variety of institutional, governmental, and professional affiliations. In sum, he has a chance to use his imagination. He needs that opportunity because he is essentially collecting materials for future use and has to project needs that have not yet been defined. Quite apart from the future, there is one present advantage which dictates complete autobiographical explorations in medicine and science. The history of medicine and science are young disciplines. The more varied the problems examined, the easier it will be to incorporate the data developed by such oral history memoirs into the corpus of traditional social, political, and economic history.

There is yet another problem that plagues those who work in oral history, and this is the problem of editing. In some programmes historians do not edit memoirs because they look upon their task as one of collecting raw data. They believe that if they edit the material they have gathered, they tamper with the truth of what has been said. My own feeling is that oral history demands very careful and special editing. This aspect of the oral historian's work is as important and demanding as interviewing. The spoken word is far different from the written word because the nature of reflection in the two processes is different. Conversation is frequently untidy, no matter how logically the historian tries to pursue a problem. Often there are unfinished sentences, repetitions, and important asides, the latter triggered by the memory of a name or an event casually mentioned. Sometimes, the interviewer and subject lapse into a conversational shorthand because of a common understanding of the subject-matter under discussion. At other times, the person interviewed does not wish to depend on memory and quotes directly from a letter or book without indicating in speech that he is quoting.

297

When such material is transcribed from the tape it may easily mis-convey to the reader what was actually said or meant unless there are editorial emendations. The oral historian's first duty is to see that the memoir says what his subject wants it to say, and to have this done as clearly as possible. I do not mean by this that the his-torian should make his subject sound grammatical if his speech is ungrammatical. Or that he should eliminate expletives if his subject uses such language. As a matter of fact, he should make every effort to keep the original inflection and nuance of speech and to remember that he is dealing with the spoken, not the written word. Nor should he correct errors of interpretation. On the contrary, if his subject makes an error in interpretation, or has misconceptions, or voices prejudices, those errors, misconceptions, and prejudices should be kept because they are revealing of the personality and beliefs of the subject. It is incumbent on the oral historian wherever he recognizes error, or is aware of the differences in interpretation of events, to note such errors and differences in footnotes. Also in footnotes he should as nearly as possible identify persons or works alluded to, but never further identified by the subject interviewed. Such editing contributes to clarity and it also adds material to the memoir that is historically useful. Editing does not preclude keeping the original transcript of the memoir. That transcript should always be kept, so that the future historian, if he wishes, can compare it with the edited version.

Research and editing take a great deal of time. It is for this reason that an oral historian should not do more than 125 hours of interviewing in any given year. If he interviews at a greater rate, he must necessarily stint on research or editing, and as a result his memoirs are necessarily poorer. There has to be an understanding at the outset of just what one expects from an oral history pro-gramme. I believe that the primary criterion must be the content and substance of what one collects, not the amount. Administrators set great store by figures, and 400 hours of interview always looks better than 125 hours in annual reports. Research and editing are the heart of the oral history process, but unfortunately they are reflected only in the content of the memoir. It should be added here that the number of double-spaced typescript pages one usually gets from an hour of interview tape, averages between twenty-two and twenty-five. On the basis of 125 hours of interview, an oral historian can produce between 2700 and 3200 pages of typescript a year. This is a good year's work for any historian, more particularly because it is in areas that have hitherto not been analysed historically. One note of caution must be sounded. Because interviews are conducted on a voluntary basis, an interviewer must frequently, and particularly at the beginning of a project, juggle two and three interviews at a time. This circumstance often makes it difficult to complete given interviews in a twelve-month period. Oral history programmes should therefore be projected over a two- to three-year period.

It is the custom in oral history projects that when interviews are over, and a memoir has been transcribed from the tape and edited, the work is regarded as having been completed. I have long felt that the completion of a memoir should not be regarded as an end in itself, but should rather serve as the signal for the beginning of another set of activities. These activities might feature special symposia, where subjects who have completed their interviews could present to their peers in medicine and science an historical summary of their careers or research. Afterwards, special commentators could be called on for a critical evaluation of the subject's historical judgements. The value of such symposia would be enormous. They would encourage physicians and scientists to engage in historical analysis of the development of their own disciplines, as well as raise new historical problems that the oral historian could pursue in future interviews. The transcripts of such symposia could moreover be used as appendices to completed memoirs and serve as yet another source for the future historian of the current beliefs of the scientific community.

One other thing might be done after a memoir has been completed. At such time, the subject and historian could sit down and prepare a half-hour videotape devoted to a discussion of an important problem in research in which the subject was involved, or else the subject might be asked to reminisce about some of his colleagues. Such videotapes could serve as the basis for the construction of a special archive of visual materials relating to the contemporary history of medicine and science, and in future be utilized for purposes of historical and scientific instruction or educational television.

In many oral history projects, because of the problems of cost, interview tapes are not kept intact. After transcription they are used for other interviews. Such procedures are inherently wasteful, because the spoken word gives fuller and better psychological insights into the character and makeup of the person being interviewed than the transcribed word can ever convey. There is yet another reason for the preservation of tape. We live in an envelope of sound. It is part and parcel of our environment, yet we have hardly begun to catalogue sound or analyse its social impact. How did Shakespeare's plays sound to his contemporaries? Did those who acted in them give special inflections to the words? Did those inflections provide nuances which modified meaning? What was the nature of sound in a nineteenth-century village or city? How did it affect the behaviour and speech of the inhabitants? By the same token the future historian might well ask about the nature and impact of sound on our own behaviour. Oral history offers us an opportunity to examine a portion of the environment, a category which we always invoke as having an effect on the development of history, and about whose many components we know little or nothing.[24]

The history and sociology of medicine and science are young disciplines. They are not only important in themselves; they are of equal importance to the medical and scientific community. They are in a sense testimony that the development of modern medicine and science has reached a point in time when physicians and scientists, as well as social scientists, must stand back and reflect on the origin and meaning of medical and scientific ideas, as well as wrestle with the burgeoning problems of the impact of science on society. In order to do this properly, the historical record of these various scientific disciplines must be assembled, preserved, and used. Physicians and scientists have long been aware that their day-to-day work has in part been historical, and that the published record of their investigations is in fact a history which serves as a fulcrum for all present and future medical and scientific activity. This record is not a complete record; it is in essence a summary of achievement. As medicine and science grow and become more specialized, that record runs in even narrower channels. It is no mistake that when an historian approaches a physician or scientist and asks him about his papers, the first material he is given is published papers. For the historian that record is but a beginning. If he wishes to probe the development and process of medicine and science and its various relationships to society, he needs a broader spectrum of records: personal correspondence, diaries, protocols of experiments, archives of hospitals, institutions, artifacts and above all the memory of physicians and scientists who can supplement these records with what has not been put to paper. Only memory can reveal the hidden detail of failures and false starts in research, the human qualities of colleagues, and the infinite variety of problems that comes with working in universities, business, and government.

IV

Perhaps the most important contribution which an oral history programme has to offer is in the future training of historians of medicine and science. Collecting the autobiographies of contemporaries in effect affords the opportunity of creating a historical laboratory, where living memory could be brought in contact with the primary and secondary materials of the recent past. The training programme I envision might be organized in the following manner. A special seminar under the direction of an oral historian could be established to examine, let us say, recent developments in medical science. During the first half-year the seminar might devote its efforts to exploring the recent growth of bacteriology. Initially, the instructor would be responsible for conducting interviews with a given bacteriologist, while the seminar engaged in collecting and immersing itself in the secondary and primary materials relevant to that bacteriologist's life and career. Each week, the seminar would be required to listen to the interviews in progress, and on the basis of their preparation in the primary and secondary materials, asked to criticize the historical relationships being developed and analysed. In this way, the student would receive an opportunity to deal critically with both primary and secondary data, and to develop an appreciation of the limitations of such sources.

In the second half-year each student would be asked to create his own memoirs of contemporary bacteriologists. In the course of such creation students would be required to collect manuscript materials relevant to the life of the person they were studying, as well as to submit their interviews to the seminar's searching criticism. The benefits of such a programme are self-evident. First, seminar members would have the singular advantage of receiving instruction in a special discipline in science by experts whose autobiographies they were collecting. Second, students would be able to exchange and share in their seminar discussions, information from an ever-increasing unique body of primary historical materials never, or hardly ever, used before. Third, students would receive practical archival training in collecting, ordering, and noting the content of manuscript material. Fourth, students would gain experience in editing, and have an opportunity to lay the foundation for future biographical or monographical studies. Nor would the advantages only accrue to the students. The university, as a result of such a programme, would become the repository of autobiographical and other source materials in the contemporary history of bacteriology, or indeed in the contemporary history of any other science, oral history seminars might want to study.

This rummaging in the past through the living requires guidance. I know of no better advice to give than that offered in a colloquy between two characters in a story by John Wyndham. Oddly enough one of these is also an historian who uses a machine to explore the past.

'History machine,' I said, 'what is a history machine?' She looked puzzled. 'It's well a history machine, you learn history with it.' 'Not lucid,' I said. 'You might as well tell me you make history with it.' 'Oh, no,' she said, 'one is not supposed to do that. It is a very serious offense.'[25]

I do not hesitate to offer this exchange as a guide for oral historians about to study the recent history of medicine and science, although I am sure that most readers will recognize John Wyndham as a science fiction writer.

REFERENCES

1   G. Sarton, *The life of science : essays in the history of civilization*, pp. 19–20, Bloomington, Ind.: Indiana University Press, 1960.
2   G. Misch, 'Conception and origin of autobiography' in *A history of autobiography in antiquity*, transl. E. W. Dickes, 2 vols., I, 1–18, London: Routledge & Kegan Paul, 1950. For an excellent discussion of the nature and role of autobiography, see also R. Pascal, *Design and truth in autobiography*, London: Routledge & Kegan Paul, 1960.

3 L. R. Grote (ed.), *Die Medizin der Gegenwart in Selbstdarstellung*, 8 vols., Leipzig: F. Meiner Verlag, 1923–29.

4 C. Murchison (ed.), *A history of psychology in autobiography*, 3 vols., Worcester: Clark University Press, 1930–36.

5 E. G. Boring, H. S. Langfeld, H. Werner and R. M. Yerkes (eds.), *A history of psychology in autobiography*, vol. 4, Worcester: Clark University Press, 1952; E. G. Boring (ed.), *A history of psychology in autobiography*, vol. 5, New York: Appleton Century Crofts, 1967.

6 See further D. K. Wilgus, *Anglo-American folksong scholarships since 1898*, New Brunswick, N.J.: Rutgers University Press, 1959, and more especially the seminal and stimulating work of I. and P. Opie, *The lore and language of school children*, Oxford: Clarendon Press, 1959.

7 G. B. Grinnell, *Pawnee hero stories and folk-tales: with notes on the origin, customs and character of the Pawnee people*, pp. v–vi, London: D. Nutt, 1893.

8 A. Nevins, *The gateway to history*, preface, New York: D. C. Heath, 1938.

9 G. Renard and G. Weulersse, *Life and work in modern Europe: 15th to 18th century*, p. 12, New York: A. Knopf, 1926.

10 H. A. Innis, *Empire and communication*, pp. 183–4, London: Oxford University Press, 1950. Innis is one of the few historians one can read over and over again with profit. He was gifted with ideas.

11 S. Benison, Appendix G. 'Note on manuscript sources, footnotes, appendices and bibliography' in *Tom Rivers: reflections on a life in medicine and science*, pp. 621–50, Cambridge, Mass.: M.I.T. Press, 1967.

12 One of the best discussions on the nature of oral materials is by the anthropologist and historian, J. Vansina, *Oral tradition: a study in historical methodology*, transl. H. M. Wright, London: Routledge & Kegan Paul, 1965.

13 See especially P. A. Shaffer and W. Coleman, 'Protein metabolism in typhoid fever', *Arch. intern. Med.* 1909, 4, 538–600; E. F. DuBois, 'The absorption of food in typhoid fever', ibid. 1912, 10, 177–95; E. F. DuBois and W. Coleman, 'Clinical calorimetry. Seventh paper. Calorimetric observations on the metabolism of typhoid patients with or without food', ibid. 1915, 15, 887–938.

14 The decline of typhoid fever in Boston was in large measure a result of the superior public health work of William T. Sedgwick. See especially his pioneer papers: W. T. Sedgwick, *A report of the biological work of the Lawrence Experimental Station by the State Board of Health of Massachusetts upon sewerage*, etc., Part 2, Boston, 1890; idem, 'Investigation of recent epidemics of typhoid fever in Massachusetts', *Annual Report of the State Board of Health of Massachusetts* 1893, 24, 664–742; W. T. Sedgwick and J. L. Batchelder, Jr, *Boston med. surg. J.* 1892, 126, 25–8.

15 For a brief résumé of the development of the medical departments at the Harvard Medical School, see brochure Anon., *The Harvard Medical School, 1782–1906*, pp. 15–30, 73–85, Boston: privately printed, n.d.; H. R. Viets, *A brief history of medicine in Massachusetts*, pp. 119–84,

Boston: Houghton Mifflin & Co., 1930. For a brief view of Shattuck as a medical educator and clinician, see E. D. Churchill (ed.), *To work in the vineyard of surgery. The reminiscences of J. Collins Warren (1842–1927)*, pp. 250–1, Boston: Harvard University Press, 1958.

16   G. Rosen, *A history of public health*, pp. 359–60, New York: M.D. Publications, 1958; C. E. A. Winslow, *The Life of Hermann Biggs*, p. 226, Philadelphia: Lea & Febiger, 1929.

17   For further details see J. Aub, 'Eugene F. DuBois', *National Academy of Science Biographical Memoirs* 1962, 36, 125–45. See also S. Benison, *The reminiscences of Joseph Aub*, chapter 2, New York: Oral History Research Office, Columbia University, 1959 [in typescript].

18   H. Harris (ed.), *Garrod's Inborn errors of metabolism*, London: Oxford University Press, 1963.

19   The best summary discussion of problems of oral history was prepared by Professor Alfred Rollins of the University of Vermont following a symposium on oral history held under the auspices of the Kennedy Library at Harvard University in the summer of 1965. Unfortunately it only exists in mimeographed form.

20   Dr Zuckerman's interviews are stored in the Oral History Research Office Archives at Columbia University, New York. Her study is soon to be published.

21   T. S. Kuhn, J. I. Heilbron, P. Forman and L. Allen, *Sources for history of quantum physics: an inventory and report*, pp. 3–6 and especially pp. 150–6, Philadelphia: American Philosophical Society, 1967.

22   R. G. Hewlett and O. E. Anderson, Jr, *The new world, 1939/1946* (vol. 1 of *A history of the United States Atomic Energy Commission*), pp. 662–4, University Park, Penn.: The Pennsylvania State University Press, 1962. See also R. G. Hewlett, 'A pilot study in contemporary scientific history', *Isis* 1962, 53, 31–8, and especially the discussion pp. 39–51.

23   R. C. Cochrane, *Measures for progress: a history of the National Bureau of Standards*, Washington, D.C.: National Bureau of Standards, U.S. Department of Commerce, 1966.

24   See the imaginative work of F. Berry, *Poetry and the physical voice*, Part I Introductory, pp. 3–43, London: Routledge & Kegan Paul, 1962; actually the whole volume bears careful study.

25   J. Wyndham, 'Chronoclasm' in *The seeds of time*, p. 20, London: Penguin Books, 1960. By permission.

The following additional references to oral history may also be of interest:

I. B. Cohen, 'An interview with Einstein', *Sci. Amer.* July 1955, pp. 69–73.

W. D. Miles, 'Usefulness of oral history in writing the story of a large scientific project', *Actes Hist. Sci.* Ithaca 1962, 1, 351–3.

'Project on the history of recent physics in the United States', *Newsletter* (American Institute of Physics) May 1964, vol. 1, No. 1 [no pagination]; see also subsequent numbers.

L. H. Berman, 'Oral history as source material for the history of the behavioral sciences', *J. Hist. Behav. Sci.* 1967, 3, 58–9.

H. Fruchtbaum, 'Scientists and the history of science' [letter], *Nature, Lond.* 1968, 219, 880.

The National Library of Medicine's Oral History Program is described in *Bull. Hist. Med.* 1968, 42, 274.

R. Blythe, *Axenfield. Portrait of an English village*, London: Allen Lane the Penguin Press, 1969. The special joy of this oral history is that it was created by a poet.

18 A Research and Teaching Collection of Primary Source Material on the History of Medicine

EDWIN CLARKE and B. I. WILLIAMS

One of the overall purposes of this book is to examine certain ways of studying the history of medicine with a view to increasing the quality of research and teaching done in the field. This can in part be brought about by reconsidering basic methods of work in the light of new approaches and techniques which are now at our disposal. Thus the object of the following paper is to report a method of handling some of the primary source material of the history of medicine and concerns the collection of Xerox copies of them. Although this may seem to be an activity worthy of little notice, it does, in fact, have at least two far-reaching and fundamental implications for the discipline.

II

The first concerns the availability of materials. The prime requisite for any historian is ready access to the primary sources which constitute the essential raw materials of his subject. Their provision is clearly his central problem, for like the chemist he must be able to analyse before he can synthesize. This is especially true in the history of medicine where many kinds of people write on its various aspects. One of the commonest failings of many of them is a tacit willingness to accept another author's citation from primary material or his interpretation of it, without having seen the original. A great deal of the so-called historical writing in medicine is, in fact, based upon secondary, tertiary or even more remote sources. At times this may incur no danger and in some instances it is the only course available, but inevitably there are many occasions when the errors in the material that is being slavishly copied or followed implicitly are transmitted with it. The widespread and iniquitous plagiarism of other historians' references to the literature without consulting the book or periodical cited, is another evil which is far too common. To avoid such happenings therefore and to help to encourage the production of sounder and more accurate writing in the history of medicine, the greater availability of primary source material is indispensable.

III

Secondly we must consider the relationship of the library and of bibliography to the history of medicine. The library is to the historian as the laboratory is to the scientist, and in each the quantity and quality of research carried out does not necessarily bear any relationship to the space or the facilities provided. Thus it is well known that certain scientists and scholars in the past have achieved revolutionary advances whilst subjected to appallingly primitive conditions of work.[1] The reverse is also true, and in the field of history there are several examples of men who, having amassed large collections of books, made little scholarly use of them themselves. As far as the history of medicine is concerned the libraries of Pybus, now in the Library of the University of Newcastle upon Tyne, of Waller, and of Henry Wellcome spring readily to mind; more recent examples are the collections of J. A. Benjamin and L. Reynolds.[2] We must, of course, be grateful, not only to the men who were able to accumulate materials which now form valuable research tools, but also to those who have helped to make them available to scholars and in some instances are still doing so; the excellent catalogues of the Wellcome Historical Medical Library now appearing indicate the extraordinary richness of one man's collection and the magnitude of his gift to scholarship.

Despite these benefits accruing from bibliophilia, it nevertheless seems that in the history of medicine, the antiquarian, as opposed to the working, library has, on the whole, played too prominent a role. There is today in some countries a conception of the historian of medicine as a multilingual expert on rare books, working exclusively in an antiquarian library and thus entirely divorced from modern medicine. There are probably several reasons for this apart from the natural need that the medical historian has for early works. The most important is the influence of such men as Osler and his disciples, who encouraged all those around them to think of the history of medicine as mainly an antiquarian, library-based study. This possibly accounts for the more frequent occurrence of this interpretation in Britain and in the United States of America, whereas in Germany, for example, where the Oslerian tradition is much less, it is rare. In addition, the dealers in antiquarian books have tended to encourage and perpetuate this state of affairs; their involvement with age and rarity are factors with which *per se* the historian is not concerned.[3]

As well as the association of medical history with the library there is another link with books, fostered by certain historians in the past, and this is bibliography. For any historical study based on primary printed sources the knowledge supplied by this technique is essential, but its association with historians of medicine has also contributed to their 'book-bound' image. This situation is seen less often in other branches of history.

On the whole it would appear that the public assessment of the historian of medicine might be enhanced by liberating him to some extent from the library, essential though his contacts with it must always be. It is becoming increasingly apparent that in certain countries in order to survive he must forge stronger links with more recent history and especially with the present; and this means with the medical school and hospital and with their staffs and students. Collections of early medical works are essential but the medical historian must not be identified with them exclusively. Basically the historian of medicine needs a working library and ready access to primary source material.

IV

To assist therefore in the improvement of work in the history of medicine and to avoid the restrictions of the antiquarian library, some way is needed of making primary source material more readily obtainable for teaching and research purposes.

Fortunately a method has become available in the last decade so that in certain fields the contents of the antiquarian library can be made more accessible. In the Sub-Department of the History of Medicine in University College London there is a scheme of collecting photocopies of primary sources. This relates, at the moment, to the history of the medical sciences and in particular to the evolution of knowledge concerning the anatomy and the physiology of the cardiovascular system.

It is hardly necessary to describe in detail a technique which must be obvious. First of all, the main contributions to the topic are selected on the basis of personal experience and on that of others. The primary sources are sought and a Xerox copy made of the relevant pages of book or periodical; in the case of a book the title-page is also copied and if necessary photographs of illustrations are prepared. These are kept in folders and stored in a filing cabinet suspension system together with secondary material dealing with the contributor himself or with an appraisal of his work, portraits of him, etc. The method of arranging the folders can be determined by the topic[4] but whichever form is chosen, alphabetical or by subject, the alternative scheme can be created on index cards. Xeroxing is the obvious method of choice for producing copies, owing to its simplicity, versatility, reliability and relative cost; in the case of the more recently published material the problem of copyright is of course taken into account.

V

There is nothing very extraordinary about this simple technique of making a collection of primary sources in the history of the medical sciences, and no doubt others have created a similar research and teaching tool. They would probably justify their activity with the same arguments that we can cite in its favour. The practical advantages are as follows:

(1) First and foremost is the advantage of ready availability. Quite often the classic contribution was printed in a periodical which is now rare and therefore difficult to procure. The same is often true of printed books and although both these and some of the classical journal articles have been republished either singly or in anthologies, the number is still small compared with the amount of material being sought; moreover certain items will never be reprinted because they will not create a commercially viable product.

In the case of rare and valuable books, their worth continues to increase and there is no indication yet that this process of escalation will not continue.[5] They will eventually be so precious that their custodians will, quite justifiably, allow them to be consulted only under strict supervision, if at all. The same is true of certain nineteenth-century items, the paper of which is becoming increasingly brittle so that handling must be reduced to a minimum if the book, journal or offprint is to survive. At the same time it is recognized that the copying process itself may result in damage to the binding of frail books and so may be inadvisable in some cases.

Research is obviously facilitated if the material needed for its execution is available immediately, instead of days or weeks later. How often does one wish to refer to the exact words of an author when one is seeking precision, but how often, if the matter is a minor one, does one wonder whether the need justifies the effort necessary to comply with this essential of scholarship?

There is a similar urgency in the case of teaching. If a contribution being discussed can be produced at once, the answers to questions may be provided without the delay that would otherwise prove unavoidable. In addition, the student sees the item, although in reproduction; the need to show him original works is, of course, recognized.

(2) The passages selected will frequently be in a language other than the reader's own and a translation will usually be necessary to make them more widely available. An organized programme of translation can therefore be established which, as well as providing a more universally convenient version of the material, provides students with excellent practice. When a translation is already available this can be copied and filed with the original version and improved upon where necessary. Eventually all the elements of the collection will be in the language of the users and for junior students without linguistic skills this will prove to be a great boon. It will allow them to make direct contact with authors otherwise denied to them.

(3) Obviously one of the most useful assets available to the owner of a reproduction, but which is absolutely denied the reader of the original work, is the possibility of adding to the text his own emendations, marginal comments, explanatory footnotes and linguistic elucidations. For the sake of future users of the system, the individual responsible must be identified so that his interpolations can be evaluated by them. Thus adequate margins should be provided and additions welcomed.

310

(4) Although manual copying from original sources is essential practice for the student in his effort to achieve absolute accuracy, the time and money saved by mechanical reproduction is one of its most important practical contributions to the techniques of scholarship. Copy typing is no longer necessary and the elimination of this stage in the process of reproduction saves not only the historian's money but also the time he would spend in checking.

(5) The copy may at times have better physical properties than the original itself because its white paper can provide a much better contrast for the black printing than the discoloured paper of an early work. This paradoxical situation recalls the fact that a reproduction is impeccably faithful and everything of the original can be duplicated except the qualities and watermark of the paper, and, in the case of a book, it tells us nothing of the binding. Fortunately these are bibliographical niceties which are only occasionally important to the historian of the medical sciences.

Further copies can, of course, be taken from the Xerox originals should it be necessary, for example, to supply a group of students with primary source material, and if copyright laws allow.

(6) The reproduction is obviously much more convenient to handle, especially when the alternative is a large and heavy volume which has to be carried to the scholar's place of work.

(7) Invariably the hours that a library is open to the research worker are limited and even if source material is suitably located for him topographically, he can study a copy at any time or place convenient to him.

VI

These are the main practical advantages of a teaching and research collection of primary sources and they are on the whole obvious enough; others probably exist. But, in addition, there are the two fundamental implications referred to above.[6] The most important of these is the emphasis this method places upon the use of primary sources. The need for their ready availability has been observed above as one of the urgent requirements for the improvement, in particular, of writing in the history of medicine. The second suggested benefit relates to the library and the problem of its role in the history of medicine. The medical historian, by providing himself with a collection of reproduced primary source material, achieves some degree of emancipation from the library. This must inevitably contribute to a process of personal rehabilitation urgently needed in certain countries today. The umbilical cord attaching him to the library and carrying literary sustenance, so to speak, is still intact but he is no longer *in utero*!

In addition there are other basic merits of the system, such as its flexibility. The material can be arranged according to the image in the historian's mind and is not bound by rigid library systems of classification.[7] On the other hand a legitimate criticism would be that scientific advances are being illustrated by a method which deals only with them and thus severs them from material dealing with their multifold background, from the exogenous factors which have so much to do with the advancement of any science. This need be no hazard if the danger is recognized and wherever possible avoided. The historical evidence for the creation and growth, or decline, of a scientific concept is handled in this system much as in an anthology of primary sources. But rather than forming a static repository, the scheme is a dynamic, ever-changing accumulation of data. As more experience and knowledge of a subject are acquired, modifications will become necessary. Some contributors may become less significant than others not included and may have to be removed; the reverse will also pertain. Supplementary secondary material can be added continuously as it is discovered or as it is published. The classification can also be modified whenever necessary. Thus all parts of the collection are amenable to change, which in most instances will, it is hoped, be in the direction of improvement and comprehensiveness.

Finally, with this system an introduction to the great pioneers of the medical sciences becomes available more readily than hitherto, and for the younger student, when the selections are in his mother tongue, this is an important and necessary exposure. Moreover, to follow the thought processes of a brilliant and original mind should be one of the principal motivations of the historian of science or medicine.

From the evidence presented, in the form of practical and then fundamental benefits, it is evident that this simple method of providing primary source materials on the history of medicine, together with the increasing volume of published reprints of classi-

312

cal works, will alter the working habits of the historian. It is hoped that it will also help to improve the quality of research and teaching in the field of medical history.

NOTES AND REFERENCES

1 F. L. Fiaux (in *L'enseignement de la médecine en Allemagne*, pp. 10 and 14–15, Paris: Germer-Baillière, 1877) mentions the miserable laboratories of Robin, Vulpian and Béclard and the sufferings of Claude Bernard, Longet and others.

2 *Catalogue of the medical history collection presented to UCLA by Dr and Mrs John A. Benjamin...* Los Angeles: University of California Library, 1964; and *Supplement,* 1966 and *Second Supplement,* 1968: *Rare books and collections of the Reynolds Historical Library. A bibliography,* University, Alabama: University of Alabama Press, 1968.

3 An excellent example of the distorted and artificial situation induced by commercialism was provided by a recent auction sale when a copy of the neglected and relatively unimportant *Inventum novum* (1761) of Auenbrugger brought a price ten times that given for the very much more significant and influential French translation of 1808.

4 In the case of the history of cardiovascular physiology it has been found convenient to adopt a chronological sequence up to Harvey and, for the moment, alphabetical thereafter. With the growth of the collection it will become necessary to break down the post-Harveian material into subject groups, such as cardiac output, cardiac muscle anatomy and physiology, electrophysiology, etc.

5 It is said that 'Values have increased 2000 per cent in the past 10 years' (T. Giles, 'The Angry Antiquarians', *Sunday Times* 30 March 1969). The 1968 Times–Sotheby Index for books (*The Times* 10 March 1969) shows that from 1951 to 1968 prices for scientific and medical books have multiplied twelve times, the biggest increase for any type of book.

6 pp. 306–8.

7 See pp. 277–85.

19 The Graphic Presentation of Data and Relationships in the History of Medicine

K. E. ROTHSCHUH

The use of drawings, either for the reproduction of experimental results in the history of medicine or as teaching aids in lectures and in textbooks on the subject, is still very uncommon. Graphic presentation is here understood to be the depiction of medico-historical data or relationships in a diagram or a semi-diagram or as a graph with one or two coordinates. For qualitative data or associations, diagrams can be used, but graphs are suitable only for results containing numerical information and measurements. There are particularly favourable areas for the application of the diagram to the material of medical history. Therefore we will first look briefly at those subjects in the history of medicine which gain in precision and clarity as a result of this technique. Secondly, the possible methods of presentation and their advantages, or perhaps their disadvantages, will be described. A few characteristic illustrations (Figs. 1–10) will indicate the various kinds of diagrams.

II

INTERPRETATION AND PURPOSE, POSSIBILITIES AND LIMITATIONS

The history of medicine, like any science, is concerned on the one hand with data, and on the other with relationships. *Data* include events, conventions, individuals, opinions, phenomena and findings. *Relationships* are the connections between the data, such as dependent factors, influences, associations, effects, changes in time and extension in space, etc. Graphic methods of presenting data and relationships have been used in many branches of medicine for a long time, for example, in descriptive and topographical anatomy, in botanical and zoological morphology and taxonomy, in geography, etc. These subjects deal with the shapes or associations in space of observable objects. A diagrammatic presentation is therefore only a summary of many pieces of information. If these were described purely *verbally*, even with an extensive account taking up considerable space, it would be very much less precise and, apart from this, less vivid, than using illustrations. In other subjects, such as physiology, physics and technology, the interest is in the *variations* of quantities due to specific influences. In precisely these areas, graphic presentation in chart, diagram or graph has established itself everywhere during the last 100 years, beginning in the second third of the nineteenth century.[1] It has, for example, summarized experimental results in diagrams of blood-clotting, of the dioptrics of the eye, of the connection between CO_2-pressure and the frequency of respiration, and of pressure volumes. It has also been used to demonstrate clearly and instructively complicated relationships, such as the structure and function of the autonomic nervous system, and to replace tables of figures with graphs. For a long time therefore in non-historical sciences, *verbal descriptions* of data *have been replaced by illustrations*, or the verbal method of presenting relationships has been completed, illustrated and enhanced by diagrams. This is equally true in both research and teaching. In historically orientated subjects, particularly in the humanities, verbal presentation is the rule and the use of the graphic method is, indeed, in many cases not possible because the diversity of facts and ideas can often only be presented in words, a method so rich in nuances. In *medical history* the reproduction of certain objects of a 'documentary' character is considered usual and no substitution is possible; this is so for portraits, buildings, title-pages, instruments, historic illustrations, and the like. Such pictures are irreplaceable in a *descriptive* history of medicine, which is more concerned with the findings at any given moment rather than with changes over a period of time. However, as the occasion offers, one can with advantage use the graphic method for the presentation of changes, of *relationships* between events, persons or ideas in place and time, or when studying the dependence on specific historical circumstances or influences of these changes. In this way descriptions can be supported, supplemented and enhanced.

An essential prerequisite for graphic presentation is *clarity* of the material to be illustrated. This is true for philosophical systems[2] or for disease systems in the history of medicine, such as the fourfold scheme of humoral pathology.[3,4] Only systems with sufficient intrinsic consistency can be shown graphically, as for example, Brown's system[5] (Fig. 9) or the principles of Schelling's *Natur-philosophie*,[6] but not, however, obscure thought complexes such as Stahl's animism. In the depiction of systems one is seeking for teaching purposes a visual demonstration of an obscure concept by working out the skeleton of thought behind it. Yet leaving out details always leads to an abstraction. Such a procedure does in some degree collect a lot of facts in *concentrated* form, and it emphasizes the important at the expense of the unimportant. It allows one to bring together the relations between the components by means of their association or grouping, and so aid teaching and learning. Illustrations, said Leibniz,[7] are 'a great remedy for the uncertainty of words'. What is more, they often summarize a considerable amount of information by pictorial conciseness; as man can only appreciate a very few facts at any one time, the simultaneousness of the linear structure of a diagram helps him to take in more quickly the significant thoughts or sequence of ideas and to impress their order on his memory. It is difficult to present and difficult to learn disorderly and obscure material, as well as that which is too complicated. Therefore it is essential in any graphic treatment to *leave out* unimportant aspects. This, of course, requires a degree of subjectivity, but *selection* and emphasis are also necessary in verbal presentation. In the pictorial handling of historical data or relationships, these act as *documentation* of experimental results or as an emphasis on certain relationships which are important for the presentation. In the *bio-ergogram*, as developed largely at the Münster Institute, the influence of events, people and publications on a scientist's life are demonstrated. Here, *leaving out the unimportant* is the most difficult problem, for judgement enters into the procedure. Every selection is therefore inevitably an *interpretation* and each diagram to some extent a curtailment of the truth. But this is also true of every verbal presentation. Normally, illustrations do not furnish proof, they try to summarize what has been discovered or proved. But this is valid for *all* sciences. A pictorial representation of the nervous system sums up what is known at the time, and changes with the growth of knowledge. One should in fairness make allowances for the *incompleteness of knowledge*, also a feature of diagrammatic presentation. But it can and must be improved. Every scientific diagram is in principle a *temporary representation*. The first primitive illustration of the reflex arc was produced about two hundred years after work on the phenomenon began and since then it has been constantly improved. Graphic art therefore appears towards the end rather than at the beginning of work in a scientific field. The expert will not expect any finality of a diagram, particularly in the case of those used for teaching. In teaching, the illustration serves more as an aid to the *memory* for the tracing and retention of relationships and ideas, rather than to the faculty of reasoning, as Leibniz said,[8] but it awakens the intellect and facilitates the acquisition of knowledge.

The *symbolic diagram* is something very different from the *scientific* or *objective* kind. Symbols are not intended to transmit knowledge, but to instigate beliefs and arouse feelings. Scientific diagrams are used to reproduce scientific information; the same is true in the case of the history of medicine. Here one may recall that in the Middle Ages pictures of plants and anatomical illustrations were chiefly of a symbolic nature and they were not intended to depict a naturalistic version of what had been observed. Robert Herrlinger[9] has convincingly worked out this change from the symbolic to the scientific type of picture as occurring at about the time of Leonardo da Vinci.

Both *qualitative* and *quantitative information* can be presented graphically. The latter can be simple statistical data, that is, numerical results, and they can be represented by means of straight lines or in columns. Or they may be arranged chronologically if, as in certain cases, they afford very clear presentations of the changes in time of particular quantities; for example the citing of classical authors[10] (Fig. 5). Over and above this, graphs can be used to present the results of *statistical investigations* of earlier periods, as for example the change in mortality or the incidence of disease as related to time. Richard H. Shryock[11] has clearly indicated the achievements in the field of hygiene by these, as well as having dealt with the history of quantification in medicine.[12] Quantitative inquiries attempt to verify or disprove subjective impressions by the use of numerical data which are as accurate as possible. The increase of publications in physiology shown as a *curve* in a graph clearly demonstrates an important phenomenon of modern science[13] (Fig. 3). The quantitative illustration for the presentation of the material of the science of science[14] is particularly valuable; for example, the money spent on the sciences, the number of research workers, etc. Many years ago Merton[15] carried out a quantitative investigation into the change in the type of subjects published in the *Philosophical Transactions* during the seventeenth century. Graphic depiction therefore imitates the method of the natural sciences in demonstrating the functional relationships between two or more amounts as accurately, objectively, and as clearly as possible, either only qualitatively, or quantitatively as the mathematical representation of causal association in natural laws. In such *diagrams* the connections between factors are presented. This is done by making geometrical relationships on the graph correspond to quantitative relations between the objects.

The graph demands a large amount of highly accurate data and as it is not often possible to achieve this with historical relationships, they are relatively rare. The following types of presentation are informative: the number of medical works translated from English into German and from German into English between 1650 and 1800;[16] Szafer's attempt[17] to determine statistically a scholar's *creativity*, or rather literary output, and to relate it to his age. Certainly the possibility of reproducing quantities graphically in the history of medicine is relatively infrequent, but it should not be forgotten when suitable opportunities occur. The language of illustration, as E. J. Marey said in 1868,[18] is a *universal language*, which replaces the confusion of words by clarity and conciseness, particularly in the case of the graph and diagram, provided that the figures given are correct.

Altogether the advantage of graphic presentation is that it forces one to be clear and *accurate*. Anything that has not been thought out lucidly cannot be translated into the clarity of geometrical coordination. Therefore it is necessary that before an illustration is planned its essential elements and the intrinsic relationships between the ideas or between the data should be understood precisely. Naturally graphic reproduction no more excludes mistakes than does verbal description.

III

A SYSTEMATIC REVIEW OF POSSIBLE TOPICS AND METHODS IN THE GRAPHIC PRESENTATION OF MEDICO-HISTORICAL MATERIAL

The simplest things to present pictorially are certain *qualitative* objects, such as apparatus, portraits, buildings and books. These illustrations appear mainly in the larger, widely-circulated text-books of medical history, for example those of Garrison,[19] Mettler,[20] and Castiglioni.[21] Moreover in medical history the tendency to document data concerning persons or material has been paramount. Equally easy to reproduce graphically is simple numerical data such as the number of quotations from specific authors or the frequency with which certain concepts appear, say in Haller's poetry.[22] The main field of graphic presentation is however the large area involving relationships and connections, qualitative or quantitative; it is only here that its possibilities can really be developed by illustrating the interrelationships of facts, with or without the inclusion of time or space dimensions.

1. *Relationships without numerical factors, which can be presented graphically*

(a) *Personal relationships:* For example, between teacher, pupils and colleagues (e.g. with J. Müller, Carl Ludwig[23]) or the 'family tree' of savants; also further personally determined and subjective relations in certain schools of research (Institutes) as with the schools of E. du Bois-Reymond[24] (Fig. 2), of Helmholtz,[25] and of Virchow.[26]

(b) *Logical relationships:* The derivation of conclusions from axioms. The presentation of philosophical systems, or of relationships in theological arguments, etc., belong here. There have been attempts to present the chief ideas in Leibniz's philosophical system[27] (Figs. 7, 8), as well as those of others. Heyde has for a long time been using such representation as teaching diagrams in lectures on philosophy,[28] for example, for the philosophies of Plato and Hegel, for the development in time of the theory of knowledge, etc.

(c) *Connections* between phenomena and groups of related phenomena. To this belong all schematic presentations of individual

319

disciplines in their general context; e.g. Galen's[29] and Fernel's[30] systems of physiology (Fig. 10); the ancient fourfold scheme of the elements,[31] qualities and humours;[32] the microcosm-macrocosm schemata;[33] the man-cosmos-model of Paracelsus.[34] The depiction of the nosological systems of earlier times belong here; also the chronological stages in the development of apparatus and instruments, perhaps of the stethoscope,[35] obstetrical forceps,[36] electrical measuring instruments, and surgical knives.[37]

(d) *Relationships of problems:* In many empirical sciences advances tend to proceed linearly, in a direct, 'autocatalytic self-expansion'. We have examples in the evolution of knowledge of the circulation in connection with William Harvey[38] and the development of research in acetylcholine in connection with Otto Loewi[39] (Fig. 6). It is also possible to show the relationship of the subjects studied by a scientist during his lifetime, as in the case of Claude Bernard.[40]

(e) *Bio-ergograms* make clearer the connections between an individual's life and work. This means the lucid, graphic presentation of the important stages, the places of work, his important encounters, and his scientific productivity. There are such bio-ergograms for Descartes,[41] Leibniz[42] (Fig. 7), de Sauvages,[43] Diderot,[44] and Daniel Voet.[45] Various modes of presentation are possible.

(f) *Extension in space and time* of ideas, knowledge, etc. Examples are the graphic presentation of the subdivision of western medicine in modern times,[46] particularly in the nineteenth century; further, the diffusion of Romantic medicine,[47] the propagation of Brownianism and the theory of irritability.[48]

(g) *Relationship between certain publications:* for example, the experiments on A. von Haller's phenomenon of irritability,[49] and the Romantic literature in the hands of Schelling.

2. Relationships presented in the form of a graph based on time or other coordinates

Data that can be calculated may illustrate certain developments very well; that is changes in time, particularly when they are shown in columns, segments of circles, graphs or in diagrams of any kind. So far there are diagrams showing the development of the number of physiological periodicals in the nineteenth century[50] (Fig. 3), the subject-matter of journals at particular times,[51] and the number of scientific discoveries in physiology[52] (Fig. 4). Further experiments are to be found in the science of science literature; this has been discussed already (p. 318).

Additional important medico-historical drawings are the graphs of deaths from specific diseases or according to age, social position or to the therapy of earlier times.

The field is capable of expansion in all directions.

The *technique of the diagrammatic form* chosen varies according to the subject. Good surveys are to be found in Weidenmüller[53] and Wlach.[54] *Qualitative associations* and relationships can be shown by means of linear connections, ramifications and the like; for example the subdivision of medicine[55] and nosological schemata.[56] The decline or supremacy of ideas (inductive, deductive derivations) can be demonstrated by spatial arrangement. The drawing of life histories as horizontal lines against time coordinates is used in the well-known synchronoptical diagrams and also in medical history.

Quantitative relationships or data can be shown clearly by means of panels, segments of circles, and straight lines with scales so that the figures can be juxtaposed for purposes of comparison. Quantitative changes in time can be reproduced discontinuously in step-diagrams (histogram) or in the continuous curve of a graph.

IV

SOME CONCRETE EXAMPLES OF THE GRAPHIC PRESENTATION OF DATA AND RELATIONSHIPS

Figure 1

Diagram of the school of Emil du Bois-Reymond (1818–96), the physiologist, indicating the individual's chosen fields of research.[57] The diagram shows first the most important pupils and colleagues, and then the names of the second generation. In addition to this, an attempt has been made to show, by means of stylized shading, the main research of those included. For example, horizontal hatching indicates a preference for electrophysiology as in the cases of du Bois-Reymond, von Bezold and Hermann. Vertical hatching represents metabolism. The combination of both themes is found in Pflüger. There are also similar diagrams of the schools of H. von Helmholtz and Rudolph Virchow.

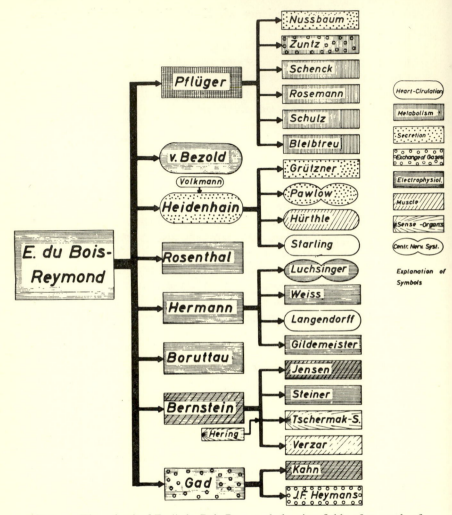

FIG. 1. The school of Emil du Bois-Reymond showing fields of research of individuals. (Fig. 7a on p. 382; see note 24.) With permission.

Figure 2

The pupils and collaborators of Emil du Bois-Reymond with a time axis, according to Marseille and Rothschuh.[58] The period of collaboration in du Bois-Reymond's Institute is shown as a horizon-

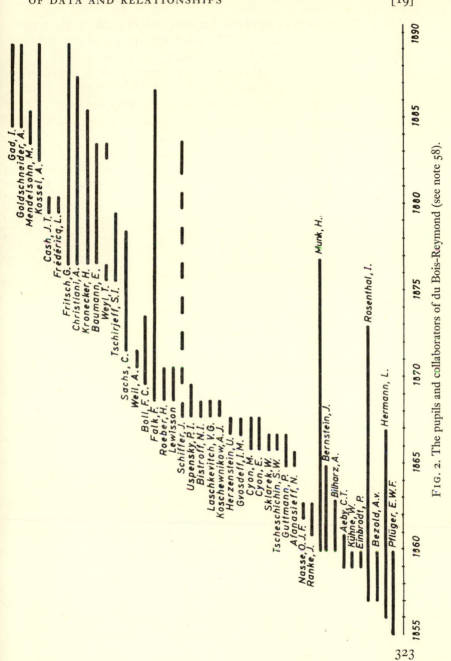

FIG. 2. The pupils and collaborators of du Bois-Reymond (see note 58).

tal line. The lower lines represent his associates of earlier years, and the later ones follow above. The long association of du Bois-Reymond with L. Hermann, I. Rosenthal, H. Munk, F. Falk, C. Sachs, E. Baumann, A. Kronecker, etc., is evident. It is also clear that a large number of Russians worked with him between 1864 and 1870. Many collaborators were with du Bois-Reymond for about a year only, as the short lines show.

Figure 3

The graph shows the growth in number of physiological journals between 1795 and 1950, according to Rothschuh and Schäfer.[59] One

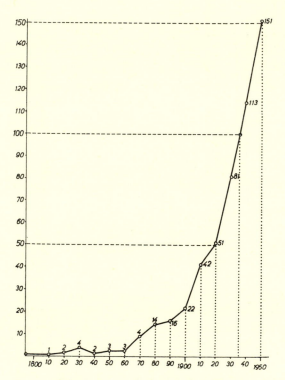

FIG. 3. The increase of physiological literature in periodicals between 1795 and 1950. (From K. E. Rothschuh, 'Die ungenutzte Wissen', *Nachrichten für Dokumentation*, Stuttgart, 6.Jg. (1955), Heft 2.) With permission.

can see the slow increase up to 1860, and the rapid climb which began thereafter. The illustration demonstrates the growing flood of literature in the field of physiology.

Figure 4

This graph gives the frequency and increase in number of important physiological discoveries in each decade between 1600 and 1900.[60] The figures are based on Rothschuh's 1952 tables.[61] The peak in the second half of the seventeenth century and the rapid increase during the nineteenth century are worthy of note.

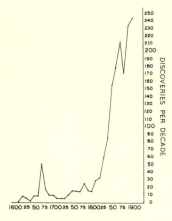

FIG. 4. The frequency and increase in number of physiological discoveries per decade since 1600. (Fig. 3 on p. 351; see note 52.) With permission.

Figure 5

The frequency with which ancient authors are cited in physiological works published between 1542 (Fernel) and 1702 (Berger), according to Rothschuh.[62] The height of the columns as related to the scale represents the percentage of classical and Arabic writers referred to out of all the authors cited (= 100). It is clear that the influence of classical antiquity is still very considerable up to the middle of the seventeenth century, until which time the ancient writers are still regarded as authorities. Then their reputation begins to decline. More and more the works of new authors with new discoveries are referred to.

325

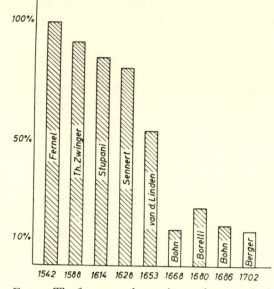

F ig. 5. The frequency that ancient authors are cited
in physiological works, 1542 to 1702. (Fig. 1 on p.
264; see note 10.) With permission.

Figure 6

The auto-generation of research subjects, shown by the history of
physiological research on acetylcholine.[63] In 1921 Otto Loewi
detected the vagus nerve's transmitting agent in the frog's heart,
acetylcholine. From this time until the middle of the century (at the
right of the illustration) new facets of the problems of physiological
analysis developed, in relation to the heart, the peripheral nerves,
the muscles and the brain. Loewi's discovery led to many new
questions being asked and discoveries made, whose subject is
characterized in each field separately. Productive research problems
tend therefore to generate again and again new ramifications of
problems and to act as a catalyst for them.

Figure 7

Bio-ergogram of G. W. Leibniz's relations with the medicine of
his time. His life is shown as a panel with a time coordinate.[64] The
most important stages and events in Leibniz's life, as well as his

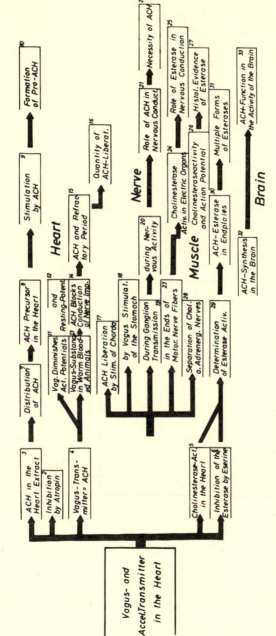
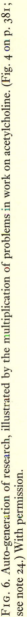

Fig. 6. Auto-generation of research, illustrated by the multiplication of problems in work on acetylcholine. (Fig. 4 on p. 38; see note 24.) With permission.

most important writings and ideas, are recorded inside the panel. To the right of it are shown the dates of the exchange of letters or ideas with important contemporary doctors and scientists, and to the left other influences bearing upon Leibniz's thought. Several bio-ergograms put side by side show inter-personal relationships.

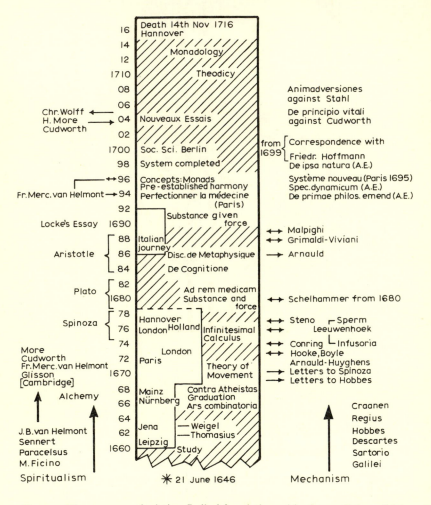

FIG. 7. Bio-ergogram depicting Leibniz's relation with the medicine of his time. (Fig. 1 on p. 865; see note 27.) With permission.

Figure 8

Leibniz's physiological system as depicted by his fundamental ideas.[65] The diagram illustrates Leibniz's concept as a development of preformed strivings according to divine plan towards God through spheres of increasing perfection of plants, animals and man. There exists a harmony, pre-established by God, between a mechanical, material world of efficient causes (outer, as a connected chain of cause and effect) and a spiritual, psychical world of ideas, aspirations and final causes (inner, as a linked chain). The monads are the metaphysical elements of the cosmos, which evolve according to a divine plan in a continuous association of phenomena.

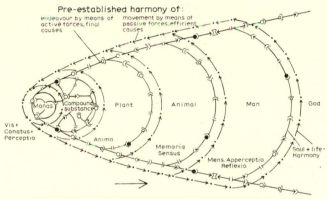

FIG. 8. Leibniz's physiological system. (Fig. 2 on p. 866; see note 27.) With permission.

Figure 9

John Brown's theory of organism and disease (1780).[66] Brown's system is extraordinarily simple. Life is a state maintained by stimuli. Strong stimuli produce strong excitation and thereby reduce the amount of excitability; with weak stimuli the reverse occurs. Stimuli which are too strong lead to sthenic illnesses, those which are too weak to asthenic ailments. Health is a balance of excitation and excitability. Therapy follows logically from this.

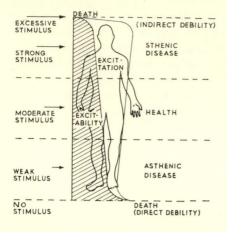

FIG. 9. John Brown's theory of organism and disease (1780). Taken, with permission, from the essay 'Geschichte der Medizin', incorporated within MEDIZIN, I, edited by Fritz Hartmann, Johannes Linzbach, Rudolf Nissen, Hans Schaefer (Das Fischer Lexicon), © Fischer Bücherei KG, Frankfurt am Main, 1959. (Fig. 13 on p. 146.)

Figure 10

Jean Fernel's physiological system according to his *De naturali parte medicinae*, 1542.[67] The picture attempts to illustrate the important ideas in Fernel's physiology. The four elements (below) are endowed with four qualities which determine their effect. Aside from this all parts have a specific anatomical structure (*partes*). The parts are brought to life by the *spiritus* and they are the mediators for the enlivening and animating faculties (*facultates*) of the soul. Their effects are the performances of the organs (*functiones*). The arrangement of the *facultates animae naturales*, *vitales* and *animales* is shown above, that of the *functiones* on the right. The system of blood circulation (centre) follows Galen's opinion, as does the theory of the digestive processes. Fernel had a comparatively well-developed conception of the building of tissues from elements, the *humores* (e.g. blood) and from the *spiritus naturales* (below in the picture). The *anima* enlivens and animates the whole.

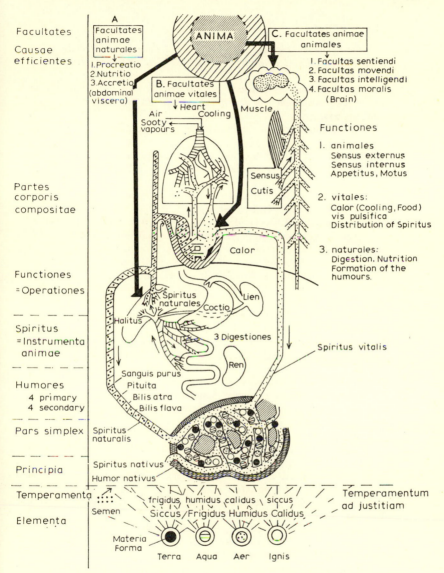

FIG. 10. The physiological system of Fernel (1542). Taken, with permission, from K. E. Rothschuh, 'Das System der Physiologie von Jean Fernel (1542) und seine Wurzeln', *Verh. XIX. int. Kongr. Geschichte der Medizin, Basel 1964*, pp. 529–36, Basel/München/New York: Karger, 1966 (Fig. 1 on p. 530).

REFERENCES

1   A. Taubert, *Die Anfänge der graphischen Darstellung in der Medizin*, Kiel, 1964, pp. 73 (*Heft I of Kieler Beiträge zur Geschichte der Medizin und Pharmazie*).

2   J. E. Heyde, *Technik des wissenschaftlichen Arbeitens mit einem ergänzenden Beitrag Dokumentation von Dr Heinz Siegel*, 9th ed., Berlin: Kiepert, 1966, pp. 272.

3   K. E. Rothschuh, *Geschichte der Physiologie*, p. 7, Fig. 2, Berlin: J. Springer, 1953.

4   R. Herrlinger in T. Meyer-Steinegg and K. Sudhoff, *Illustrierte Geschichte der Medizin*, 5th ed. by R. Herrlinger and F. Kudlien, p. 90, Fig. 56, Stuttgart: G. Fischer, 1965.

5   K. E. Rothschuh, 'Geschichte der Medizin' in *Fischer-Lexicon Medizin*, I, 146, Frankfurt a.M.: G. Fischer, 1959.

6   K. E. Rothschuh, 'Ansteckende Ideen in der Wissenschaftsgeschichte, gezeigt an der Entstehung und Ausbreitung der romantischen Physiologie', *Dtsch. med. Wschr.* 1961, 86, 396–402, see Fig. 1 on p. 397.

7   G. W. Leibnitz, *Nouveaux essais sur l'entendement humain*, 2 vols., II, p. 299, para. 19, ed. W. von Engelhardt and H. H. Holz, Frankfurt a.M.: Insel-Verlag, 1961.

8   Ibid., p. 301, para. 20.

9   R. Herrlinger, *Geschichte der medizinischen Abbildung, von der Antike bis um 1600*, I, 180, Munich: H. Moos, 1967.

10   K. E. Rothschuh, 'Ein quantitatives Hilfsverfahren zur Charakterisierung medizinhistorischer Quellen (Autorenzitate)', *Sudhoffs Arch.* 1966, 50, 259–66.

11   R. H. Shryock, *The development of modern medicine. An interpretation of the social and scientific factors involved*, London: V. Gollancz, 1948, pp. 384.

12   R. H. Shryock, 'The history of quantification in medical science', *Isis* 1961, 52, 214–37.

13   K. E. Rothschuh and A. Schäfer, 'Quantitative Untersuchungen über die Entwicklung des physiologischen Fachschrifttums (Periodica) in den letzten 150 Jahren', *Centaurus* 1955, 4, 63–6.

14   D. J. de Solla Price, *Little science. Big science*, New York: Columbia University Press, 1963, pp. 119.

15   R. K. Merton, 'Science, technology and society in seventeenth century England', *Osiris* 1938, 4 360–632.

16   E. A. Underwood, 'The relations between British and German medicine from 1650 to 1800' in *Verhandlungen des XX. Internationalen Kongresses für Geschichte der Medizin, Berlin, 22.–27. August 1966*, pp. 22–8, Hildesheim: G. Olms, 1968.

17   W. Szafer, 'Creativity in a scientist's life: an attempt of analysis from the standpoint of the science of science', *Organon*, Warsaw 1968, 5, 1–39.

18   E. J. Marey, *Du mouvement dans les fonctions de la vie*, Paris: G. Baillière, 1968, pp. v–vi, 'Par l'emploi de la méthode graphique disparaissent les

illusions de l'observateur, la lenteur des descriptions, la confusion des foits. Ces deux qualités dominantes, clarté, et concision, devenaient chaque jour plus désirable en présence du développement énorme que prennent les publications biologiques.'

19 F. H. Garrison, *An introduction to the history of medicine*, Philadelphia and London: W. B. Saunders, 1929.

20 C. Mettler, *History of medicine*, ed. F. A. Mettler, Philadelphia: Blakiston, 1947.

21 A. Castiglioni, *A history of medicine*, transl. from Italian and ed. E. B. Krumbhaar, New York: A. A. Knopf, 1958.

22 R. Toellner, *Über die Einheit im Denken Albrecht von Hallers*, in press.

23 Rothschuh, 1953, op. cit. (above, note 3), p. 151.

24 K. E. Rothschuh, 'Dynamische Momente in der Entfaltung der Wissenschaft, gezeigt an der Geschichte der Physiologie', *Naturwiss. Rundschau* 1961, 14, 379–84.

25 Ibid.

26 B. Denhardt, *Rudolf Virchow und seine Schüler. Eine Untersuchung über die deutschen Pathologenschulen im Anschluss an Rudolf Virchow*, Diss. Med., Münster, 1966.

27 K. E. Rothschuh, 'Die Beziehungen zwischen Leibniz und der Medizin seiner Zeit', *Hippokrates* 1966, 37, 864–70.

28 Personal communication.

29 Rothschuh, 1953, op. cit. (above, note 3), p. 16.

30 K. E. Rothschuh, 'Das System der Physiologie von Jean Fernel (1542) und seine Wurzeln' in *Aktuelle Probleme aus der Geschichte der Medizin. Verhandlungen des XIX. Internationalen Kongresses für Geschichte der Medizin, Basel, 7.–11. September 1964*, pp. 529–36, Basel: S. Karger, 1966.

31 Cf. notes 3 and 4.

32 R. Herrlinger, 'Die Rolle von Idee und Technik in der Geschichte der Anatomie', *Sudhoffs Arch.* 1962, 46, 1–16.

33 K. E. Rothschuh, *Physiologie. Der Wandel ihrer Konzepte, Probleme und Methoden vom 16. bis zum 19. Jahrhundert*, Freiburg and München: K. Alber, 1968, pp. 407, see p. 98.

34 Rothschuh, 1959, op. cit. (above, note 5), p. 139.

35 E. G. H.-G. Ingerslev, *Die Geburtszange: eine geburtshülfliche Studie*, Stuttgart: F. Enke, 1891, pp. 146.

36 Herrlinger, 1965, op. cit. (above, note 4), p. 287, Fig. 192.

37 J. Genner, 'Die Geschichte des chirurgischen Messers' in op. cit. (above, note 16), pp. 682–93.

38 K. E. Rothschuh, 'Die Entwicklung der Kreislauflehre im Anschluss an William Harvey', *Kl. Wschr.* 1957, 35, 605–12.

39 Rothschuh, 1961, op. cit. (above, note 24).

40 Ibid.

41 K. E. Rothschuh, 'René Descartes und die Theorie der Lebenserscheinungen', *Sudhoffs Arch.* 1966, 50, 25–42, see p. 29.

42 Rothschuh, 1966, op. cit. (above, note 27).
43 K. E. Rothschuh, 'Spontaneität und Zwangsläufigkeit im Erkenntnisfort-schritt, gezeigt an der Geschichte der Medizin und Physiologie' in H. W. Hetzler, *Entwicklungstendenzen in der Forschung*, pp. 87–108, see p. 92, Dortmund: Werkstattgespräche, 1966 (Publ. d. Sozialforschungsstelle Dortmund).
44 G. Rudolph, 'Diderots Elemente der Physiologie', *Gesnerus* 1967, 24, 24–45.
45 C. Dieckhöfer, *Daniel Voet. 1630–1660. Ein 'Neoaristoteliker' des 17. Jahrhunderts*, Diss. Med., Münster, 1968.
46 Rothschuh, 1959, op. cit. (above, note 5), p. 143, and also in K. E. Rothschuh, *Prinzipien der Medizin*, pp. 32–3, Munich: Urban & Schwarzenberg, 1965.
47 Rothschuh, 1961, op. cit. (above, note 6), p. 398.
48 K. E. Rothschuh, 'Von der Idee bis zum Nachweis der tierischen Elektrizität', *Sudhoffs Arch.* 1960, 44, 25–44.
49 G. Rudolph, 'Hallers Lehre von der Irritabilität und Sensibilität' in K. E. Rothschuh (ed.), *Von Boerhaave bis Berger*, pp. 14–34, see Fig. 4 on p. 19, Stuttgart: G. Fischer, 1964.
50 Rothschuh, 1955, op. cit. (above, note 13).
51 A. Tobüren, *Das erste Archiv für Physiologie. Darstellung seiner thematischen Entwicklung nach quantitativer Methode*, Diss. Med., Münster, 1968.
52 K. E. Rothschuh, 'Ursprünge und Wandlungen der physiologischen Denkweisen im 19. Jahrhundert', *Technikgeschichte*, 1966, 33, 329–55.
53 W. Weidenmüller, *Die graphische Darstellung im Unterricht* [=Die Ernte. Heft 8], Ansbach (no date, c. 1925), pp. 55.
54 F. Wlach, 'Organisationstechnische Darstellung. Ihre Aufgabe und ihre bisherige Entwicklung', *Z. Organisation* 1927, 1, 429–41.
55 Rothschuh, op. cit. (above, note 46).
56 Unpublished data.
57 Rothschuh, 1961, op. cit. (above, note 24).
58 J. Marseille, *Das physiologische Lebenswerk von Emil du Bois-Reymond mit besonderer Berücksichtigung seiner Schüler*, Diss. Med., Münster, 1968.
59 Rothschuh and Schäfer, 1955, op. cit. (above, note 13), in Rothschuh, 1966, op. cit. (above, note 52), p. 352.
60 Rothschuh, 1966, op. cit. (above, note 52), p. 351.
61 K. E. Rothschuh, *Entwicklungsgeschichte physiologischer Probleme in Tabellenform*, Munich and Berlin: Urban & Schwarzenberg, 1952.
62 Rothschuh, 1966, op. cit. (above, note 10).
63 Rothschuh, 1961, op. cit. (above, note 24).
64 Rothschuh, 1966, op. cit. (above, note 27).
65 Ibid.
66 Rothschuh, 1959, op. cit. (above, note 5).
67 Rothschuh, 1966, op. cit. (above, note 30).

20 The Mapping of Disease in History

G. MELVYN HOWE

Maps provide an efficient and unique method of demonstrating distributions of phenomena in space. Some may be an end in themselves, designed to show essential features of a country or district, independent of the uses which may be made of them, though drawn mindful of the range and varied interests of their likely users. This is broadly true of the maps in a general world atlas which show the arrangement of countries with respect to one another and the configuration of their boundaries. There are other maps, however, of a different character, used by scientists concerned with the causes and effects of the distributions of phenomena in space, in such disciplines as meteorology, climatology, geology, geomorphology, pedology, oceanography, ecology, economics, the social sciences and geography. Though constructed primarily to show facts, to show spatial distributions with an accuracy which cannot be attained in pages of description or statistics, their prime importance is as research tools. They record observations in succinct form; they aid analysis; they stimulate ideas and aid in the formulation of working hypotheses; they make it possible to communicate findings.

The mapping of disease falls into the last category although it cannot be claimed that its early use was necessarily intended to further epidemiological research. Rather were early disease maps adjuncts to reports and intended to supplement literary descriptions of disease morbidity or mortality. It is the purpose of this paper to survey the history of medical maps and to indicate how they may be used in the historiography of medicine.

II

Gilbert[1] was of the opinion that 'the great outbreaks of cholera in the first half of the nineteenth century seem to have been the factor

335

which first stimulated cartographic work...' on disease and Winslow considered John Snow's famous map of the historic Broad Street (London) cholera epidemic, which appeared in 1855,[2] to be 'the first use of the spot map[3] in epidemiology'.[4] It would appear however that the mapping of disease, and also the employment of the spot or dot technique, was first used in North America at the close of the eighteenth century. Stevenson[5] draws attention to several spot maps prepared in the context of yellow fever on the eastern seaboard of the United States at the end of the eighteenth century at the time of the debate between contagionists and anti-contagionists. Two spot maps (Fig. 1) were used by Valentine Seaman[6] to illustrate a paper on yellow fever in New York. As Stevenson admitted, 'Except as he unwittingly described circumstances which were apt for the breeding of mosquitoes, and demonstrated, somewhat reluctantly it must be confessed, the exotic origins of the fever, he proved little or nothing if his work is examined from our present viewpoint.'[7] Seemingly all that distinguished Seaman's paper from contemporary writings on the same theme was his use of maps.

In 1820, twenty-two years after Seaman's spot maps were published, Felix Pascalis-Ouvière[8] drew a careful spot map to show the distribution of cases of yellow fever in New York, in an effort to establish causative factors. The map was larger than the one prepared by Seaman and very much easier to read.

Both Seaman and Pascalis-Ouvière were anti-contagionists and at that time the map was, in large measure, the weapon of this faction. It was used to exhibit a concentration of cases in one restricted area, characterized by a specific set of environmental factors, thus giving support to a local origin for disease. A map was made use of in 1826 by another anti-contagionist, S. A. Cartwright, with the object of focusing attention on a particular locality, Natchez, in Mississippi, which had suffered an epidemic of yellow fever in 1823. 'The extension of the epidemic, as shown on the map, was facilitated in Cartwright's view, by the insalubrious state of things Under the Hill [a part of the town]. A damp climate, an eighty-degree temperature...combined with the special effluvia of rotting pork and oysters to envelop the community in a sort of pathogenic mist. The inevitable consequence was widespread yellow fever.'[9]

Early writers on geographical pathology (geographical medicine or medical geography) rarely furnished their studies with distribution

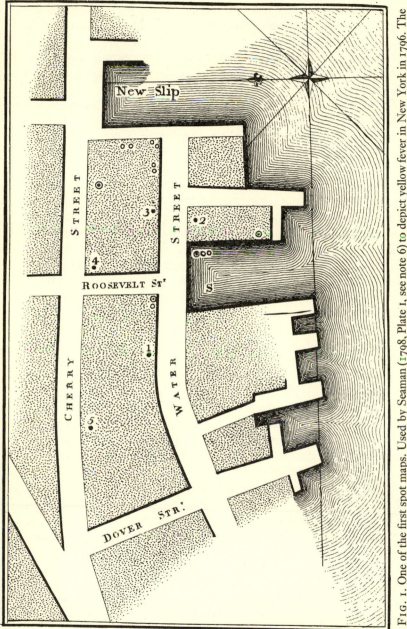

FIG. 1. One of the first spot maps. Used by Seaman (1798, Plate I, see note 6) to depict yellow fever in New York in 1796. The numbers 1 to 5 represent fatal cases; ⊙ represents a near-fatal case; ○ a mild case of fever. The disease incidence was greatest around the Roosevelt Street drain's outflow into the Water Street inlet. (By courtesy of the Wellcome Trustees.)

maps. William Harty's map of Ireland marking the dates of the commencement of the epidemic in the principal towns from 1816 to 1818[10] (Fig. 2), however, was a beginning and depicted cases of 'contagious fever'. In most cases it showed the month, but in the remainder only the season, when the epidemic commenced in the named towns.

Born largely of experience with yellow fever in the United States and with cholera in Britain, disease mapping became relatively commonplace in the course of the next thirty or forty years. Reports on the several outbreaks of cholera in Britain in the nineteenth century were often accompanied by maps showing the general distribution of deaths. Thus a better example of the use of the cartographic technique than that of Harty is the cholera plan of Leeds which accompanied Dr Robert Baker's *Report of the Leeds Board of Health of 1833*.[11] It indicated by hatching[12] the districts in which cholera prevailed but it did not show the precise location of individual cases or of deaths. Gilbert draws attention to Baker's observation of '...how exceedingly the disease has prevailed in those parts of the town where there is a deficiency, often an extreme want, of sewage, drainage and paving'.[13]

In 1849 Shapter published a book which included a dot map of the distribution of deaths caused by cholera in Exeter from 1832 to 1834.[14] This map is important in the history of disease mapping for it was published six years before the famous one of Snow (Fig. 3). By means of differently shaped red symbols for each year, it shows the localities where deaths took place and it also marks the places where clothes were destroyed, the cholera burying grounds, the druggists, the soup kitchens, etc. It demonstrates that a large proportion of the deaths occurred in the low-lying, south-eastern quarter of the old walled city.

Augustus Petermann, the distinguished German geographer, while working in London from 1847 to 1854, made significant experiments in various techniques of thematic[15] mapping. These included differential shading to indicate population density, as used by Harness[16] and also by the Irish Census Commission of 1841.[17] In his population map from the 1851 Census of Great Britain Petermann employed graduated dots or circles, proportional approximately to the population and the average extent of ground covered by the town, a technique also practised by Harness. In 1852,

338

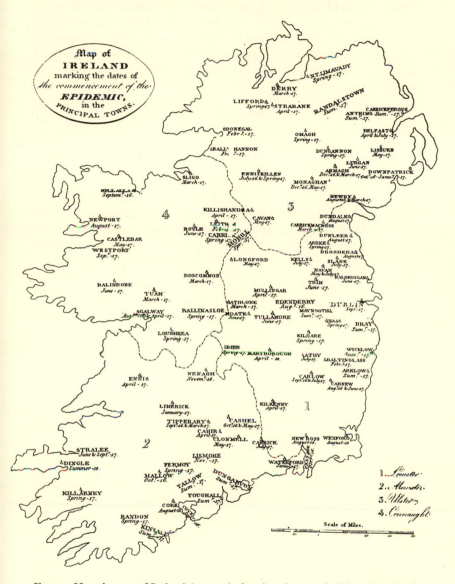

Fig. 2. Harty's map of Ireland (note 10) showing dates and places of outbreak of 'contagious fever', 1816–18. Probably the first disease map used in U.K.

Petermann brought out a cholera map of the British Isles showing the districts attacked in 1831, 1832 and 1833,[18] and his stated object in constructing this map, together with an inset plan of London in which six different tints of red and pink are used to indicate the varying proportions of deaths from cholera to total population in the 1832 outbreak, was,

...to obtain a view of the Geographical extent of the ravages of this disease, and to discover the local conditions that might influence its progress and its degree of fatality.

For such a purpose, Geographical delineation is of the utmost value, and even indispensable; for while the symbols of the masses of statistical data in figures, however clearly they might be arranged in Systematic Tables, present but a uniform appearance, the same data, embodied in a Map, will convey at once the relative bearing and proportion of the single data, together with their position, extent, and distance, and thus, a Map will make visible to the eye the development and nature of any phenomenon in regard to its Geographical distribution. (p. 2)

The year 1855 saw the publication of the second edition of John Snow's essay *On the mode of communication of cholera*, first published in 1849.[19] This substantial enlargement of his original pamphlet includes a map of the distribution of deaths from cholera near Golden Square in London during September 1854 (Fig. 3).

The most terrible outbreak of cholera which ever occurred in this kingdom, is probably that which took place in Broad Street, Golden Square, and the adjoining streets, a few weeks ago. Within two hundred and fifty yards of the spot where Cambridge Street joins Broad Street, there were upwards of five hundred fatal attacks of cholera in ten days. The mortality in this limited area probably equals any that was ever caused in this country, even by the plague; and it was much more sudden, as the greater number of cases terminated in a few hours. (p. 38)

The scale of the map is 30 inches to 1 mile and deaths are shown by black rectangles; water pumps are also marked. Snow is thought to have proved that cholera was a water-borne disease and to have traced the highest mortality to the low-lying areas served around Broad Street by the Southwark and Vauxhall Water Company. The incidence of cholera was highest among persons who drank from the Broad Street pump, but the numbers of new and subsequently fatal cases during the critical fortnight of August to September

1854 suggest that the outbreak was already limiting itself and that the value of removing the pump handle was largely symbolic.[20] The weight of positive evidence was provided by the distribution map, aided by observations such as that of the case of the widow of a percussion-cap maker, aged 59, who lived in the Hampstead district; '...and it was the custom to take out a large bottle of the water from the pump in the Broad Street, as she preferred it',[21] and without having visited Broad Street, caught the cholera.

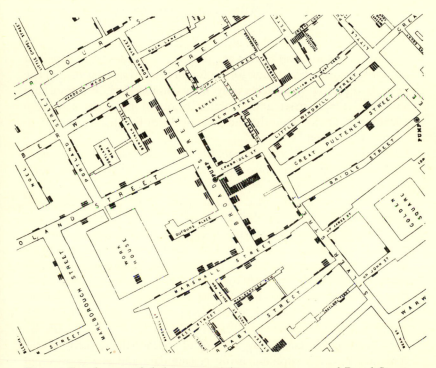

F IG. 3. Snow's map of cholera cases and water pumps around Broad Street, London in 1854 (notes 2 and 19).

A year later Acland produced his *Memoir on the cholera at Oxford in the year 1854*[22] which contains a map of the city on which cases of cholera are represented by symbols of different shapes and colours in order to differentiate the cases in the 1832, 1849 and 1854 epidemics and to distinguish cases of cholera from those of 'choleraic diarrhoea'. It is Gilbert's view that Acland's plan of Oxford is the most elaborate in the whole series of cholera maps.[23]

An interesting map, in which dots showing deaths from cholera in London in 1866 (27 June to 21 July) are superimposed on a map of the geological formations, is contained in the *Report of the Medical Officer of the Privy Council* for 1866.[24]

The first edition of Haviland's book published in 1872[25] contains coloured plates to show the distribution in 1851 to 1860 of heart disease, dropsy, cancer (females only) and phthisis (females only) in the eleven registration divisions and in the forty-four registration counties (North and South Wales being reckoned as two) of England and Wales. Crude death rates are mapped in shades of red for low mortality and shades of blue for high mortality. The first part of the second edition of 1892 deals only with Cumberland, Westmorland and the Lake District and contains coloured plates to show the distribution of the same three causes of death for the years 1851 to 1870 in these areas.

During the 1880's the British Medical Association sponsored a collective investigation into the incidence in Britain of several diseases and a number of reports were published.[26] In 1889 a set of coloured maps was compiled by Isambard Owen to illustrate these reports, but none was published. Maps of England and Wales and of Scotland, on an approximate scale of 1 inch to 10 miles, show the geographical distribution of rickets, acute and sub-acute rheumatism, chorea, cancer and, for the Orkney and Shetland Isles and Channel Isles only, urinary calculus. The several reports from general practitioners and health officers indicate where the disease was stated to be of common, uncommon or doubtful incidence.

The systematic survey of social conditions in London made by Charles Booth[27] assisted by a team of investigators, incorporates statistical research supplementing census data and is accompanied by a series of 'poverty maps'. In the latter, seven colours are used to indicate the distributions of differentially graded states of poverty or wealth. One map describes London poverty by districts, with each district classified according to the percentage of poverty therein. This percentage is represented on the map by varying shades of mauve. A second map, divided into four sections, shows London poverty, street by street. On each section, street frontages are

coloured according to the inhabitants' standards of living, of which
there are seven classes:

Class	Description	Colour representation
Lowest class	Vicious, semi-criminal	Black
Very poor, casual	Chronic want	Dark blue
Poor	18s. to 21s. a week for a moderate family	Light blue
Mixed	Some comfortable, others poor	Mauve
Fairly comfortable	Good ordinary earnings	Pink
Well-to-do	Middle class	Red
Upper-middle and upper classes	Wealthy	Yellow

A combination of colours indicates mixed proportions of each of the
classes represented by the respective colours.

The *Survey gazetteer of the British Isles* published in 1904[28]
contains a useful series of specially prepared coloured maps to illustrate the most interesting geographical features. The demographic
maps are based on the 1901 census and include for England and
Wales, (a) average total death rate per 1000, (b) average death rate
of children under one year, (c) average death rate from phthisis per
million, and (d) average death rate from 'zymotic diseases'. Different
ranges of colours are employed in each case. No differentiation of
the sexes is attempted and the employment of crude death rates
inevitably leads to erroneous conclusions.

Percy Stocks, Medical Statistician at the General Register Office,
London, was one of the first to attempt to overcome the limitations
of the crude death rate in the study of geographical distributions of
disease within a country. Mortality is so greatly dependent upon
the relative proportion of old people in the population that, in his
contribution to the London Cancer Conference of 1928,[29] he made
corrections for differences in age, sex and urban distribution in his
examination of mean cancer rates for 1919 to 1923 for the separate
counties of England and Wales and for the 1921 to 1925 rates for
each county borough. He illustrated the results with a map (Fig. 4)
and concluded that the mortalities '...vary over such wide limits and
the counties group themselves into such definite regions of high

343

and low prevalence, that there can be no question that geographical influences are in some way concerned' (p. 518). A more
detailed study by Stocks, in collaboration with Karn,[30] of the
distribution of cancer and tuberculosis in England and Wales
from 1921 to 1926, employed a comparative mortality figure for

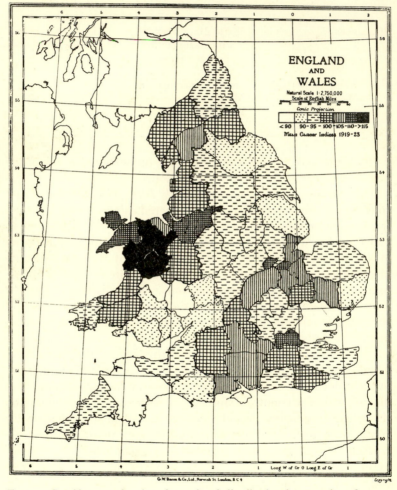

FIG. 4. Stock's map showing the regional distribution by counties of cancer
prevalence in England and Wales, 1919–23 (see note 29). The first of many
such maps. (With permission of Dr P. Stocks, The Empire Cancer Campaign
for Research and J. Wright & Sons Ltd.)

344

the series of sixteen maps presented. The 1921 to 1926 mortality in each county aggregate of districts, expected on the basis of the age and sex distribution of its population in 1921, was taken as a thousand in each case and the actual mortality was expressed in terms of this. More refined methods for comparing mortality in the different geographical parts of Britain became possible, and in his contributions to the 1936, 1937 and 1939 *Annual Reports* of the British Empire Cancer Campaign, Stocks[31] presented a series of seventy-four maps to show by means of standardized mortality ratios[32] the distribution in England and Wales of cancer of various organs in different age-groups for each sex.

During World War II German epidemiologists, under the direction of Zeiss, prepared the *Seuchen Atlas*.[33] In this atlas, multi-coloured maps were employed to illustrate relationships between variations in the prevalence of epidemic diseases and peculiarities in the geographical environment, but only those diseases and areas such as Europe, the Near East and North and West Africa, which were then of military significance to Germany, were included. The atlas was, however, the forerunner of the elaborate and impressive *Weltseuchenatlas*.[34] Edited by E. Rodenwaldt and H. H. Jusatz under the sponsorship of the Heidelberger Akademie der Wissenschaften, this atlas amply demonstrates the possibilities of the graphic recording of epidemic diseases. Maps show the world distribution of various epidemic diseases and numerous cartographic devices are used for superimposition of a maximum amount of epidemiological data. Each map is accompanied by an explanatory and descriptive comment in German and English.

Jacques M. May produced an *Atlas of diseases* on behalf of the American Geographical Society.[35] This is in the form of separate, coloured folding maps, illustrating the distribution of, for example, poliomyelitis from 1900 to 1950, cholera from 1916 to 1950, malaria vectors, helminthiases, rickettsial diseases, and spirochaetal diseases (yaws, pinta, bejel, relapsing fever). Each map contains notes on the epidemiology of the disease in question, basic sources of information and also those epidemiological features which can be presented geographically in the limited space of the maps. Of particular interest are two maps related to a study in human starvation, the first dealing with sources of selected foods, and the second with diets and deficiency diseases (beri-beri, pellagra, scurvy, rickets, etc.).

345

A. T. A. Learmonth, well known for his medico-geographical studies in India and Pakistan, evolved an ingenious method of plotting on the same map health or disease data concerning both intensity and variability of incidence.[36] The method, illustrated by maps of cholera (Fig. 5), involved the calculation of mean mortality rates for the period 1921 to 1940 in respect of each administrative district. These were then arranged in descending order and classified as 'high', 'medium' or 'low'. Variability rates were also calculated and similarly classified. The three grades of intensity of incidence and the three grades of variability were plotted on the map by grades of

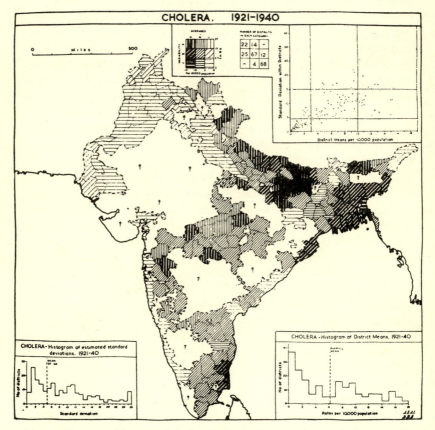

FIG. 5. Learmonth's map of cholera in India, 1921–40 (note 36). See text for explanation. (With permission.)

346

intensity of strokes to yield nine combinations, from high incidence with high variability to low incidence with low variability. While the method of classification was generally arbitrary and based on extremely inaccurate records the resulting maps indicated in a suggestive way the areas which might provisionally be regarded as epidemic or endemic in varying degrees of severity. The same author used the isopleth technique[37] to show urban infant mortality rates in the Indian subcontinent for the year 1958.[38] So did Élisabeth Carpentier to indicate the dates of arrival of the Black Death in West and Central Europe in the fourteenth century (Fig. 6).[39]

Brown used the proportional circles technique to demonstrate the distribution in Nigeria of cerebrospinal meningitis in 1950, sleeping sickness in 1949, and relapsing fever in 1948.[40] That cerebrospinal meningitis cases are especially typical of the Sudan zone, while human sleeping sickness cases show a marked localization in the central sector of the Middle Belt, is well revealed by the maps, but there is no reference to the distribution of 'population at risk'.

The world and continental scale of the maps in the atlases of Rodenwaldt[34] and of May[35] and of the maps by Learmonth,[36,38] Brown,[40] and others, means that geographically large areas, such as whole countries, are used as units for mapping. Inevitably these large units lack homogeneity both in the prevalence of disease and in the factors relating thereto. Problems also arise concerning medically 'unexplored' areas for which significant data for satisfactory mapping are not available, and of the many countries where the available statistics of mortality by cause are not yet complete or reliable. Nevertheless, for some diseases, international differences and relationships not readily apparent on a more restricted regional basis have been demonstrated in the world atlases. World-scale maps should ideally be built up from regional or national maps on which a more detailed presentation of the data is possible. Into this category comes the *National atlas of disease mortality in the United Kingdom* prepared by the present author on behalf of the Royal Geographical Society.[41] In Britain the existence of a comprehensive National Health Service means that medical and statistical facilities extend to all classes of society with a high degree of equality. In the case of death, for instance, causes are classified according to an internationally agreed system and are listed according to the area of usual residence of the deceased and not to the hospital in which the death

347

occurred, unless the deceased had been there for more than six
months. With such data, and making due allowances for differences
in local age[42] and sex structure of the population and for degree of
urbanization, Howe calculated standardized mortality ratios for
thirteen major causes of death in Britain (e.g. arteriosclerotic heart
disease, including coronary disease; vascular lesions affecting the
central nervous system; bronchitis; lung cancer) in 320 administrative units for the period 1954 to 1958. The results were plotted on
to a geographical base map (Fig. 7).

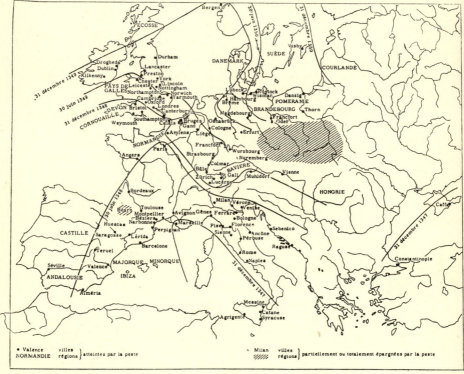

ESSAI DE REPRÉSENTATION DE LA PESTE NOIRE EN EUROPE OCCIDENTALE ET CENTRALE

N.B. - Les courbes ne délimitent pas de zones précises, mais ont été tracées pour souligner l'évolution de l'épidémie de six mois en six mois.

FIG. 6. The extension of the Black Death across Europe, 1347–50; see Carpentier, note 39. (With permission.)

In 1970 the author published an enlarged and revised edition of
the *National atlas of disease mortality* based on mortality data for the

348

period 1959 to 1963.[43] This edition differs from the earlier *National atlas* in that a demographic base map is employed for the presentation of areal data. The geographical base maps used in the first edition were found to give undue prominence to mortality data of extensive, sparsely and unevenly populated areas of the United Kingdom but provided insufficient weighting in the case of limited

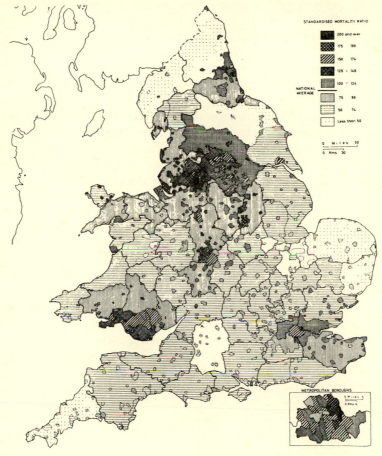

BRONCHITIS (MALES)

FIG. 7. From Howe's *National atlas of disease mortality in the United Kingdom* (1963). (See note 41 and text.) S.M.R.s (see note 32) for deaths due to bronchitis in England and Wales in 320 administrative units, 1954–58. (With permission of the Royal Geographical Society and T. Nelson & Sons Ltd.)

349

and localised areas of dense population associated with towns and cities. Incorrect visual impressions of regional intensities of mortality were thereby created. The demographic base map used in the revised edition relates disease ratios to local populations 'at risk' to disease. A system of 'squares' representing urban populations and 'diamonds' representing rural populations is employed so that main centres of population concentration assume increased proportions while large counties with numerically small populations are reduced in area relative to the United Kingdom as a whole. A stylistic coastline is added to assist in reading the maps (Fig. 8). The first edition of the atlas is essentially a geography of death, but the revised edition provides, in addition, possible explanations for the mortality distributions shown.

Computer graphics, the most recent development in map-making, is the construction of maps and diagrams by means of the electronic computer. Such lengthy and repetitive processes as the calculation of attack rates, fatality rates, standardized mortality ratios and other disease indices are performed by the computer in a fraction of the time taken by other means and the information so obtained is plotted directly on to a map. The result is an excellent working map which, if necessary, can be used for the drafting of more refined pieces of cartography. R. W. Armstrong used computer graphics to show the 1959 to 1961 distribution of deaths from 'All causes' for the population of Illinois, U.S.A., by county units.[44] The same technique has been employed by Howe to study the 1959 to 1963 distribution of standardized mortality ratios for arteriosclerotic heart disease, including coronary disease, for the male population of Glasgow by wards.[45] Standardized mortality ratios were calculated, arranged in order of magnitude and then broken into categories. Symbols representing categories appropriate to the particular wards were plotted according to Cartesian co-ordinates on to a demographic base map.[46]

III

For international studies, the medical data necessary for comprehensive mapping are either not available or fall far short of the levels of accuracy and detail required. On the other hand, where the data are available and reliable, the foregoing, arbitrarily and severely selected

350

examples of dot, choropleth and computer graphic maps, provide
some indication of the improvement in quality and sophistication of

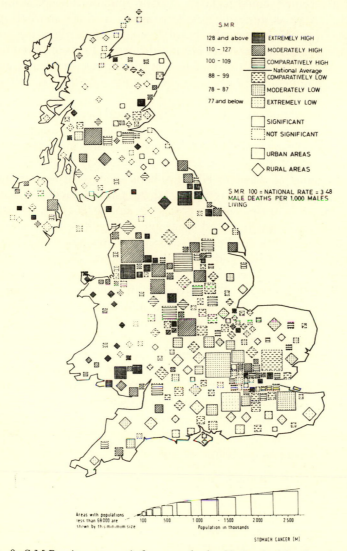

FIG. 8. S.M.R.s (see note 32) for 1959–63 in *National Atlas* (1970). (See
note 43 and text.) (With permission of the Royal Geographical Society and
T. Nelson & Sons Ltd.)

cartographic techniques which has taken place. Maps are valuable aids or research tools for the epidemiologist or public health worker, but cognizance should be taken of their limitations. Correlations in space can be as misleading as correlations in time, and data provided by maps will usually be of this character. Maps may offer pointers to possible answers but not the proof. Proof of causation in the ordinary sense of the phrase must still require detailed evidence of the conjunction of cause and effect *in the individual* as well as in the community.

The association of disease with topographical factors of aetiology has been recognized since the earliest days of medical practice and its history has been reviewed briefly by Sigerist,[47] and more recently by Ackerknecht.[48] But despite several contributions to this field, the most famous of which is Hirsch's book on historico-geographical pathology first published 1860–64,[49] there is still a great deal of work to be done. As Sigerist suggested as long ago as 1933,[50] each disease must be studied in time and space and, to facilitate this, maps will be essential. Those of Senf,[51] Liebscher,[52] Ackerknecht,[53] Stevenson[5] and Carpentier[39] in particular, illustrate the value of this technique. Maps as convenient methods of indicating the location of phenomena in space have therefore an important role to play in the historiography of medicine, and new cartographic techniques will facilitate their production. They will be a vital element in future studies of the history of disease, of historical demographical data, and of other human events of medico-historical importance. As Rosen has recently stated, '…one of the next assignments for medical historians is to put disease on the map',[54] or, as the late Sir Dudley Stamp said more tersely, 'Put it on a map.'[55]

REFERENCES AND NOTES

1   E. W. Gilbert, 'Pioneer maps of health and disease in England', *Geogrl. J.* 1958, 124, 172–83.

2   J. Snow, *On the mode of communication of cholera*, 1st ed., London: J. Churchill, 1849; this has no maps. The 2nd ed., London, 1855, has the map facing p. 45. See note 19.

3   Spot or dot maps show the density of distribution of cases or deaths—individual or otherwise—by means of dots of uniform size. The size of the dots and the value for which they stand is fixed so that the dots

coalesce in a solid mass at the place of greatest density and in other places they are proportionately distributed,

4   C.-E. A. Winslow, *The conquest of epidemic disease: a chapter in the history of ideas*, p. 274, Princeton, N.J.: Princeton University Press, 1943.

5   L. G. Stevenson, 'Putting disease on the map: the early use of spot maps in the study of yellow fever', *J. Hist. Med.* 1965, **20**, 226–61.

6   V. Seaman, 'An inquiry into the cause of the prevalence of the yellow fever in New-York', *The Medical Repository*, New York, 1798, 1, 315–32.

7   Stevenson, op. cit. (above, note 5), p. 237.

8   F. Pascalis-Ouvière, *Statement on the occurrences during malignant yellow fever in the City of New York*. Cited by Stevenson, op. cit. (above, note 5), pp. 242–4, who adds that 'A generous extract, twenty-eight pages all told, appeared in *The Medical Repository* in 1820, accompanied by a reissue of the fold-out map' (p. 243).

9   S. A. Cartwright, 'A series of essays on the causes, symptoms, morbid anatomy, and treatment of some of the principal diseases of the southern states', *Medical Recorder* 1826, 9, (3–44, 225–67), 4–7. Cited by Stevenson, op. cit. (above, note 5), p. 250.

10 W. Harty, *An historic sketch of the causes, progress, extent, and mortality of the contagious fever epidemic in Ireland during the years 1817, 1818, and 1819: with numerous tables, official documents, and private communications, illustrative of its general history and of the system of management adopted for its suppression*, Dublin: Hodges & M'Arthur, 1820.

11 R. Baker, *Report of the Leeds Board of Health*, Leeds, 1833. (Cited by Stevenson, op. cit. (above, note 5), p. 228.) Accompanied by a map, *Cholera plan of Leeds*, surveyed by Charles Fowler, Leeds, January 1833.

12 The hatching or tinting of civil divisions or areas with graduated lines or with colours, the degree of darkness of which is proportionate to the intensity or value represented, is a simple and effective method of showing statistical data on maps to which the term 'choropleth' (i.e. quantity in area) is applied.

13 Gilbert, op. cit. (above, note 1), p. 175.

14 T. Shapter, *The history of the cholera in Exeter in 1832*, London: J. Churchill, 1849.

15 'Thematic' or 'special' maps represent the data of various sciences in their distribution and interrelationship on the surface of the earth.

16 H. D. Harness, *Atlas to accompany the Second Report of the Commissioners appointed to consider and recommend a general system of railways for Ireland*, Dublin: Her Majesty's Stationery Office, 1838.
    Saul Jarcho ('The contributions of Heinrich and Hermann Berghaus to medical cartography', *J. Hist. Med.* 1969, **24**, 412–15) claims that Berghaus's maps (H. Berghaus, *Physikalischer Atlas*, Gotha, 2nd ed., 1852) '...are apparently the first medical maps which form part of an atlas, all discoverable predecessors being either unpublished or else issued as part of medical writings'. Dr Jarcho's excellent little article cites several maps

not mentioned by us, nor by Stevenson (op. cit. above, note 5) which helps to emphasize the need for a thorough investigation of medical cartography as a historiographical technique. His most recent paper, 'Yellow fever, cholera, and the beginnings of medical cartography,' ibid., 1970, 25, 131–42, lists 36 cholera maps, 1820–38.

17 *Report of the Commissioners appointed to take the census of Ireland for the year 1841*, Dublin: Her Majesty's Stationery Office, 1843 (*Reports from Commissioners 1843*, vol. 13).

18 A. H. Petermann, *Cholera map of the British Isles, showing the districts attacked in 1831, 1832 and 1833. Constructed from official documents*, London: John Betts, 1852. The map is accompanied by *Statistical notes to the cholera map of the British Isles*, etc., pp. 8, which is of considerable geographical, historical and medical interest.

19 Snow, op. cit. (above, note 2). See also *Snow on cholera: being a reprint of two papers by John Snow, M.D., together with a biographical memoir by B. W. Richardson, M.D. and an introduction by W. H. Frost*, New York: The Commonwealth Fund, 1936. Only the second edition (1855) is reprinted here.

There are also cholera maps of various kinds in *Appendix A to the Report of the General Board of Health on the epidemic cholera of 1848 and 1849*, report by Dr Sutherland, London: Her Majesty's Stationery Office, 1850. They are of London and Hamburg.

20 See for example Lord Cohen of Birkenhead, 'John Snow—"The autumn loiterer"?', *Proc. R. Soc. Med. (Sect. Hist. Med.)* 1969, 62, 99–106, see Table 1.

21 Snow, 1855, op. cit. (above, note 2), p. 44.

22 H. W. Acland, *Memoir on the cholera at Oxford in the year 1854*, London: J. Churchill, 1856. The map (scale approximately 10 inches to 1 mile) was based on an unpublished survey by Robert Syer Hoggar, an engineer. It displays an original system of contouring. Instead of working upwards from a base level, Hoggar worked downwards from Carfax (the centre of the town of Oxford, at the junction of High Street, Cornmarket Street, Queen Street, and St Aldates Street) drawing contours every 5 feet below its summit. The resulting contours reveal with unusual clarity the siting of the old town of Oxford on the highest land.

23 Gilbert, op. cit. (above, note 1), p. 181.

24 This (Map I) accompanies an article by Mr J. Netten Radcliffe on 'Cholera in London, and especially in the Eastern Districts', which appeared on pp. 264–368 as Report 7f in *Public Health. Ninth Report of the Medical Officer of the Privy Council. With Appendix. 1866*, London: Her Majesty's Stationery Office, 1867.

25 A. Haviland, *The geographical distribution of heart disease and dropsy, cancer in females and phthisis in females in England and Wales*, London: Swan Sonnenschein, 1875. Part I of the second edition ('Cumberland, Westmorland, and the Lake District; their climatology, geology, and disease distribution') was published in London in 1892 with the title

The geographical distribution of disease in Great Britain, but Part II ('The climatology, geology, and disease distribution of the basin of the Thames') does not seem to have ever appeared.

26 G. M. Humphry and F. A. Mahomed (eds.), *British Medical Association Collective Investigation Committee, Collective Investigation Record*, London 1883, 1884, 1887 and 1888.

vol. I (1883)   Reports on phthisis, acute pneumonia, chorea, acute rheumatism and on diphtheria.

vol. II (1884)   Reports on acute pneumonia.

vol. III (1887) Reports on chorea, cancer of the breast, old age, and on centenarians.

vol. IV (1888)   Reports of acute rheumatism, maladies of old people, and of the inquiry into the connection of disease with intemperance.

Folders with maps were compiled by Isambard Owen to show the geographical distribution of disease (see 'Reports of the Collective Investigation Committee of the British Medical Association. Geographical distribution of rickets, acute and subacute rheumatism, chorea, cancer, and urinary calculus. In the British Isles', *Br. med. J.*, 1889, 1, 113–16):

I   Rickets (England and Wales, Manchester District, Glasgow, Edinburgh, Channel Islands, Orkneys and Shetlands).

II   Acute and subacute rheumatism (England and Wales, Manchester District, Glasgow, Edinburgh, Channel Islands, Orkneys and Shetlands).

III   Chorea (England and Wales, Manchester District, Edinburgh, Glasgow).

IV   Cancer (England and Wales, Manchester District, Edinburgh).

Also urinary calculus for Orkney and Shetland Isles and Channel Isles.

27 C. Booth, *London life and labour*, London: Williams & Norgate, 1889.

28 J. G. Bartholomew (ed.), *The survey gazetteer of the British Isles, topographical, statistical and commercial. Compiled from the 1901 Census of Britain and the latest official returns, with appendices and special maps*, London: Bartholomew, 1904.

29 P. Stocks, 'On the evidence for a regional distribution of cancer prevalence in England and Wales', *Report of the International Conference on Cancer, London—17th–20th July 1928*, pp. 508–19 (one map), London: British Empire Cancer Campaign, 1928.

30 P. Stocks and M. N. Karn, 'The distribution of cancer and tuberculosis mortality in England and Wales', *Ann. Eugen.* 1931, 4, 341–61 (16 maps).

31 P. Stocks, 'Distribution in England and Wales of cancer of various organs', *British Empire Cancer Campaign, Thirteenth Annual Report... 23-11-[19]36*, pp. 239–80 [17 maps]; ibid., *Fourteenth Annual Report... 30-11-[19]37*, pp. 198–223 [24 maps]; ibid., *Sixteenth Annual Report* [1939], pp. 308–43 [33 maps].

32 The standardized mortality ratio (S.M.R.) expresses the mortality of a local administrative area as a percentage of that of the country as a whole

which is taken as 100. The use of the S.M.R. avoids erroneous conclusions concerning regional or local mortality.

33 H. Zeiss (ed.), *Seuchen Atlas*, Gotha: Justus Perthes [name changed in 1954 to VEB. Hermann Haack Geographisch-Kartographische Anstalt], 1941–45.

34 E. Rodenwaldt (ed., Parts I–III) and H. H. Jusatz (ed., Parts II–III), *Weltseuchenatlas*, Hamburg: Falk, 1952, 1956, and 1966.

35 J. M. May, *Atlas of diseases*, New York: American Geographical Society, 1950–55. Seventeen sheets to be used with idem., *Studies in medical geography*, 3 vols., ibid., 1958–61.

36 A. T. A. Learmonth, 'A method of plotting on the same map health data on both intensity and variability of incidence, illustrated by three maps of cholera in Indo-Pakistan', *Ann. trop. Med. Parasit.* 1954, 48, 345–8.

37 An isopleth or isoline is a line drawn through places having the same value of a certain element. Such lines show the geographical distribution of the element. Familiar examples of isopleth are isotherms, isobars and isohyets.

38 A. T. A. Learmonth, *Health in the Indian sub-Continent 1955–64. A geographer's review of some medical literature*, pp. 80 (Occasional Papers No. 2), Canberra: Department of Geography, A.N.U. School of General Studies, Australian National University, April 1965.

39 Élisabeth Carpentier, 'Autour de la peste noire: famines et épidémies dans l'histoire du XIVe siècle', *Annales. Economies. Sociétés. Civilisations* 1962, 17, 1062–92.

40 A. Brown, 'Disease as an element in the Nigerian environment', pp. 41–57, in K. M. Buchanan and J. C. Pugh, *Land and people in Nigeria*, London: University of London Press, 1964.

41 G. Melvyn Howe (ed.), *National atlas of disease mortality in the United Kingdom*, prepared on behalf of the Royal Geographical Society, London: T. Nelson, 1963.

42 The much older age structure of the population of certain parts of the country gives an apparent mortality disadvantage for those areas. Conversely there is an apparent mortality advantage for those parts where the population has a relatively young age composition.

43 G. Melvyn Howe (ed.), op. cit. (above, note 41). Revised and enlarged edition, London: T. Nelson, 1970.

44 R. W. Armstrong, 'Computer graphics in medical geography' in *Proceedings of the International Geographical Union, Latin American Regional Conference*, pp. 69–74 [in Spanish], 1966, Mexico City, vol. 6, *Special Commission on Medical Geography*.

45 G. Melvyn Howe, 'The geography of death', *New Scientist* 12 December 1968, 40, 612–14, see Fig. 3.

46 The areas of the 'squares' are proportional to the populations at risk at the time of the 1961 census.

47 H. E. Sigerist, 'Problems of the history of geography and disease', pp. 66–85 of *A history of medicine: I Primitive and archaic medicine*, vol. 1, London: Oxford University Press, 1951.

48 E. H. Ackerknecht, *History and geography of the most important diseases*, New York and London: Hafner, 1965, 8 maps.

49 A. Hirsch, *Handbuch der historisch-geographischen Pathologie*, 2 vols., Erlangen: F. Enke, 1860–64. 2nd ed., 2 vols., Stuttgart; F. Enke, 1881–1886. English transl., *Handbook of geographical and historical pathology*, 3 vols., transl. C. Creighton from the 2nd German ed., London: The New Sydenham Society, 1883–86.

H. J. Jusatz ('Zur Entwicklungsgeschichte der medizinisch-geographischen Karten in Deutschland', *Mitt. Reichsamts Landesaufn.* 1939, 11–22. Cited by Stevenson, op. cit. (above, note 4), p. 228, footnote 4) has reviewed the history of disease maps in Germany.

50 H. E. Sigerist, 'Problems of historical-geographical pathology', *Bull. Hist. Med.* 1933, 1, 10–18.

51 H. Senf, 'Ein kartographischer Beitrag zur Geschichte des englischen Schweisses', *Kyklos* Leipzig 1930, 3, 273–91, 8 maps.

52 H. Leibscher, *Ein kartographischer Beitrag zur Geschichte der Tanzwut*, Inaugural-Dissertation, Leipzig, 1931, 4 maps.

53 E. H. Ackerknecht, *Malaria in the Upper Mississippi Valley, 1760–1900*, Baltimore: Johns Hopkins Press, 1945, 6 maps (Suppl. 4 of *Bull. Hist. Med.*).

54 G. Rosen, 'People, disease and emotion: some newer problems for research in medical history', *Bull. Hist. Med.* 1967, 41, 5–23, see p. 20.

55 L. Dudley Stamp, *Some aspects of medical geography*, p. 96, London: Oxford University Press, 1964.

21 Practical History. The Role of Experimentation in Medical History

EDWIN CLARKE and J. G. BEARN

Whether history is an art or a science was a subject of keen controversy some decades ago.[1] Today this debate is largely irrelevant and it can be accepted that although the purposes, functions, and subject-matter of history and science are distinct enough, the intellectual processes they require are identical and their methodologies do have certain similarities. Nevertheless, most would claim that whereas the scientist uses both laboratory and library, the historian's workshop is only the library and he does not indulge in practical experiments. He does not, it is said, use the experimental method of science. In certain parts of history such an evaluation of historiography, however, is not correct and it is the purpose of this paper to indicate how the historian in general, but the historian of medicine in particular, can occasionally adopt an experimental approach to his data by the use of what has been called *practical history*.[2] This term is not entirely satisfactory, but a better one has yet to be suggested.

II

The historian can be restricted in his analyses and interpretations by the very nature of the material upon which he must base them, the written record. Fortunately this is usually adequate, but when insufficient, obscure or contradictory there may be no way of remedying the deficiency and certain passages must, it seems, remain enigmatical to test the ingenuity of generations of scholars. Admittedly there are ancillary aids such as a search through the rest of the author's writings for clues, or enlisting the help of his friends and contemporaries and of those succeeding him, who may have provided the missing key in their works. In the case of descriptive material, accompanying illustrations may lead to a solution, and a wide knowledge of ideas current at the time the author was writing and of contemporary events, can help.

However, even by employing these and other techniques, a solution may not be forthcoming. Thus in the history of anatomy there are writers who have recorded statements incomprehensible to the modern investigator. When Aristotle writes that '...the brain lies in the front part of the head...'[3] and that, 'The back of the head is with all animals empty and hollow...'[4] there seems to be no means of understanding him. There are no surviving illustrations, his assertions are the same in all his biological writings, and commentators, while remarking on the curiosity of the statements, have consistently failed to provide elucidation. A similar enigma occurs with Malpighi's essay on the cortex of the brain.[5] His description of the microscopical appearances of grey matter is obscure and there are no illustrations; furthermore a study of the author's other works helps little in detecting the precise nature of the structures Malpighi called 'glands'. Rather than leaving this as an unsolved problem, the majority of historians have interpreted the 'glands' in the light of modern knowledge and have concluded that they must represent the nerve cell bodies of the grey matter. Whereas the Aristotle puzzle evoked in historians no reaction other than wonderment, this unhistorical approach to Malpighi's work represents a type of response much to be deprecated. The only possible attitude to historical, literary obscurities must, like that of the competent clinician, be one of watchful expectancy. Until fresh evidence provided by new data or techniques is available, unwarranted speculation must be avoided in history as much as in science.

As well as the historian's desire to evaluate observations recorded by a previous author, he may wish to assess a practice, a custom, a tradition or a body of anonymous historical knowledge. Again he will be restricted to the available written, pictorial, oral or artefactual material. Thus, in the case of an ancient therapeutic agent or procedure he may have the precise details for its preparation or use, and also of its reported effects, which very likely may never have been critically tested. He must therefore accept the paucity of information and review the problem when and if further data materialize.

III

On a number of occasions in the past, historical problems have been tackled in a practical, scientific fashion. If a modern scientist wishes to assess another investigator's work he will attempt to repeat the reported experiment and so hope to be able to confirm or refute the results. Much the same approach can be adopted in certain areas of history. The only difference is the time scale because the record of the events under examination is either of recent origin, as in the case of the scientist, or it is from the 'historical' past. But in each instance the scientist or the historian is attempting to reproduce a past event or situation so that he may analyse the work of an earlier investigator and so be able to check on this person's interpretations as well as on his results. Each is trying to put himself in the original participant's situation or is attempting 'to look over his shoulder'. Each is attempting to inquire further into a predecessor's ideas and the manner in which they were conceived. Or a past custom or tradition is being recreated and then examined and, it is hoped, elucidated.

This is the technique of *practical history*, which in special instances can help the historian to understand earlier happenings or situations better. It may be of value in comprehending past scientific research, or in solving other historical problems such as those concerning a custom, tradition, or anonymous historical data. Basically it is an attempt to recreate and then study a past event or situation, whether it be an experiment, an observation, or a custom.

The sequence of events is the same in the various types of problems to which it may be applied and can be analysed as follows. In each, a piece of information is accepted at some point in history: the report of an experiment or observation is published and is received favourably, or the reverse; the method of preparing a chemical drug is recorded and used; the recipe for an effective remedy is written down; a custom is established and transmitted, perhaps only orally. Some time later, after years or even millennia, a person questions the piece of information and proceeds to assess the situation afresh. He therefore repeats the experiment or observations, or he produces the chemical or remedy according to the instructions, or he tests out the custom or tradition practically and critically. There are two possible outcomes of his research. He will perhaps disprove the results and interpretations of earlier observers concerning experiments, observations, preparations, customs, etc., and will demonstrate conclusively that everyone, including the originator, if one is known, has been incorrect in his conclusions. On the other hand he may demonstrate the reverse, that they were correct. In the case of the second, which is a less common result, there may be a persuasive argument for reintroducing for example a drug or practice which, although now obsolete, has been shown nevertheless to be effective; as will be seen below, the discovery of the drug Rauwolfia and the swaddling of infants are examples of this.

As a general historical method and as far as the historian is concerned, practical history is the physical counterpart of his indispensable state of mind whereby he must divorce himself mentally from all his present-day knowledge and surroundings in order to recreate the conditions and concepts contemporary with the individual or phenomenon he is studying. He must be aware of, and scrupulously avoid, all the various anachronistic hazards this method is likely to evoke. Practical history may therefore be difficult to practise but its end-results can often repay richly the efforts expended. The data it supplies may permit a more critical appraisal of a man's work and it may allow the historian to penetrate for the first time into portions of the subject's writings which have previously been inaccessible. He thus achieves a deeper insight into the intellectual processes of the individual as he repeats and observes the progression of ideas. Or it may allow the investigator to evaluate a problem, a custom or a theory, or to interpret a particular development with a much-increased perception which is denied the scholar whose activities are restricted to the passive examination of written, pictorial, and arte-factual historical material. Finally there is the contribution that a practical approach makes to the teaching of history in facilitating the comprehension and retention of complex technical details. Moreover the actual recreation of historical events or situations will invariably heighten one's appreciation of, and interest in, the past.

It is possible that practical history can be made use of in a wide variety of historical research and no doubt has been so employed. The naval historian can construct model ships to help solve problems otherwise lacking solution, and the military historian can do the same with scale models of battlefields. A biographer can retrace his subject's travels or other activities in order to tackle questions otherwise unanswerable. The historian of printing or of literature may wish to reconstruct an early press to study perplexing aspects of printing techniques,[6] and the same is true with the evaluation of many situations in the history of technology. Its value in philology for the elucidation of obscure passages in medical writings will be referred to below; no doubt it has been employed in the case of texts on other subjects.

Many anthropological and ethnological problems can be tackled from the practical point of view and the epic of the Kon-Tiki is a classical example of how a tradition was put to the test.[7] A number of similar experiments must have been undertaken, perhaps less heroic but nevertheless occasionally with potential hazards for the investigator, as was the case with an 'ethnographic feed-in' conducted by anthropologists wishing to understand more closely primitive methods of food preparation and to appreciate more fully, and in a direct way, some of the everyday problems of primitive or early man.[8] Leakey has also used the practical approach to show how efficient a simple stone implement can be in the preparation of food.[9]

IV

In the history of science, practical history can, on certain occasions, be particularly rewarding. Likewise in the history of medicine it has a definite role to play, for there are in the literature numerous instances of its use, each testifying to the new dimension which the method provides in solving long-standing problems or providing new historical data. We can cite only a few examples here but there must be many more recorded in the literature which we have not encountered.

Professor L. Belloni of Milan has paid special attention to practical history as applied to certain problems in the history of medicine and of science, especially in anatomy. Thus he states, 'This, so to speak, experimental method of investigation makes easier our efforts to achieve a history of science which is a history of facts and ideas and which at the same time elucidates the influences one upon the other...'[10]

1. *Anatomy*

The two instances of insoluble medico-historical problems cited above, found in the works of Aristotle and of Malpighi, relate to morphological and to microscopical anatomy, respectively, and they illustrate fields of knowledge where practical history can be of especial value.

(i) *Morphological anatomy*. The only way to tackle Aristotle's enigma of the location of the brain in the cranial cavity was to look more closely at his dissecting experience. There is, in fact, considerable evidence to suggest that his curious and apparently inexplicable statements were based on the dissection of a marine creature. The dissection of a turtle's skull and brain was the contribution of practical history to this hypothesis and from it one may assume that Aristotle was applying his knowledge of turtle anatomy to man and other animals.[11]

As mentioned already practical history has proved useful in philology. In the case of anatomical texts the translator using the practical approach is recreating a situation by carrying out elucidatory dissections, just as the writer or illustrator had done when compiling his book or preparing his drawings. Thus Singer facilitated his translation of the first portion of Galen's *Anatomical procedures* by dissecting the ape to elucidate obscure passages.[12] Similarly Woollam[13] and Millen and Woollam[14] have drawn attention to the need to interpret Galen's account of the cerebral ventricular system from a knowledge of the ox and not the human brain. This is also essential for a full understanding of other parts of his writings on brain anatomy and is best accomplished by dissecting an ox brain whilst grappling with difficult passages. Temkin and Straus also carried out dissections to help with the elucidation of Galen's anatomy and in the case of the muscles moving the forearm they used the monkey.[15]

(ii) *Microscopical anatomy*. The problem created by Malpighi's account of the 'glands' he had seen in the grey matter of the brain was resolved by the repetition of experiments. Belloni repeated his preparations and concluded that the 'glands' were an artefact, which he then argued was vascular in origin.[16] These findings have been conclusively verified by Clarke and Bearn who were able to reproduce and photograph the artefact that had deceived Malpighi; they could demonstrate that it is produced by the capillary network of the cortex.[17]

The field of the history of microscopical anatomy is especially suitable for the application to it of practical history, mainly because of the microscope and the various associated histological techniques. In the past, apart from rare but important exceptions,[18] interest in early microscopes has been limited to their appearance, whereas their capabilities have received less attention. Bradbury,[19] however, has used them to look at and photograph objects and Clarke and Bearn have shown that a primitive microscope can still be employed today for the examination of animal and plant material.[20] The historian of microscopical anatomy is thus provided with a most important tool. For example, a seventeenth-century instrument has been used to produce photomicrographs[20] and, in the case of the study of Malpighi's essay on the cerebral cortex, a preliminary and fundamental step was to determine the probable aid given him by a microscope.[17]

Belloni has pioneered the application of practical history to problems of anatomy, especially microscopic, but prefers to use the expression 'ripezione delle ricerche'.[16] During the last ten years or so he and his colleagues have employed it successfully in a number of important investigations. The studies of Belloni on Malpighi's histological treatises,[16,21] the studies of Randelli on bone structure,[22] those of Iurato on the organ of Corti,[23] those of Zanobio on Fontana's investigations of the nerve,[24] and those of Grondona on the kidney,[25] are among the several outstanding contributions of the Italian school to this part of practical history. The purposes of these investigations were not, however, always the same. Thus Iurato[23] was confirming Corti's ingenious techniques and correct observations, whereas the work on Malpighi's brain 'glands' was aimed at the elucidation of incomprehensible textual statements.

The remarkable studies carried out by Leeuwenhoek have always attracted attention, both concerning his microscopes[26] and the materials he examined. In the case of the latter, Svihla was able to reproduce lenses very similar to those used by Leeuwenhoek and with them he examined yeast.[27] He concluded that the globules described by the Dutch microscopist were ascospores, whereas Chapman,[28] who had also repeated these observations, thought them to be yeast cells. Many more uses of practical history are needed here, although the technical problems are likely to be immense because few modern investigators could hope to equal Leeuwenhoek's remarkable abilities.

Many problems in cytology and histology await study by means of practical history. For example, explanations for the artefacts observed, particularly by the eighteenth-century microscopists, have yet to be formulated and there is no method of tackling these problems other than by means of an experimental approach. Thus Zanobio[29] has carried out an excellent study of a peculiar microscopic artefact reported by Fontana (1781), Alexander Monro II (1783), and other eighteenth- and nineteenth-century microscopists, and Belloni has investigated 'animalculae' due to optical deception.[30] The 'globule' theory which preceded the cell theory of animal life, is another problem of early microscopy which so far has not been accounted for adequately. In fact, a comprehensive history of histology, with a practical evaluation of observations, interpretations, instruments and techniques, has yet to be produced.

2. *Physiology*

In physiology, ancient experiments have been repeated by historians seeking an explanation for obscurities or paradoxes in recorded observations or interpretations. Thus Forrester[31] carried out Galen's famous experiment on the artery, which attempted to show the means by which the pulse is conducted. Although it did not account with certainty for the anomalous results described by Galen, a better understanding of the problems, and certain hypotheses, resulted. Amacher,[32] and Malato and Scarano,[33] seemingly unaware of this earlier work, made the same use of practical history. McKusick and Wiskind also investigated a problem in cardiovascular physiology.[34] The contribution of the horse to cardiovascular research has been investigated by Geddes, Hoff and McCrady[35] and they have repeated several of the classical experiments, including, of course, that of Stephen Hales,[36] in order to understand more thoroughly the problems, observations and interpretations of early physiologists. Their work illustrates another aspect of practical history for they used modern apparatus, in particular the technique of telemetry. A purposeful combination of old and new methods has also been employed elsewhere, as for example by Randelli in an investigation of Troja's experiments on the periosteal regeneration of bone,[22] and in the chemical procedures to be reported below. In microscopical anatomy a comparison of results, using early and modern microscopes, is often necessary. The anachronistic hazards of the technique are considerable but if recognized they can be avoided.

3. Clinical examples of practical history

(i) *Therapeutic and toxic agents.* The evaluation of a time-honoured remedy is also an example of the use of practical history and this field of study is one of the largest. Unlike the recorded experiment or observation, the origins of a treatment may be unknown but nevertheless it may have been accepted as an apparently useful therapeutic measure. This is the popular assessment, just as the experiment has been judged correct and therefore useful. Practical history allows the critical student to reproduce the experiment, the observation or the therapeutic procedure and to evaluate each accordingly. He will be able to either confirm or deny the earlier conclusions and in the case of the latter he will if possible have to find out why they were faulty. Thus bleeding dates from prehistoric times but was not examined critically until early in the nineteenth century when Louis applied the numerical method to it and found it wanting as a universal beneficial measure; he made similar assessments of emetics and counter-irritants.[37] Thus he subjected historically accepted facts to the rigours of experiment and statistical analysis.

Obviously more precise information concerning drugs and other therapeutic measures employed in the past, including the preparation, effects and uses of them, would be of the greatest value to the medical historian. An early example is the work of Richardson who attempted to assess the properties of mandragora by observing the effects of a vinous preparation on animals and man, including himself.[38] With a similar objective, Deffarge,[39] amongst others, has used practical history to investigate the supposed anaesthetic properties of the soporific sponge.

The only way to determine the therapeutic effectiveness of ancient preparations, providing their exact composition is known, is to analyse their contents and to test the pharmacological activity of each. In India the ancient Hindu ayurvedic writings have been examined in this way[40] and provide an example of a previous

practice being proved useful; the Rauwolfia alkaloids were discovered by these investigations and introduced to the West as
tranquillizers in the mid-1950's.[41] A similar exploit, to discover the
nature of paricá, a snuff used by certain South American Indians
and said to have a narcotic effect, has been reported.[42] The search
for exotic remedies and panaceas, hidden perhaps amongst the
remedies of primitive peoples, continues.[43]

A classical example of putting to the test pharmacological properties claimed for a substance in earlier times, is the experimental
approach by Strong and McCawley to a contraceptive preparation
mentioned in the sixteenth-century Voynich Manuscript.[44] The
main ingredient is oil of spindle which they could prove has a
spermicidal effect due to its acidic properties. As the authors concluded, there is need for the same approach to comparable problems,
of which there are many.[45]

Also to be recorded here is the practical approach to the history
of anaesthetics. Smith has shown that certain aspects of the evolution of nitrous oxide anaesthesia can only be understood by the
experimental approach.[46] This has involved him in the reproduction of original apparatus, and this technique must be applied in
any aspect of practical history if the early material has not survived
and where adequate technical details are available to allow of its
reconstruction. Smith, like Richardson,[47] is an example of an
auto-experimenter, often a necessary and occasionally a hazardous
accomplishment of the practical historian.

Assessment of toxic agents also presents many practical historical
situations and examples are plentiful. Take for example the recent
suggestion that the smoke from Roman lamps produced abortion,
and the comparable events in animals exposed to pheromones.[48]
This historical problem could be partially solved by animal experimentation although as with many pharmacological enigmas a full
elucidation is unlikely in view of the human involvement.

Another important use of the laboratory in the historical evaluation of therapeutic agents is the work carried out at the institute
for the history of pharmacy at the technical university of Braunschweig and reported by Hickel in a paper entitled 'The laboratory
as an adjunct to historical research'.[49] A systematic study of phar-
macopoeial chemical products is at present in progress and it
involves their identification, the investigation of their purity, the

rationality of the given formula, their adulterations, the differences in quality of various commercial samples of them, and the fluctuation in their composition over periods of time. First, the chemicals were prepared according to the old formulas with, of course, the use of contemporary apparatus and they were then examined by modern methods of analytical chemistry. One of the most striking discoveries has been the lack of purity of alkaloids when prepared by early methods. In one experiment when the directions for the production of morphine taken from a pharmacopoeia of 1827 were followed, only narcotine was obtained. Early quinine always contained quinidine, and strychnine was contaminated with brucine. In this field too, extensive studies await the practical historian of medicine and the results, like these, may be of the greatest importance for the history of therapy. Hickel concludes with a statement that can be applied to all aspects of medical history where practical techniques are applied:

'Thus, in combining laboratory methods with the more common literature studies, the history of drugs can be given a valuable additional dimension' (p. 108).

In the case of surgery, superseded techniques occasionally may be reproduced at operation and assessed; for example Shepherd reports his evaluation of J. Y. Simpson's 'acupressure', a method of controlling bleeding vessels during operations.[50]

(ii) *Bacteriology*. The results obtained in experimental work carried out by Bastian in defence of the ancient concept of spontaneous generation and against Pasteur's theories, have never been satisfactorily explained and the only way of assessing them would be to repeat his experiments.[51] Hare has recently reconstructed Fleming's discovery of penicillin by the repetition of his early experiments.[52] It is likely that other puzzling results in early microbiology should be examined in this way.

(iii) *Diagnosis*. In the history of clinical medicine, practical history may be of value in assessing the contributions made by early diagnostic methods. Thus an audiographic study of early stethoscopes or a practical investigation of early thermometers would be possible. Here the experiments of Crane concerning Hauksbee's pioneer work in 1709 on the electrical excitation of a vacuum, which led eventually to the X-rays, radio, neon lighting, etc., should be included.[53]

368

(iv) *Strait-waistcoat.* Hunter and Widdicombe have ingeniously suggested[54] that the belief held in the eighteenth and nineteenth centuries that pulmonary tuberculosis and madness were incompatible can be explained on the then current use of the strait-waistcoat which constitutes a form of collapse therapy. They were able to prove experimentally that the garment reduced functional residual lung capacity similar to that of an artificial pneumoperitoneum. Thus the restrained psychotic suffering from pulmonary tuberculosis was, unknowingly, being treated for his pulmonary disease.

(v) *Swaddling.* The experimental investigation of a similar problem, that of swaddling in infants, has also been reported.[55] Rather than limiting themselves to speculating on its possible effects and to consulting ancient writers on the subject, the authors showed experimentally that the '...motor restraint is largely responsible for the effect of swaddling' (p. 562), and that this maintains a state of subdued physiological activity, beneficial to child and parents. It seems likely that certain other practices now mostly unused or completely obsolete should be studied in this way. As in the case of Rauwolfia, swaddling is another example of how the data derived from practical history may confirm the value of a remedy or procedure introduced empirically in the first instance.

4. *Teaching*

The introduction of practical history into the teaching of medical history concerns us less here but this has been practised frequently in the past. Two of the best-known examples are Temkin's dissection of the monkey and pig to illustrate for students Galen's anatomical studies,[56] and the use of dissections and experiments in a film to accompany Harvey's elucidation of the circulation of the blood. Clearly there are many instances of this technique, and books on classical experiments in the history of science allow easy access to the experimental protocols.[57]

VI

On the evidence produced here, it would seem to be wise to remember practical history whenever traditional historical sources and methods have failed; it is certain that there are more uses for it than have been discussed. In addition to shedding light on a previously obscure problem, however, the method makes the historian acutely aware of the potential anachronistic pitfalls and so helps to heighten his historical sense.

Moreover there is another aspect of practical history which was demonstrated in our papers on an early microscope[58] and on Malpighi's cortical 'glands'.[59] The data accumulated in this type of historical investigation are essentially experimental in nature and therefore are suitable for publication in the form used in a scientific article. Thus the traditional sequence of headings can be employed: introduction with clear statement of problem and research intent, materials and methods, experiments and results, discussion and conclusions. It might seem that this presentation can be adopted only for scientific reports, as those concerning the results of practical history generally are. There may however be a case for using it in a modified form for the publication of other types of historical information. It would certainly demand that the historian should marshal his facts and evidence in a clear, precise and sequential fashion; this alone is a salutary exercise for any researcher, and should lead to greater clarity of thought. If in addition the scientist could acquire some of the historian's prose skills there could be universal satisfaction. It is usually considered that history should be written with a graceful literary style and in general this is unchallengeable. There are, however, parts of history, for example the history of the medical sciences, where accuracy and clarity may be of greater value to the writer and to his reader. A combination of techniques is clearly the objective that should be sought.

Those who have represented history as a science have echoed Bury's words: '...though she [history] may supply material for literary art or philosophical speculation, she is herself simply a science, no less and no more' (p. 223),[60] and even Trevelyan, the dauntless opponent of this view, has begrudgingly and sarcastically allowed that '...in collecting and weighing evidence as to facts, something of the scientific spirit is required for an historian, just as it is for a detective or a politician' (p. 229).[61] There can be little doubt, however, that practical history is an important addition to the historian's techniques. Its use, together with the presentation of the data it provides, introduces an element of scientific method into history which can only be for the good of the subject.

REFERENCES AND NOTES

1 Selections from the works of the earlier contestants are in F. Stern (ed.), *The varieties of history from Voltaire to the present*, London: Thames & Hudson, 1957, pp. 427.

2 E. Clarke, 'Practical historical medicine', *Verhandlungen des XX. Internationalen Kongresses für Geschichte des medizin Berlin, 22.–27. August 1966*, pp. 352–5, Hildesheim: G. Olms, 1968.

3 *Historia animalium*, I, 16, 494 b 25, *The works of Aristotle...*, vol. IV, *Historia animalium*, transl. D'Arcy W. Thompson, Oxford: Clarendon Press, 1910.

4 Ibid., I, 16, 494 b 30.

5 M. Malpighi, *De viscerum structura exercitatio anatomica*, 'De cerebri cortice', pp. 50–72, Bologna: J. Monti, 1666.

6 A modern facsimile of an Elizabethan type printing press built by the late Professor A. H. Smith of University College London allowed students to 'learn the methods by which Shakespeare's plays and other books of the sixteenth and seventeenth centuries were printed'. See *University College London* [a descriptive handbook, published in 1952], photographs following p. 48.

7 The expedition is described in detail by T. Heyerdahl in *American Indians in the Pacific: the theory behind the Kon-Tiki Expedition*, Oslo: Gyldendal Norsk Forlag, 1952, and idem, *The Kon-Tiki Expedition: by raft across the South Seas*, transl. F. H. Lyon, London: Allen & Unwin, 1950. However, data in support of this theory diminish, as shown by B. Pickersgill and A. H. Bunting ('Cultivated plants and the Kon-Tiki theory', *Nature, Lond.* 1969, **222**, 225–7) when reviewing the botanical evidence. This does not seem to support the theory that American Indians crossed the Pacific to Polynesia before Columbus made his discovery. He has recently put another theory to the test: whether the Ancient Egyptians could have reached central America in a papyrus boat (see *The Times* 30 January; 26, 27, 29 May; 2, 3, 7, 11, 20 June; 10, 11, 15–17, 19, 23 July 1969, 14 July 1970). Similar navigational exploits have been made and more will no doubt be attempted in the future.

8 'Ethnographic feed-in', *The Times* 4 May 1968.

9 This he clearly demonstrated in a film. A practical study involving the reproduction and use of stone tools and weapons is reported by S. A. Semenov, *Prehistoric technology: an experimental study of the oldest tools and artefacts from traces of manufacture and wear*, transl. M. W. Thompson, London: Cory Adams & Mackay, 1964.

10 L. Belloni, 'Auf dem Wege zur Elementardrüse als Sekretionsmaschine. Forschungen des Kreises um Borelli (Auberius, Bellini—Zambeccari, Malpighi)' in *Medizingeschichte im Spektrum*, Festschrift zum 65. Geburtstag von Johannes Steudel, *Sudhoffs Arch.* 1966, Beiheft 7, pp. 11–29, see p. 28. See in particular his excellent survey of the technique in 'The

repetition of experiments and observations: its value in studying the history of medicine (and science)'. *J. Hist. Med.* 1970, **25**, 158–67.

11 E. Clarke and J. Stannard, 'Aristotle on the anatomy of the brain', *J. Hist. Med.* 1963, **18**, 130–48.

12 C. Singer, *Galen on anatomical procedures*, p. xxi, London: Wellcome Historical Medical Museum, 1956.

13 D. H. M. Woollam, 'Concepts of the brain and its functions in classical antiquity' in *The history and philosophy of knowledge of the brain and its functions*, pp. 5–18, Oxford: Blackwell, 1958.

14 J. W. Millen and D. H. M. Woollam, *The anatomy of the cerebrospinal fluid*, pp. 8–9, London: Oxford University Press, 1962.

15 O. Temkin and W. L. Straus, Jr., 'Galen's dissection of the liver and of the muscles moving the forearm translated from "The anatomical procedures" ', *Bull. Hist. Med.* 1946, **19**, 167–76.

16 L. Belloni, 'I trattati di M. Malpighi sulla struttura della lingua e della cute ("De lingua"—"De externo tactus organo")', *Physis* 1965, **7**, 431–75, see pp. 435–6. He considers this in greater detail in 'La neuroanatomia di Marcello Malpighi', *Physis* 1966, **8**, 253–66, and in 'Die Neuroanatomie von Marcello Malpighi' in G. Scherz (ed.), *The historical aspects of brain research in the 17th century*, pp. 193–206, Oxford: Pergamon, 1968 (*Analecta Medico-Historica*, 3).

17 E. Clarke and J. G. Bearn, 'The brain "glands" of Malpighi elucidated by practical history', *J. Hist. Med.* 1968, **23**, 309–30.

18 P. H. van Cittert, *Descriptive catalogue of the collection of microscopes in charge of the Utrecht University Museum*, Groningen: Noordhoff, 1934; S. Bradbury and G. L'E. Turner, 'An electron microscopical examination of Nobert's ten-band test-plate', *J. microscop. Soc.* 1965, **84**, 65–75; S. Bradbury, 'The quality of the image produced by the compound microscope: 1700–1840' in S. Bradbury and G. L'E. Turner (eds.), *Historical aspects of microscopy*, pp. 151–73, Cambridge: W. Heffer, 1967; G. L'E. Turner, 'The microscope as a technical frontier in science', ibid., pp. 175–99.

19 S. Bradbury, ibid.

20 E. Clarke and J. G. Bearn, 'A seventeenth century microscope', *Med. Biol. Ill.* 1967, **17**, 74–80.

21 L. Belloni, 'I capillari sanguigni nelle tavole del Malpighi', *Physis* 1963, **5**, 70–7; 'I trattati di M. Malpighi sulla struttura della lingua e della cute ("De lingua"—"De externo tactus organo")', *Physis* 1965, **7**, 431–75.

22 M. Randelli, 'La "Anatome ossium" di Domenico Gagliardi', *Physis* 1960, **2**, 223–31; 'Ripetizione degli esperimenti di Michele Troja sulla rigenerazione delle ossa', *Physis* 1964, **6**, 45–64.

23 S. Iurato, 'The neurological work of Alfonso Corti' in L. Belloni (ed.), *Essays on the history of Italian neurology*, Proceedings of the International Symposium on the History of Neurology, Varenna, 1961, Milan, 1963, pp. 165–77.

24 B. Zanobio, 'Le osservazioni microscopiche di Felice Fontana sulla struttura dei nervi', *Physis* 1959, 1, 307–20.

25 F. Grondona, 'Strutturistica renale da Galeno al Highmore', *Physis* 1963, 5, 173–95; 'L'esercitazione anatomica di Lorenzo Bellini sulla struttura e funzione dei reni', ibid., pp. 423–63; 'Il "De renibus" di Marcello Malpighi', ibid. 1964, 6, 385–431; 'La struttura dei reni da F. Ruysch a W. Bowman', ibid. 1965, 7, 281–316.

26 P. H. van Cittert, 'The "Van Leeuwenhoek microscope" in possession of the University of Utrecht', *Konink. Akad. Wetenschappen Amsterdam. (Proc. Sect. Sciences)* 1932, 35, 1062–3, and Part II, ibid. 1933, 36, 194–6.

27 G. Svihla, 'The yeast cell: what did Leeuwenhoek see?', *The Microscope and Crystal Front* Brighton, Sussex, 1967, 15, 289–300.

28 A. C. Chapman, 'The yeast cell: what did Leeuwenhoek see?', *J. Inst. Brewing* 1931, 37, 433–6.

29 B. Zanobio, 'L'immagine filamentoso—reticolare nell'anatomia microscopica dal XVII al XIX secelo', *Physis* 1960, 2, 299–317.

30 L. Belloni, 'Micrografia illusoria e "animalcula" ', *Physis* 1962, 4, 65–73.

31 J. M. Forrester, 'An experiment of Galen's repeated', *Proc. roy. Soc. med. (Sect. Hist. Med.)* 1954, 47, 241–4.

32 M. P. Amacher, 'Galen's experiments on the arterial pulse and the experiment repeated', *Sudhoffs Arch.* 1964, 48, 177–80.

33 M. T. Malato and G. B. Scarano, 'Su di un esperimento di Galeno piu' volte ripetuto e non àncora concluso', *Riv. Storia Med.* 1966, 10, 194–205.

34 V. A. McKusick and H. K. Wiskind, 'Osborne Reynolds of Manchester: contributions of an engineer to the understanding of cardiovascular sound', *Bull. Hist. Med.* 1959, 33, 116–36.

35 L. A. Geddes, H. E. Hoff and J. D. McCrady, 'Some aspects of the cardiovascular physiology of the horse', *Cardiovascular Research Center Bulletin* 1965, 3, 80–96.

36 H. E. Hoff, L. A. Geddes and J. D. McCrady, 'The contributions of the horse to knowledge of the heart and circulation. I. Stephen Hales and the measurement of blood pressure', *Conn. Med.* 1965, 29, 795–800. See also L. A. Geddes, J. D. McCrady and H. E. Hoff, 'The contributions of the horse to knowledge of the heart and circulation. II. Cardiac catheterization and ventricular dynamics', ibid., pp. 864–76; H. E. Hoff, L. A. Geddes and J. D. McCrady, 'The contributions of the horse to knowledge of the heart and circulation. III. James Mackenzie, Thomas Lewis and the nature of atrial fibrillation', ibid. 1966, 30, 43–8.

37 P. C. A. Louis, *Recherches sur les effets de la saignée dans quelques maladies inflammatoires, et sur l'action de l'émétique et des vésicatoires dans la pneumonie*, Paris: J. B. Baillière, 1835.

38 B. W. Richardson, 'A history of some original researches in therapeutics. Atropa mandragora', *The Asclepiad* 1888, 5, 174–83.

39 A. Deffarge, *Les éponges somnifères à base de drogues végétales (histoire critique)*, Thèse de Bordeaux, 1928, chap. III, 'Étude pharmacodynamique des diverses éponges somnifères utilisées par les anciens', pp. 257–62.

40 'Institute of History of Medicine, Hamdard Waqf Laboratories, Delhi, formulate scheme', *Spem* Nov.–Dec. 1960, No. 25–8, pp. 2–2a and 14.

41 H. Schadewaldt, 'Zur Geschichte der Rauwolfia', *Veröff. int. Ges. Gesch. Pharm.* 1958, N.F 13, 139–55.

42 S. H. Wassen and B. Holmstedt, 'The use of paricá, an ethnological and pharmacological review', *Ethnos* Stockholm 1963, 1, 5–45. They cite similar articles in their bibliography.

43 A recent study by R. E. Schultes ('Hallucinogens of plant origin. Interdisciplinary studies of plants sacred in primitive cultures yield results of academic and practical interest', *Science* 1969, 163, 245–54) deals with hallucinogens. There must by now be a large literature on primitive cures examined by modern techniques; the author cites some of it.

44 L. C. Strong and E. L. McCawley, 'A verification of a hitherto unknown prescription of the 16th century', *Bull. Hist. Med.* 1947, 21, 898–904.

45 At times the outcome of this type of study may be only personally satisfying as for example the recipe for marmalade discovered by Gweneth Whitteridge in a medieval manuscript and found to make a most palatable product (personal communication).

46 W. D. A. Smith, K. Siebold, M. D. Hargreaves and A. Pegg, 'The development of nitrous oxide anaesthesia and a comparison of anaesthetic techniques', *Progress in Anaesthesiology. Proceedings of the World Congress of Anaesthesiologists, 1968,* London, 1970, pp. 208–13 (*Excerpta Medica International Congress Series* No. 200). Smith has exploited practical history to the extent of reproducing a music-hall scene with the singing of a nineteenth-century ballad on 'laughing gas' and recording it with colour cinematography!

47 Richardson, 1888, op. cit. (above, note 38).

48 A. Montagu, 'Those smelly Roman lamps' [letter], *Science* 1969, 163, 1271; see a textual solution by H. McCully, 'Pliny's pheromonic abortifacients' [letter], *Science* 1969, 165, 236–7.

49 E. Hickel, 'The laboratory as an adjunct to historical research', *Pharmacy in History*, Madison, Wisc. 1968, 10, 105–8. The author provides a list of publications of her colleagues on this theme.

50 J. A. Shepherd, *Simpson and Syme of Edinburgh*, p. 276 n. 170, Edinburgh and London: E. & S. Livingstone, 1969.

51 G. Belyavin, personal communication, 1967.

52 R. Hare, *The birth of penicillin and the disarming of microbes*, London: Allen & Unwin, 1970.

53 A. W. Crane, 'Francis Hauksbee. Did he, in 1709, see his hand through sealing-wax and pitch? (with a repetition of the experiments)', *Am. J. Roentgenol.* 1933, 29, 671–87.

54 R. A. Hunter and J. G. Widdicombe, 'The strait-waistcoat. An early unrecognized form of collapse therapy', *Brit. J. Tuberc.* 1957, 51, 146–50; also published in more detail in 'Tuberculosis and insanity. Historical and experimental observations on the strait-waistcoat as collapse therapy', *St. Bart's Hosp. J.* 1957, 61, 113–19.

55 E. L. Lipton, A. Steinschneider and J. B. Richmond, 'Swaddling, a child care practice: historical, cultural and experimental observations', Supplement to *Pediatrics* 1965, 35, 521–67.

56 O. and C. L. Temkin, 'Some extracts from Galen's "Anatomical procedures" ', *Bull. Hist. Med.* 1936, 4, 466–76.

57 M. L. Gabriel and S. Fogel (eds.), *Great experiments in biology*, Englewood Cliffs, N.J.: Prentice-Hall, 1955, pp. 317; M. H. Shamos (ed.), *Great experiments in physics*, New York: H. Holt, 1960, pp. 370.

58 Clarke and Bearn, 1967, op. cit (above, note 20).

59 Clarke and Bearn, 1968, op. cit. (above, note 17).

60 J. B. Bury, 'History as a science' in op. cit. (above, note 1), pp. 209–23.

61 G. M. Trevelyan, 'Clio rediscovered' in op. cit. (above, note 1), pp. 227–45.

Index

Italic numerals in figure numbers represent chapter numbers.

376

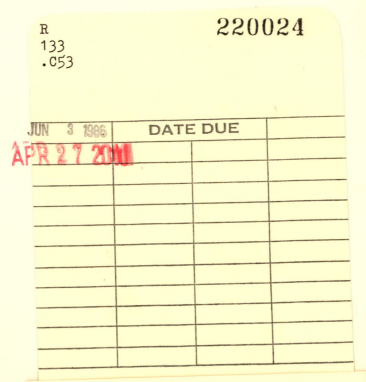